P9-CQF-288

LECTURE NOTES ON
RESPIRATORY DISEASE

LECTURE NOTES ON
RESPIRATORY DISEASE

WRITTEN AND ILLUSTRATED BY

R.A.L. BREWIS
MD, FRCP

Consultant Physician,
Royal Victoria Infirmary,
Newcastle upon Tyne
Senior Lecturer in Medicine,
University of Newcastle upon Tyne

THIRD EDITION

BLACKWELL SCIENTIFIC PUBLICATIONS

OXFORD LONDON EDINBURGH

BOSTON PALO ALTO MELBOURNE

© 1975, 1980, 1985 by
Blackwell Scientific Publications
Editorial offices:
Osney Mead, Oxford, OX2 0EL
8 John Street, London, WC1N 2ES
23 Ainslie Place, Edinburgh, EH3 6AJ
52 Beacon Street, Boston
  Massachusetts 02108, USA
667 Lytton Avenue, Palo Alto
  California 94301, USA
107 Barry Street, Carlton
  Victoria 3053, Australia

All rights reserved. No part of this
publication may be reproduced, stored
in a retrieval system, or transmitted,
in any form or by any means,
electronic, mechanical, photocopying,
recording or otherwise
without the prior permission of
the copyright owner

First published 1975
Revised reprint 1976
Reprinted 1977, 1978
Second edition 1980
Spanish edition 1980
Third edition 1985

Photoset by Enset (Photosetting)
Midsomer Norton, Bath, Avon
and printed and bound
in Great Britain by
Biddles Ltd,
Guildford and King's Lynn

DISTRIBUTORS

USA and Canada
  Blackwell Scientific Publications Inc
  PO Box 50009, Palo Alto
  California 94303

Australia
  Blackwell Scientific Book Distributors
  31 Advantage Road, Highett
  Victoria 3190

British Library
Cataloguing in Publication Data

Brewis, R.A.L.
  Lecture notes on respiratory diseases.—
  3rd ed.
  1. Respiratory organs—Diseases
  I. Title
  616.2   RC731

ISBN 0-632-01412-1

CONTENTS

PREFACE TO THE THIRD EDITION

The aims and structure remain the same as in the previous editions but the whole text has been reviewed and updated, and seventeen new figures have been added. As a result the book has become a little larger. There are two new chapters—on Defences of the Lung and Cystic Fibrosis—and there has been expansion elsewhere to include topics such as the flow–volume curve, bronchoalveolar lavage, combination chemotherapy of small-cell cancer, long-term oxygen therapy and improvements in aerosol administration. The emphasis remains clinical and biased towards the commoner conditions so that, compared with previous editions, the book has become rather more of a clinical handbook in some parts. This seems to me to reflect the needs of the students and young doctors that I come into contact with—as well as my own interests! I am grateful to the students, young doctors and to many others for stimulation and encouragement.

R.A.L.B.

Newcastle upon Tyne, 1985

PREFACE TO THE FIRST EDITION

The aim of this book is to present a concise review of respiratory disease. In addition to offering the medical student an alternative to attending lectures it is hoped that this book might provide the MRCP candidate with his basic minimum requirements in the respiratory field and the more mature general medical reader with a painless refresher course.

The emphasis throughout is on information which is useful and relevant to everyday clinical medicine. In reviewing pulmonary physiology and the assessment of pulmonary function all unnecessary complexities, symbols and equations have been avoided and attention has been focused on concepts and investigations which are in everyday use. A number of rare conditions receive little or no mention but the practical aspects of management of the commoner disorders are dealt with in some detail.

Numerous teachers, colleagues, students and patients have played a part in the development of my interest in respiratory disease but I owe a particular debt to Professor Jack Howell for opening my eyes to some of the special fascinations of the subject. I am grateful to Miss Veronica Downey for help with typing; without her watchful eye on my other commitments it would have been impossible to attend to the business of writing. I am grateful to Dr Martin Farebrother for reading parts of the manuscript and to Mr Per Saugman for his encouragement and courtesy. I hope to express my gratitude to my wife and family by seeing a little more of them.

R.A.L.B.

Newcastle upon Tyne, 1974

CHAPTER 1 / REVIEW OF ANATOMY OF THE LUNG

The essential function of the lung is exchange of oxygen and carbon dioxide between the blood and the atmosphere. This takes place by a process of molecular diffusion across the alveolar membrane. A very large surface area is necessary to achieve this gaseous exchange—in an adult man it is estimated that the surface area of the alveoli is about 60 square metres. The structure of the lung represents an evolutionary solution to the problems of accommodating this huge membrane, moving air and blood to and from its surfaces and protecting it from external insults.

Surface anatomy

The position of the lungs and some useful external landmarks are indicated in Fig. 1.1. A few points are worthy of special mention.
1   The apices of the lungs extend well above the clavicles.
2   The posterior surface of the lungs extends further downwards than the anterior surface.
3   The upper lobes are situated *in front of* the lower lobes so that the lung immediately below the anterior chest wall is largely derived from the upper lobe and that beneath the posterior chest wall is mainly lower lobe.
4   The diaphragm, in its resting position, rises quite high into the thorax—a fact readily confirmed on any standard chest X-ray but commonly overlooked during examination of the patient.

Subdivisions of the lung

The lungs are divided into **lobes**—three on the right and two on the left—which are separated by slit-like invaginations of the pleural space. Each lobe has its own lobar bronchus. Each lobe is further subdivided by incomplete fibrous septa which extend inwards from the pleural surface into **bronchopulmonary segments**. Each bronchopulmonary segment is supplied by its own segmental bronchus and the usual arrangement of the segmental bronchi is shown in Fig. 1.2. Some pathological processes may be limited to particular segments which may be identified

1

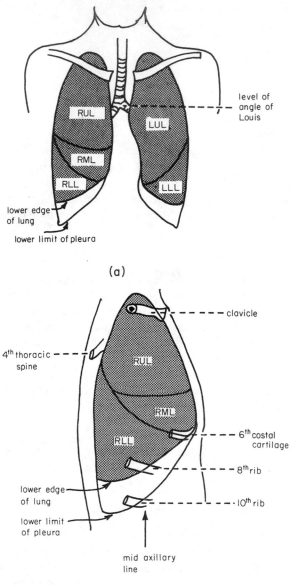

(a)

(b)

Fig. 1.1. *Surface anatomy.* (a) Anterior view of the lungs. (b) Laterial view of right side of chest at resting end-expiratory position. RUL, right upper lobe; RML, right middle lobe; RLL, right lower lobe; LUL, left upper lobe; LLL, left lower lobe.

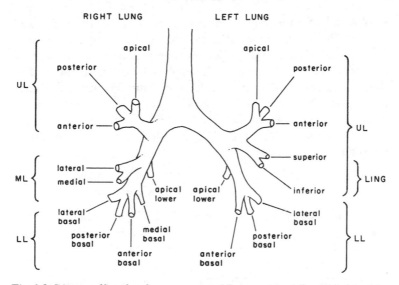

Fig. 1.2. *Diagram of bronchopulmonary segments.* UL, upper lobe; ML, middle lobe; LL, lower lobe; LING, lingula.

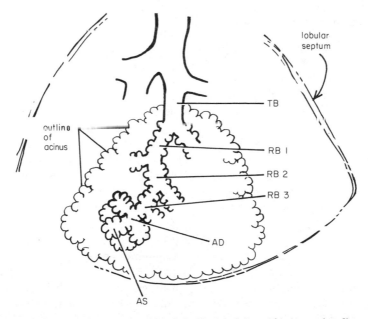

Fig. 1.3. *Diagram of the anatomy of the lobule.* The lobule lies within incomplete fibrous

radiologically. Smaller incomplete fibrous septa are present within each segment which outline individual **lobules**. Lobules are about 1 cm in diameter and of variable shape but generally they are pyramidal with the apex towards the bronchiole which supplies them. The anatomy of the lobule is illustrated in Fig. 1.3. Each lobule contains three to five **acini**, each supplied by a terminal bronchiole. Acini are sometimes visualized on the chest X-ray when they are filled with secretions or broncho-graphic contrast medium producing a blotchy appearance sometimes referred to as acinar pattern.

Branching of the airways

The trachea divides into two main bronchi. The left main bronchus is longer than the right and comes off at a more abrupt angle. The right main bronchus is more directly in line with the trachea so that inhaled material tends to enter the right lung more readily than the left. The main bronchi divide into lobar and then segmental bronchi as shown in Fig. 1.2. Further divisions occur in an uneven dichotomous fashion; that is, the branches at a division are not necessarily of the same size.

Bronchi and bronchioles

Bronchi are airways with cartilage in their walls. There are about 10 divisions of bronchi beyond the tracheal bifurcation. Smaller airways without cartilage in their walls are referred to as **bronchioles**. The term **respiratory bronchiole** refers to the peripheral bronchioles with alveoli in their walls. The bronchiole immediately proximal to the appearance of alveoli is known as the **terminal bronchiole**. The number of divisions between the bifurcation of the trachea and the terminal bronchiole varies between about 9 and 32. In general there are fewer branches to acini near the hilum and more branches to the peripherally-situated acini.

The total cross-sectional area of the airways increases at each sub-division so that it is enormously greater at, say, 14 divisions from the trachea than it is in the trachea itself (Fig. 1.4). This means that rate of airflow also diminishes strikingly as air penetrates more deeply into the lungs. This distribution of cross-sectional area and hence rate of airflow has important implications when considering the site of resistance to airflow in health and disease (p. 15) and also when considering mech-anisms of deposition of inhaled particulate matter (p. 39).

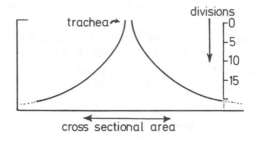

Fig. 1.4. *Diagrammatic representation of the increase in total cross-sectional area of the airways at successive divisions.*

Collateral ventilation

Holes in the alveolar walls known as pores of Kohn allow communication between parts of the lobule supplied by different respiratory bronchioles. There is a variable degree of communication at alveolar level between neighbouring lobules. Collateral ventilation through these communications is of importance in panacinar emphysema. In this condition they are increased in size and number as part of the parenchymal destructive process.

Pulmonary vasculature

Pulmonary artery

The pulmonary artery divides into left and right pulmonary arteries which provide branches accompanying the branches of the bronchial tree. The arteries accompanying bronchi are elastic but only have their muscular coats. The arteries accompanying bronchioles have well-developed medial muscular coats which become thinner peripherally. The **arterioles** accompanying terminal and respiratory bronchioles are thin walled and contain little smooth muscle.

Capillary network

The capillary network in the alveolar walls is very dense and provides a very large surface area.

Pulmonary venules

The pulmonary venules do not accompany the arterioles but drain laterally to the periphery of lobules and then pass centrally in the interlobular and intersegmental septa, ultimately joining to form the four main pulmonary veins which empty into the left atrium.

The bronchial circulation (Fig. 1.5)

Small bronchial arteries usually arise from the descending aorta and travel in the outer layers of the bronchi and bronchioles supplying the tissues of the airways down to the level of the respiratory bronchiole.

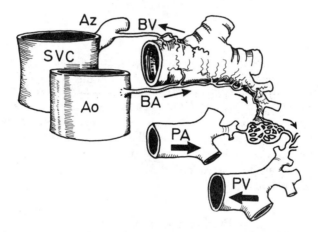

Fig. 1.5. *The bronchial circulation.* Three or more bronchial arteries (BA) arise from the aorta (Ao) and supply the bronchi down to the level of the terminal bronchiole. They also supply the vessel walls of pulmonary arteries (PA) and veins (PV). The bronchial supply to the large bronchi drains to the right atrium via bronchial veins (BV), the azygos or hemiazygos veins (Az) and the superior vena cava (SVC). Most of the bronchial arterial blood, however, drains to the left atrium via the pulmonary veins; there are plexuses linking the two circulations in the lung periphery.

Most of the blood drains into radicles of the pulmonary vein contributing a small amount of desaturated blood which accounts for part of the 'physiological shunt' observed in normal individuals. The bronchial arteries may be much enlarged in some diseases (e.g. severe bronchiectasis, pulmonary fibrosis).

Structure of the airways

Trachea

The trachea has cartilaginous horseshoe-shaped 'rings' supporting anterior and lateral walls. The posterior wall is flaccid and during coughing, when intrathoracic pressure is raised and the glottis opens, this soft posterior segment billows forwards reducing the lumen of the trachea to a U-shaped slit. This results in a high linear velocity of air-flow which produces a shearing effect, hastening the clearance of any excess of secretions. The trachea is lined with ciliated epithelium which contains goblet cells.

Bronchi

The bronchi have irregular plates of cartilage in their walls. Smooth muscle is arranged in spiral fashion internal to the cartilaginous plates and attached to them. The muscle coat becomes more complete distally as the cartilaginous plates become more fragmentary.

The epithelial lining is ciliated and includes goblet cells which become less numerous peripherally. Larger bronchi also have acinar mucus-secreting glands in the sub-mucosa. Hypertrophy of these glands is one of the more striking features of chronic bronchitis.

Bronchioles

The bronchioles have no cartilage in their walls. The muscular layer becomes progressively thinner peripherally but some strands of smooth muscle persist to the level of respiratory bronchioles and possibly beyond. Bronchial smooth muscle and bronchial innervation is considered on p. 157. The epithelium is made up of a single layer of ciliated cells with only very occasional goblet cells. A granulated cell known as the Clara cell appears in the wall of distal bronchioles and this cell is suspected of possessing secretory properties. It may contribute mucus to alveolar fluid making up the foundation of the mucous blanket which is propelled upwards by ciliary action.

Other cells are present in distal bronchioles which have a brush border. These are suspected of having a role connected with salt and water regulation of the fluid secretions passed upwards from the alveoli.

Ciliated epithelium

Ciliated epithelial cells possess about 200 cilia each 3–6 μm in length.
Cilia beat with a whip-like action very rapidly (the beat frequency is
about 20 per second), organized waves of contraction passing regularly
from cell to cell. The structure of each cilium is complex. (Fig. 1.6).

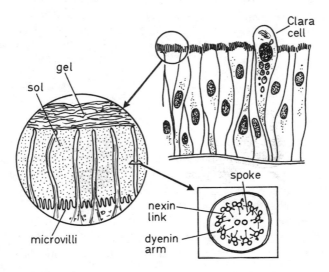

Fig. 1.6. *Ciliated epithelium in a bronchiole.* The cilia beat in the thin (sol) layer beneath the
raft of sticky mucus (gel layer). The sol layer is about 5 μm thick and its water and
electrolyte content is regulated by the brush border (microvilli) present on many cells. The
main features of a cross-section of a cilium are shown in the rectangle. Cells are about
0.2 μm in diameter.

Normal cilia contain longitudinal tubules which are arranged as nine
pairs of tubules in an outer circle with a pair of central tubules. The
peripheral tubules are connected to each other by structures referred to
as nexin links and to the central tubules by radial 'spokes'. One of each
pair of outer tubules carries two additional links referred to as dyenin
arms. These appear to be responsible for the contractile properties of
the cilium. They are absent in some forms of the immotile cilia syndrome where there is gross deficiency of pulmonary mucociliary
clearance.

Mucociliary clearance is discussed in Chapter 4.

Alveolar structure

Alveoli are about 0.1–0.2 mm in diameter and take up a variety of shapes depending on the arrangement of adjacent alveoli. The structure of the alveolar wall is represented diagrammatically in Fig. 1.7. The capillaries are completely lined by flattened endothelial cells resting on a complete basement membrane. The alveoli are completely lined by a layer of alveolar cells which are of two types.

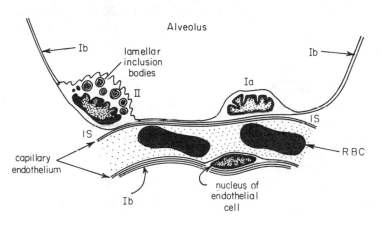

Fig. 1.7. *Structure of the alveolar wall as revealed by electron microscopy.* Ia, Type I pneumocyte; Ib, Flattened extension of Type I pneumocyte covering most of the internal surface of the alveolus. II, Type II pneumocyte with lamellar inclusion bodies which are probably the site of surfactant formation. IS, Interstitial space. RBC, red blood corpuscle. Pneumocytes and endothelial cells rest upon thin continuous basement membranes which are not shown.

Type I pneumocyte

These cells have extensive flattened processes which extend to cover most of the internal surface of the alveoli. Only the nuclei of these cells are evident on light microscopy.

Type II pneumocyte

These cells are less numerous and more globular than the type I pneumocytes. Electron microscopy reveals that these cells contain bodies with a concentric lamellated structure. It is now generally agreed that these bodies are concerned with the manufacture or storage of surfactant and that the type II pneumocyte is the principal source of surfactant (p.32).

Alveoli contain phagocytic macrophages and other cells (p. 213).

Interstitial space

There is a potential space between the alveolar cells and the capillary basement membrane which is only apparent in disease states when it may contain fluid, fibrous tissue or a cellular infiltrate. It is continuous with the interstitial space surrounding bronchi and blood vessels (p. 280).

Lymphatic vessels

Lymphatic channels are present in the interstitial space. They accompany the bronchial tree at least as far as the level of the respiratory bronchioles and supply the walls of the airway as well as the pulmonary interstitium. Lymphatics are also found in the interlobular septa and are abundant beneath the pleural surface. Drainage of lymph is towards the intrapulmonary lymph nodes adjacent to the proximal bronchi (hilar lymph nodes) and thereafter to the mediastinal lymph nodes.

CHAPTER 2 / REVIEW OF
RESPIRATORY PHYSIOLOGY

MECHANICAL CONSIDERATIONS

Breathing

Inspiration is brought about by descent of the diaphragm, by movement of the lower ribs upwards and outwards and by movement of the upper ribs and sternum upwards and forwards. Although the principal effect of diaphragmatic contraction is to cause it to descend, thereby increasing the vertical dimension of the pleural cavity, it also has a variable action on the lower ribs causing them to be elevated. This effect is probably controlled by the degree of contraction of the abdominal musculature (Fig. 2.1). If descent of the diaphragm is opposed by significant abdominal muscular contraction during inspiration then shortening of the elevated diaphragm causes elevation of the lower ribs. Forward and outward movement also takes place as the downward sloping ribs adopt

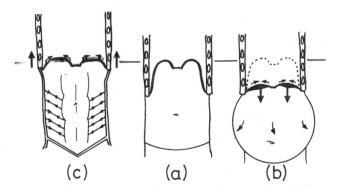

(c)   (a)   (b)

Fig. 2.1. *Effects of diaphragmatic contraction.* Diagram of the rib cage, abdominal cavity and diaphragm showing (a) the position at the end of resting expiration. If, when the diaphragm contracts, the abdominal wall is lax and atonic, the diaphragm will descend on inspiration (b) and the abdominal wall will move outwards. If, however, the abdominal muscles are in a state of active contraction during inspiration, the diaphragm is unable to descend and shortening of the diaphragm causes the ribs to be elevated (c) braced by the tense abdominal contents. The extent to which the diaphragm distends the abdomen or encourages elevation of the ribs is modulated by the degree of abdominal muscle contraction.

11

a more horizontal orientation (the bucket handle effect). The effect of the diaphragm in raising the lower ribs is most marked at low lung volumes when the peripheral part of the diaphragm is in a vertically dependent position and there is a large area of apposition of the diaphragmatic and costal pleural surfaces (Fig. 2.1). When the diaphragm descends the abdomen moves outwards. There is a close relationship between the anteroposterior movement of the thorax and that of the abdomen. Changes in breathing pattern which increase one component have an almost equal diminishing effect on the other, and vice versa.

Elevation of the upper ribs and sternum is achieved by contraction of the scalene muscles. These muscles were for a long time regarded as 'accessory muscles' of respiration but electromyographic studies suggest that they are active even in ordinary quiet breathing.

The intercostal muscles play an important part in ensuring that the influences on upper and lower ribs are conducted to all of the ribs. The parasternal intercostal muscles in particular act in concert with the scalene muscles in bringing about elevation of the chest. The intercostal muscles also exert a bracing effect on the chest, countering distortion by external pressure and resisting undue collapse or bulging of the intercostal spaces when significant negative or positive intrathoracic pressures are generated. It was at one time thought that the internal and external intercostal muscles had specific and different effects on expiration and inspiration, but this view is now less widely held.

Inspiration is thus achieved by active muscular contraction. Expiration by comparison is a relatively passive procedure. Inspiratory muscles continue, however, to act during expiration—gradually lessening their force of contraction. The action of the inspiratory muscles during breathing has been likened to a seaman hauling on a rope (inspiration) and then gradually 'paying off' (expiration), rather than merely letting go of the rope.

The abdominal musculature, apart from determining the precise effect of diaphragmatic contraction, has important actions in inspiration and expiration during fast breathing and is the principal driving force in coughing and in achieving extreme expiration (residual volume).

Lung compliance

The inherent elastic property of the lungs causes them to tend to retract from the chest wall causing a negative intrapleural pressure. The strength of the retractive force is related to the degree of stretching of the lung tissue—that is to lung volume. At high lung volumes the

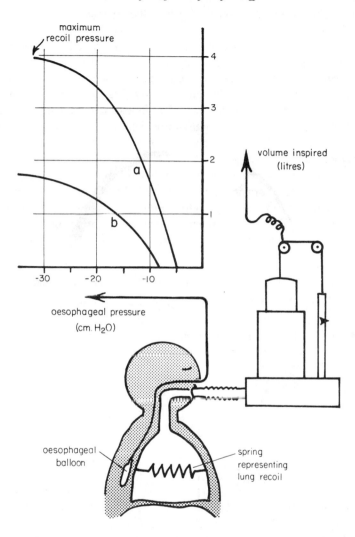

Fig. 2.2. *Lung compliance.* Oesophageal pressure is noted at a number of different volumes (each held momentarily with glottis open). The relationship between transpulmonary pressure and volume of air inspired is plotted for two individuals, a and b. Lung compliance is an expression of the change in lung volume which accompanied unit change in transpulmonary pressure (lung recoil). In the case of a, lung compliance is normal (= 0.25 1/cm H_2O approx. or 2.5 1.kPa^{-1}). In the case of b, a smaller change in volume accompanies each unit change in pressure and compliance is low (= 0.1 1/cm H_2O approx. or 1.0 1.kPa^{-1}). Note that lung compliance becomes progressively less as lung volume increases.

intrapleural pressure is more negative than at low lung volumes. The term lung compliance refers to the relationship between this retractive force and lung volume. Lung compliance is expressed as **the change in lung volume brought about by unit change in transpulmonary (intrapleural) pressure** and the units employed are litres per kilopascal or litres per centimetre of water. Fig. 2.2 shows intrapleural pressure at varying lung volumes. The slope of the line represents lung compliance. It will be seen that compliance becomes less at high lung volumes (i.e. smaller volume changes follow changes in pressure at high lung volume).

The retractive forces of the lung are balanced by the semi-rigid elastic structure of the thoracic cage and the action of the respiratory muscles. At the end of a quiet expiration the retractive force exerted by the lungs is nicely balanced by the tendency of the chest wall to spring outwards and the respiratory muscles are at rest.

Airways resistance

During breathing, bigger changes in intrapleural pressure are observed than would be explained by lung retractive forces alone and this is because of the resistance to airflow offered by the respiratory passages (Fig. 2.3). The additional pressure change depends upon the calibre of

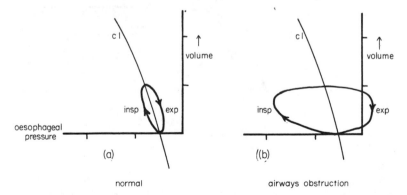

Fig. 2.3. *Change in intrapleural (oesophageal) pressure during quiet breathing.* (a) In a normal individual. During inspiration the pressure is more negative and during expiration more positive than would be expected from consideration of lung compliance: c.l., compliance line. The excessive pressure change is that required to overcome the resistance of the airways. (b) An individual with airways obstruction. Here the pressure changes are even more marked. During expiration oesophageal pressure is actually above atmospheric, indicating compression of the lungs by expiratory musculature.

the airways and also upon the rate of airflow. The greater part of the total airways resistance is situated in the large airway—main bronchi, trachea and larynx—as this is where linear velocity of airflow is highest (p. 3, Fig. 1.3). When breathing through the nose, about a third of the total resistance to flow may be imposed by the nasal passages themselves. Although the large airways and upper airway are the site of most resistance, increased resistance occurring in disease generally originates in more peripheral airways. The effects of such increased distal resistance may, however, be complex, perhaps being expressed by collapse of the larger airways in expiration.

The airways behave differently during inspiration and expiration. During inspiration pulmonary elastic recoil causes the airways to open. During expiration the pull on the walls of the airways diminishes so that there is an increasing tendency towards closure of the airways.

The flow-limiting mechnism

Consider the model of the lung described in Fig. 2.4. During expiration the resistance of the distal airway (Res) will cause a drop in pressure between a and b so that the floppy segment will tend to collapse. It will be protected from collapse by the retractive force of the surrounding lung parenchyma (Rec). The extent of the pressure drop from a to b is proportional to the rate of airflow. There will be a critical rate of airflow which results in b being so much lower than a that the retractive force of the lung is overcome and the floppy segment closes. The closure limits the airflow, leading to less dramatic pressure drop from a to b which permits some re-opening of the floppy segment. It will be apparent that the system will control the maximum rate of airflow to a level determined by lung recoil (assuming that the resistance of the upstream segment (Res) remains constant). Lung recoil depends upon how stretched the lungs are and it should now be clear why high expiratory flow rates are obtainable at high lung volumes, but as lung volume decreases during expiration the maximum flow rate progressively diminishes. For each lung volume there is a particular maximum flow rate which cannot be exceeded no matter how great the expiratory effort (p. 68).

The shape of the forced expiratory spirogram (Fig. 7.6) is thus determined by inherent mechanical properties of the lung and is to a large extent independent of effort above a certain level. This explains its very remarkable reproducibility.

When airways resistance is increased in disease a much greater pressure-drop occurs between a and b (Fig. 2.4) so that the supporting

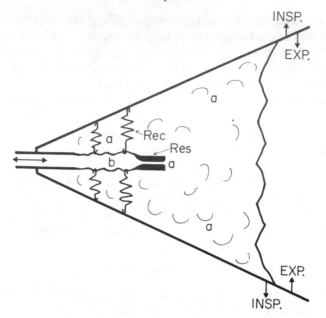

Fig. 2.4. *Model of the lung to demonstrate the flow-limiting mechanism (see text).* The chest is represented as a bellows. The airways of the lungs are represented collectively as having a distal resistive segment (Res) and a more proximal collapsible or 'floppy' segment. The walls of the floppy segment are kept apart by the retractive force of lung recoil (Rec). EXP, expiration; INSP, inspiration.

effect of recoil pressure (Rec) tends to be overcome at more modest rates of expiratory airflow than in the normal. In this situation there is obvious advantage in breathing at a high lung volume which results in a greater lung recoil (Rec).

Forced expiration is discussed further in Chapter 7 (p. 60) in the context of spirometry and the flow–volume loop.

Where does the air go?

During an inspiration the distribution of air within the lungs is uneven because the compliance of different parts of the lungs is not uniform and because the resistance of the airways is also uneven. One of the most obvious causes of the uneven distribution of lung compliance is the effect of gravity. The weight of the lungs causes the upper parts to be kept under a greater stretch than the more dependent zones and the upper parts are thus less compliant. During inspiration more air tends to pass into the lower zones. The uppermost parts of the lungs may be regarded as already almost fully stretched and thus less 'receptive'. The analogy of a suspended spring may help to make the effect of gravity clearer (Fig. 2.5). The greater ventilation of the lower zones during quiet breathing is not inappropriate because gravity also directs pulmonary blood flow preferentially to the lower zones.

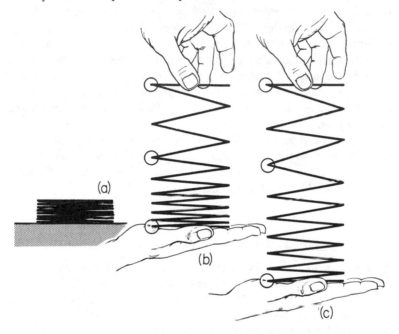

Fig. 2.5. *Gravity and regional ventilation.* The 'Slinky' spring used to demonstrate greater ventilation of the bases in the normal upright lung. (a) The 'Slinky' spring in its resting condition. (b) The spring extended upwards to represent the normal lung suspended within the pleural cavity in a stretched condition by the effect of atmospheric pressure. The circles mark the top, middle and bottom of the spring (lung) under these conditions. (c) The bottom hand has been lowered to represent inspiration. Most of the increase in length has been contributed by the lower part of the spring; the upper part was already at almost full stretch before 'inspiration'. In the lung the upper zones are relatively more stretched than the lower zones and their compliance is thus less. During inspiration under such conditions more air goes to the bases. This is appropriate since the bases are relatively better perfused than the upper zones.

The 'Slinky' spring also permits exploration of the effects of gravity in abnormal lungs. (i) When lung volume is progressively reduced it is evident that collapse is much more likely to occur in the lower zones. (ii) Lung recoil is evidently lower in the lower zones so that the smaller airways are not held open so forcibly. In the presence of diffuse airways obstruction the obstruction tends to be more severe in the lower zones. Many airways in the lower zones close on expiration and ventilation is directed more to the upper zones.

Unevenness of ventilation is also present within the lungs on a more miniature scale—adjacent lobules and even adjacent alveoli may have different compliances and, in response to a change of intrapleural pressure, may accept more or less air than expected. Local differences of airways resistance will also cause some unevenness in the distribution of inspired air. The effect of an increase in airways resistance is to reduce the rate of airflow produced by a given change in intrapleural pressure; that is, to delay filling of the lung or part of the lung. During extremely slow breathing the effect of increased airways resistance will be very small and air will pass into the most receptive (most compliant) parts of the lungs. But when breathing is more rapid, local increase in airways resistance will hamper the acceptance of air by the part of the lung in question because there may be insufficient time for proper filling of the region.

The local differences referred to are probably small in the healthy lung as the network of the lung parenchyma distributes forces fairly evenly, but local differences become important in disease of the lung parenchyma which tend to be patchy in distribution.

Where does the blood go?
(haemodynamics of the pulmonary circulation)

The pulmonary circulation normally offers a much lower resistance to perfusion than the systemic circulation and it operates at a lower perfusion pressure. The difference between the mean pulmonary artery pressure and left atrial pressure in the resting individual is only of the order of 15 mmHg—or less than one-sixth of the effective perfusion pressure of the systemic circulation.

At rest in the erect position gravity exerts a major effect upon the distribution of blood within the lungs. Blood passes predominantly to the bases and there is barely any perfusion of the apices—the pulmonary circulation is not 'full' (Fig. 2.6). If pulmonary artery pressure rises either through an increase in pulmonary vascular resistance or an increase in cardiac output then more of the pulmonary circulation in the upper zones is brought into play.

An increase in left atrial pressure secondary to left-sided cardiac disease will dam back blood in the lungs raising pulmonary venous pressure so that veins further up the lungs become filled. Pulmonary artery pressure must increase if the circulation is to be maintained so that in these circumstances more of the circulation in the upper zones is opened up.

In addition to the major regional effect of gravity there are other factors which affect the distribution of blood within the lungs and these may be quite localized.

HYPOXIA

Hypoxia is a potent pulmonary vasoconstrictor, which seems to be a directed response of arterial smooth muscle to low oxygen tension in the lung surrounding it. By this means blood tends to be diverted away from underventilated areas of the lungs—a process which may be looked upon as a form of autoregulation of pulmonary blood distribution.

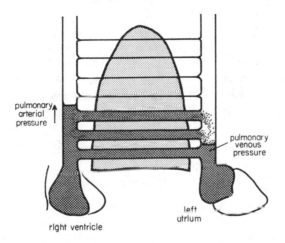

Fig. 2.6. *Model of the pulmonary circulation.* At rest in the erect position the bulk of the cardiac output passes through the bases and the apices are virtually unperfused because pulmonary artery pressure is not sufficiently high. If pulmonary artery pressure rises because of increased cardiac output, increased pulmonary vascular resistance or increased pulmonary venous pressure then more of the pulmonary circulation will be filled.

ALVEOLAR PRESSURE

The pulmonary capillaries are capable of being compressed as they pass through the alveolar walls if alveolar pressure rises above capillary pressure. Under certain circumstances local increases in alveolar pressure may develop and have an effect upon the distribution of blood flow.

GAS EXCHANGE AND VENTILATION PERFUSION RELATIONSHIPS

Overall gas exchange

During steady-state conditions the relationship between the amount of CO_2 produced by the body and the amount of oxygen absorbed depends upon the metabolic activity of the body as a whole and is referred to as the Respiratory Quotient (RQ or R).

$$RQ = \frac{CO_2 \text{ produced}}{O_2 \text{ absorbed}}$$

The actual value is dependent upon the principal metabolic substrate of the body at the time. RQ varies from about 0.7 during pure fat metabolism to 1.0 during pure carbohydrate metabolism and is usually found to be about 0.8 at rest during the day. Overall RQ is important but consideration of gas exchange in the lung is made much easier if its value is assumed to be 1.0. Oxygen and CO_2 are exchanged in equal amounts in this situation.

Alveolar ventilation

It is obvious that not all of the air drawn into the lungs reaches the alveoli. The volume of air filling the airways down to the level of the terminal bronchiole at the end of an inspiration is termed the anatomical deadspace. It is less obvious that even in the normal lung not all of the inspired air which actually reaches the alveoli participates evenly in gas exchange. Some alveoli are relatively overventilated and some are underventilated relative to the blood flow they receive. To overcome the difficulties of analysing such a complicated state of affairs the expired air can be regarded as being derived from two hypothetical sources: (i) ideal alveoli all of which contain alveolar air with the same PCO_2 as arterial blood and (ii) other areas of lung which do not participate in gas exchange at all. These two components of the total ventilation are termed alveolar ventilation and deadspace ventilation. Alveolar ventilation is effective ventilation. Deadspace ventilation is ineffective ventilation. Deadspace ventilation is normally less than a quarter of the total but the proportion varies with breathing frequency, exercise and other influences.

Effect of changing alveolar ventilation

For the moment discussion will be limited to the situation which exists in an idealized normal lung in which all of the units have well-matched ventilation and perfusion, and all behave identically.

CARBON DIOXIDE

If CO_2 is being produced by the tissues of the body at a constant rate the P_{CO_2} of alveolar air depends only upon the amount of outside air that the CO_2 is mixed with in the alveoli; that is, the P_{CO_2} depends only upon alveolar ventilation. If alveolar ventilation is high, the P_{CO_2} will be low; if alveolar ventilation falls the P_{CO_2} will rise. Alveolar P_{CO_2} is inversely proportional to alveolar ventilation.

OXYGEN

The level of alveolar P_{O_2} also varies with alveolar ventilation. If alveolar ventilation is greatly increased the steady uptake of oxygen by the body will only slightly reduce the alveolar P_{O_2} below the level in the outside air. On the other hand, if alveolar ventilation is very low then the alveolar P_{O_2} will fall to a low level. Alveolar (or arterial) P_{O_2} varies directly with alveolar ventilation. Measurement of arterial P_{O_2} is less reliable than measurement of P_{CO_2} as an index of alveolar ventilation because it is profoundly affected by regional changes in ventilation: perfusion ratio as will be shown below.

Measurement of alveolar or arterial P_{CO_2} is the only reliable guide to the adequacy of alveolar ventilation

The changes in alveolar ventilation just described are examples of changes in the ventilation: perfusion ratio (V/Q) of the lungs as a whole.

EFFECT OF OVERALL INCREASE IN V/Q

If alveolar ventilation increases in relation to perfusion then alveolar P_{CO_2} will fall and alveolar P_{O_2} will rise.

EFFECTS OF OVERALL FALL IN V/Q

If alveolar ventilation falls in relation to perfusion, alveolar P_{CO_2} will rise and alveolar P_{O_2} will fall.

In the model under discussion, all of the alveoli behave identically and the arterial blood therefore shows the same changes in P_{CO_2} and P_{O_2} as the alveolar air.

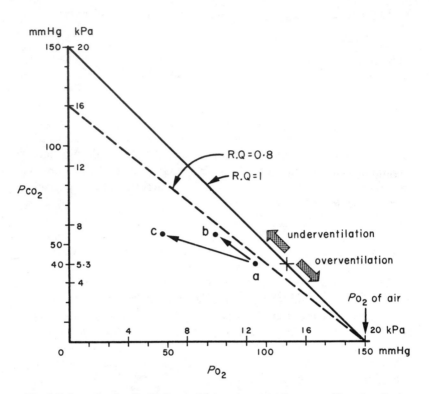

Fig. 2.7. *Oxygen-carbon dioxide diagram.* The continuous and interrupted lines describe the possible combinations of P_{CO_2} and P_{O_2} in alveolar air when the RQ is 1.0 and 0.8 respectively. (a) A hypothetical sample of arterial blood. (b) Progressive underventilation. (c) P_{O_2} lower than can be accounted for by underventilation alone.

RELATIONSHIP BETWEEN P_{CO_2} AND P_{O_2}

The possible combinations of P_{CO_2} and P_{O_2} can be explored with the help of the diagram shown in Fig. 2.7. Moist atmospheric air at 37°C has a P_{O_2} of about 20 kPa (150 mmHg). In our model, oxygen could be exchanged with CO_2 in the alveoli to produce any combination of P_{O_2} and P_{CO_2} described by the oblique line which joins P_{O_2} 20 kPa (150 mmHg) and P_{CO_2} 20 kPa (150 mmHg). The position of the cross on this line represents the composition of a hypothetical sample of alveolar air. A fall in alveolar ventilation would result in an upwards movement of this point along the line and conversely an increase in alveolar ventilation would result in a downward movement of the point.

In practice the RQ is rarely 1.0 and it is nearer the truth to say

$$\text{Alveolar } P_{O_2} + (\text{alveolar } P_{CO_2}/RQ) = 20 \text{ kPa } (150 \text{ mmHg}).$$

The interrupted oblique line represents the combinations of P_{CO_2} and P_{O_2} encountered when the RQ is 0.8. Point *a* represents the P_{CO_2} and P_{O_2} of arterial blood (it lies a little to the left of the RQ 0.8 line because of the small normal alveolar–arterial oxygen tension difference). Point *b* represents the arterial gas tension after a period of underventilation.

This relationship between P_{CO_2} and P_{O_2} is very useful clinically. For example, if the arterial P_{CO_2} and P_{O_2} were those represented by point *c*, it would be clear that the fall in P_{O_2} was more than could be accounted for on the grounds of reduced alveolar ventilation. An appreciation of the relationship between P_{CO_2} and P_{O_2} provides some safeguard against certain errors in blood gas measurement. Even when the RQ is 1.0 the sum of P_{CO_2} and P_{O_2} should not exceed 20 kPa (150 mmHg) when breathing air.

Review of the carriage of CO_2 and O_2 by blood

The quantity of a gas which blood will carry when exposed to different partial pressures of the gas is described by the dissociation curve. The dissociation curves of oxygen and CO_2 are shown together on the same scale in Fig. 2.8. The most important points to be noted are:

1   The amount of CO_2 carried by blood is roughly proportional to the P_{CO_2} prevailing (over the range normally encountered).
2   The quantity of oxygen carried is roughly proportional to the P_{O_2} only over a very limited range—from about 2.7 to 6.7 kPa (20–50 mmHg).
3   Above this level there is less additional oxygen carried with each increase in P_{O_2} and above 13.3 kPa (100 mmHg) the haemoglobin is fully saturated and hardly any additional oxygen is carried.

Effect of local differences in V/Q

In the normal lung the vast majority of alveoli receive ventilation and perfusion in about the right proportion (*a* in Fig. 2.9). In diffuse disease of the lung, however, it is usual for ventilation and perfusion to be irregularly distributed so that a greater scatter of V/Q ratios is encountered (*b* in Fig. 2.9). Even if the *overall V/Q* remains normal there is a wide local variation in V/Q. Looking at Fig. 2.9 it is tempting to suppose that the effects of the alveoli with low V/Q might be nicely

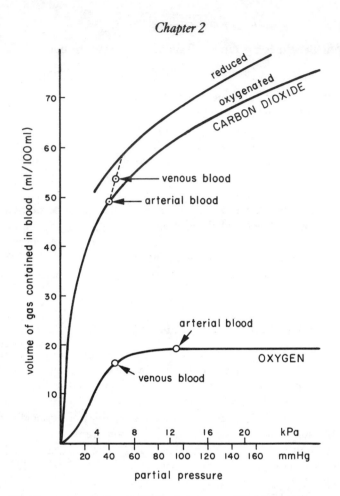

Fig. 2.8. *The oxygen and carbon dioxide dissociation curves of blood drawn to the same scale.*

balanced by the alveoli with high V/Q. In fact this is not the case: the increased range of V/Q within the lung affects the transport of CO_2 and O_2 differently.

In Fig. 2.10 (b) and (c) are regions of low and high V/Q respectively and the result of mixing blood from these two regions is shown at (d) where arterial CO_2 and O_2 content are represented.

EFFECT UPON ARTERIAL CO_2 CONTENT
Blood with a high CO_2 content returning from low V/Q areas mixes with blood with a low CO_2 content returning from high V/Q areas and the net

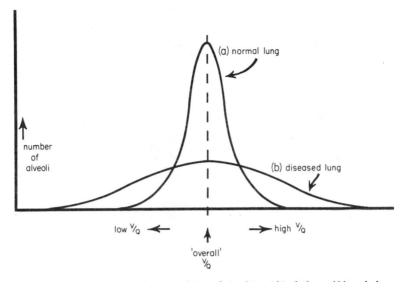

Fig. 2.9. *Distribution of ventilation–perfusion relationships within the lungs.* Although the overall ventilation: perfusion (V/Q) ratio is the same in the two examples shown, the increased spread of V/Q ratios within the diseased lung (b) will result in a lower arterial oxygen tension and content than in the normal lung (a). Arterial P_{CO_2} will be similar in the two situations shown.

CO_2 content of arterial blood may be nearly normal as the two balance out.

EFFECT UPON ARTERIAL O_2 CONTENT

Here the situation is different. Blood returning from low V/Q areas has a low P_{O_2} and a low O_2 content but there is a limit to which this deficit can be made good by mixture with blood returning from high V/Q areas which, although it has a high P_{O_2}, cannot carry more than the 'normal' quantity of oxygen as its O_2 content is limited by saturation of the haemoglobin.

1   Areas of low V/Q result in a rise in arterial CO_2 content and a fall in arterial O_2 content.

2   Increased ventilation of areas of high V/Q may balance the effect upon CO_2 content but will only partly correct the reduction in O_2 content of arterial blood; a degree of hypoxaemia is inevitable.

3   It follows that where arterial oxygen levels are lower than would be expected from consideration of the P_{CO_2} there are probably local areas of low V/Q present in the lungs.

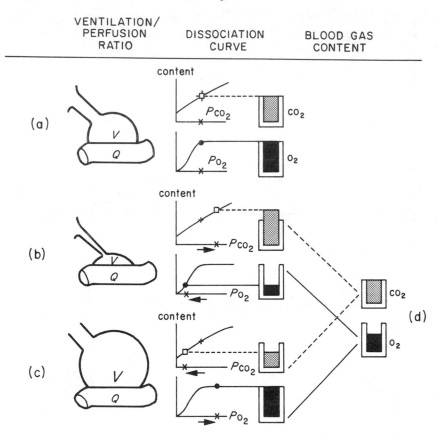

Fig. 2.10. The effect of ventilation–perfusion imbalance. (a) **Appropriate V/Q.** The
ventilation (V)/perfusion (Q) ratio is shown diagrammatically on the left. When ventilation
is appropriately matched to perfusion in an alveolus or in the lung as a whole the PCO_2 is
about 40 mmHg and the PO_2 is about 95 mmHg. The dissocation curves shown in the
centre of the diagram describe the relationship between the blood gas tension and the
amount of gas carried by the blood. The normal blood gas contents are represented very
diagramatically on the right.
(b) **Low V/Q.** Reduced ventilation relative to blood flow results in a rise in PCO_2 and a fall
in PO_2. Reference to the dissociation curves shows that this produces a rise in arterial CO_2
content and a fall in oxygen content.
(c) **High V/Q.** Increased ventilation relative to blood flow results in a fall in PCO_2 and a
rise in PO_2. Reference to the dissociation curves shows that this results in a fall in CO_2
content below the normal level but in the case of oxygen there is no increase in content
above the normal level.
     In health the vast majority of alveoli have an appropriate balance of ventilation and
perfusion and the arterial blood has a normal CO_2 and oxygen content as shown in (a). In

CONTROL OF BREATHING

The main elements involved in the control of breathing are outlined in Fig. 2.11. The respiratory centre is an anatomically ill-defined group of interconnected neurones, responsible for generating phasic motor discharges which ultimately pass by phrenic and intercostal nerves to the respiratory musculature. The medullary discharge is integrated at spinal level and the final output is matched to the mechanical loading of the lungs and chest through the operation of muscle spindles.

Chemical factors in the control of ventilation

Carbon dioxide

The P_{CO_2} of arterial blood is the most important factor in the regulation of ventilation. Normal individuals maintain an arterial P_{CO_2} very close to 5.3 kPa (40 mmHg) and an increase above this level provokes hyperventilation. Arterial P_{CO_2} exerts its effect upon the respiratory centre by stimulating sensitive areas on the surface of the medulla which are bathed by CSF. CO_2 may act on these sensitive areas directly and also by diffusing into the CSF which has less efficient buffering properties than blood. Change in CSF P_{CO_2} produces a greater change in $[H^+]$ than that which occurs in blood. The CSF-mediated effect is probably more potent than the direct effect and this may account for certain anomalies encountered in clinical practice. When longstanding disorders of acid–base balance are corrected the ventilatory control may lag behind despite improvement in the acid–base status of the arterial blood.

many disease states the V/Q ratio varies widely between areas. Such variation always results in disturbance of blood gas content. The effects of areas of low V/Q are not corrected by areas of high V/Q. The result of mixing blood from areas of low and high V/Q is shown diagrammatically on the extreme right of the diagram (d). It will be seen that with respect to CO_2 content the high content of blood from underventilated areas is balanced by the low content of blood from overventilated areas. However in the case of oxygen, the low content of blood from underventilated areas cannot be compensated for by an equivalent increase in the oxygen content of blood from overventilated areas. *Arterial hypoxaemia is inevitable if there are areas of low V/Q* (relative underventilation or overperfusion).

Hydrogen ion [H⁺]

Increase in $[H^+]$ (fall in pH) stimulates ventilation. P_{CO_2} and $[H^+]$ are able to stimulate ventilation independently. $[H^+]$ probably exerts its influence by stimulation of the carotid and aortic bodies.

Oxygen

A fall in arterial oxygen tension stimulates ventilation. The effect of oxygen tension is very small above a P_{O_2} of about 8 kPa (60 mmHg). Hypoxia sensitizes the respiratory centre to CO_2 and the effects of a fall in P_{O_2} and an increase in P_{CO_2} are more than merely additive. Hypoxia exerts its effects by stimulating the carotid and aortic bodies. These receptors are senstitive to reduced oxygen delivery arising from circulatory failure as well as that due to reduced arterial oxygen tension.

Neurogenic factors

1 Higher centres

Sleep and coma of whatever cause reduce the response to the normal ventilatory stimuli. Alarm and excitement tend to stimulate ventilation. Part of the ventilatory response to exercise may be initiated by higher centres as hyperventilation commonly precedes the actual start of exercise. Voluntary control can of course over-ride the normal automatic control of breathing.

2 Brain stem

Breathing is interrupted during coughing, swallowing, phonation and other semi-automatic activities. Damage to the brain stem may cause hyperventilation, hypoventilation or other disturbances of control.

3 Vagus

The vagus carries afferent stimuli from the respiratory tract which may influence breathing.

INFLATION REFLEX (HERING–BREUER)

In animals, stretching of the lungs causes reflex inhibition of subsequent inspiration. This effect is difficult to demonstrate in man and probably unimportant.

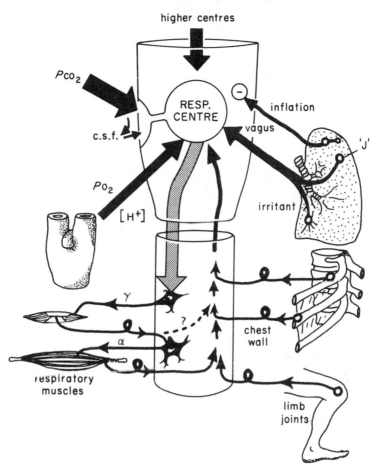

higher centres

Pco_2

RESP. CENTRE

inflation

c.s.f.

vagus

'J'

Po_2

irritant

$[H^+]$

γ

?

chest wall

α

respiratory muscles

limb joints

Fig. 2.11.*Control of ventilation.* Diagram showing some of the more important factors involved (see text).

J RECEPTORS

These are situated deep in the parenchyma of the lung and excitation stimulates ventilation. Pulmonary embolism and pulmonary oedema are among the conditions thought to excite the receptors.

IRRITANT RECEPTORS

These receptors are probably situated in the distal bronchioles. Irritation and local distortion are thought to stimulate them and this results in increased ventilation. It is possible that these receptors may play a part in the production of the hyperventilation which accompanies asthma, inhalation of irritant vapours and gases, pulmonary embolism, pneumonia, etc. Bronchoconstriction appears to be a part of the reflex response.

COUGH RECEPTORS

The larger bronchi and the trachea possess vagally innervated receptors which are sensitive to contact and irritants. Stimulation provokes the cough reflex and a variable degree of bronchoconstriction.

4 Spinal cord

Stretch receptors in muscle tendons and joint position receptors are stimulated by chest movement and may be particularly sensitive to chest deformation caused by increased respiratory effort. The central effect of this sensory information is uncertain. Stimulation of joint receptors in the limbs enhances ventilation and this may be a contributory cause of the hyperpnoea of exercise.

5 Exercise

Ventilation increases in direct proportion to work during exercise. P_{CO_2}, P_{O_2} and $[H^+]$ generally remain normal and cannot explain the ventilatory response. Psychic factors and the limb joint reflex already mentioned are similarly inadequate explanations. A number of hypotheses have been suggested which explain the observed facts but no comprehensive analysis of the control of ventilation has attained general acceptance.

Respiratory sensations

An awareness of the behaviour of the lungs and of the act of breathing may be compiled from several sources. These include vision, hearing, the sensation of movement and temperature change in the upper respiratory tract, sensations originating in vagal irritant and cough receptors, and sensations of chest wall movement.

Appreciation of breath-size and resistance to breathing is probably mainly derived from muscle tendon and joint receptors in the thorax, although the skin receptors may contribute some information. Muscle spindles may provide further sensory signals. Afferent discharge from the spindles enhances the main spinal motor discharge to the muscle when there is a mis-match between the length set by the spindle and that achieved by the muscle. It is not known whether this afferent traffic from the spindle is accessible to higher centres as an index of muscular achievement.

Dyspnoea

This is one of the most important symptoms of respiratory disease and its mode of production is probably complex. It may be defined as an awareness of increased respiratory effort which is unpleasant and recognized as inappropriate. Dyspnoea is NOT:

HYPERVENTILATION
This term is reserved for breathing which is in excess of the body's needs and which therefore results in a lowering of alveolar and arterial P_{CO_2}.

HYPERPNOEA
This merely indicates an increased level of ventilation, such as occurs during exercise: it is appropriate to the situation and not unpleasant.

TACHYPNOEA
This refers to increased rate of breathing.

Experimental work using such techniques as curarization and local anaesthesia of the vagi and chest wall suggest that vagal input, muscular action, chest-wall movement and other sensations are probably all important in the genesis of dyspnoea. There is little to suggest a single source or pathway.

Appreciation of dyspnoea involves recognition of an unsatisfactory ventilatory movement relative to the drive to breathe or an excessive drive to breathe relative to the prevailing circumstances or both. Breathing movements, drive and circumstances are in some way compared with the integrated past experience of each.

CHAPTER 3 / SURFACE TENSION
AND ALVEOLAR STABILITY

Surface tension and small bubbles

Surface tension acting at the curved internal surface of a bubble tends to cause it to decrease in size. The smaller the bubble, the greater this contracting force; small bubbles tend to empty into bigger ones (Fig. 3.1a). Very small bubbles are very unstable and tend to collapse completely. Alveoli are essentially small bubbles and surface tension would make the lungs impossibly difficult to distend if it were not for the presence of surfactant.

Surfactant

Source and nature of surfactant

Surfactant is almost certainly derived from the type II pneumocyte. It is composed of lipoprotein, largely dipalmitoyl lecithin, which is insoluble and forms a thin (probably monomolecular) layer at the air–fluid interface. The molecules probably change their orientation relative to the surfce with change in the surface area of the film.

Action of surfactant

Surfactant modifies the surface tension of the alveolar fluid film. Whereas the tendency of a bubble to collapse increases as the bubble becomes smaller, surfactant has the effect of causing surface tension to fall off markedly as the size of the surface is reduced so that a small bubble remains quite stable. Small bubbles no longer empty into bigger ones but there is instead a tendency for bubbles to adjust to the same size (Fig. 3.1c). Fluid surfaces with surfactant activity exhibit hysteresis— the surface tension-lowering effect of surfactant is improved by a transient increase in size of the surface. During quiet breathing there may be a tendency for occasional alveoli to be underventilated and gradually decrease in size. A deep breath re-expands such alveoli and restores the performance of the surfactant layer. Occasional deep breaths or sighs are a feature of normal breathing and there is some

32

evidence that minute areas of collapse may develop if sighing is prevented. In normal individuals restriction of movement of the chest wall
with strapping results in the development of patchy radiological collapse

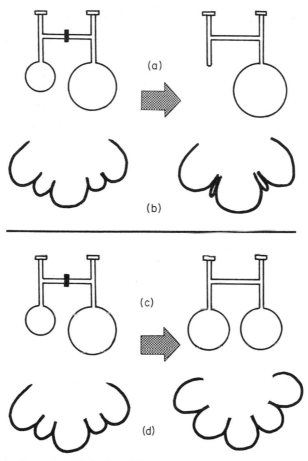

Fig. 3.1. *Surface tension and alveolar stability.*
(a) *No surfactant.* Small bubbles exert greater retractive force than larger bubbles. In a
closed system such as that illustrated small bubbles tend to empty into larger ones.
(b) Diagram of the equivalent situation at alveolar level. Although alveoli are not
interconnected by a closed system they exert retractive forces on each other by virtue of
their side-by-side and back-to-back arrangement in the lung.
(c) *Surfactant present.* Surfactant reduces surface tension as the surface area is reduced.
Small bubbles then exert only a small retractive force. Larger bubbles tend to empty into
them until the bubbles are of similar size.
(d) Equivalent situation at alveolar level. Small alveoli are now stable and there is a
tendency for alveoli to adopt a uniform size.

and an increase in intrapulmonary shunting over the course of some hours. These effects are reversed by one or two deep breaths.

Significance of surfactant in pulmonary disease

It is difficult to measure surfactant activity quantitatively. Surfactant activity is undoubtedly defective in a number of parenchymal lung disorders but in most of these the defect is probably a consequence of lung damage rather than the cause. Defective surfactant activity plays a central role in respiratory distress syndrome of the newborn and may play some part in the evolution and recovery from pulmonary oedema, lung collapse, pneumonia etc.

Patients with painful abdominal wounds, fractured ribs or thoracic cage deformity and patients on long-term artificial ventilation may have shallow tidal breathing and be prevented from taking adequate sighs. All are prone to patchy lung collapse particularly at the lung bases. It seems possible that failure to maintain surfactant activity may have some part to play in the evolution of the collapse.

Production of surfactant is impaired if pulmonary perfusion is severely reduced and this may explain the collapse associated with pulmonary embolism. A number of other factors including the presence of blood in the alveoli appear to impair surfactant activity or production.

Surfactant and the neonate

The first breath

At birth the lungs are filled with amniotic fluid. The first breaths draw the fluid–air interface into the lungs. For the infant to be able to inflate the lungs the fluid surface must have a low surface tension when the surface area is small (small bubbles must be stable). Otherwise the lungs will tend to collapse completely at every expiration. The fluid within the lungs is absorbed via the pulmonary lymphatics in the first hours of life and this is also dependent on the surface tension of the fluid being low.

Respiratory distress syndrome of the newborn (RDN, hyaline membrane disease)

PATHOGENESIS OF RDN

The syndrome is due to deficient surfactant activity usually because of prematurity. Surfactant activity is normally developed at around 32–35 weeks of gestation. In affected infants the alveoli have no stability and the lungs tend to collapse almost completely at the end of each expiration. Lung compliance is extremely low and the infant is unable to maintain adequate ventilation. Severe hypoxia results from underventilation, shunting of blood through airless parts of the lungs and from the reopening of foetal right to left shunts as a consequence of hypoxic pulmonary vasoconstriction.

Autopsy specimens of lung are largely airless. Some alveolar ducts may be aerated and contain a layer of proteinaceous material—hyaline membrane—probably derived from plasma proteins which have leaked from damaged alveolar capillaries.

CLINICAL FEATURES

Signs of respiratory distress—tachypnoea, sternal recession, grunting, cyanosis and tachycardia—are sometimes evident from the first few minutes but may not develop until after an hour or two. The tendency is towards gradual deterioration and without treatment the mortality is very high.

MANAGEMENT

This requires specialist skills. In moderately affected babies oxygenation can be achieved by oxygen administration in an incubator. Severely affected babies require IPPV by cuffed endotracheal tube. Some improvement in results has been achieved with the use of various devices designed to maintain a slight positive pressure in the airways throughout the breathing cycle. The concentration of oxygen employed requires careful control. Sustained levels of Po_2 above 20 kPa (150 mmHg) may cause retrolental fibroplasia and pulmonary oxygen toxicity may be produced with inspired concentration in excess of 50%. Repeated measurements of arterial or capillary blood gas levels are usually necessary. Control of temperature, pH, fluid intake and feeding all require detailed attention. Progress is reflected by the concentration of oxygen required to maintain a Po_2 of about 8 kPa (60 mmHg) and by other parameters such as radiological appearances, ease of ventilation of the lungs, etc.

CHAPTER 4 / DEFENCE MECHANISMS PROTECTING THE LUNG

The lungs bring the whole of the cardiac output into intimate relationship with the outside world and therefore offer the opportunity for immediate potentially devastating access by noxious agents of all sorts: particles, toxic vapours, micro-organisms, etc. A variety of mechanisms oppose such invasion and these merit separate consideration, not least since breakdown of any of them may be associated with pulmonary disease.

Nose

The nose plays an important part. Both smell and non-olfactory detection of irritants in the air can lead to the avoidance of harmful inhalation. Nose breathing removes an important proportion of inhaled particles of all sizes and can remove virtually all particles above about 20 μm. The nose and pharynx 'condition' the inspired air so that over a very wide range of combinations of external temperature and humidity the air in the trachea is fully saturated and at normal body temperature. This prevents drying of the airways which would otherwise lead to crusting of mucus and failure of the mucociliary escalator.

Larynx

Proper sensory and motor function of the larynx is crucial to the protection of the airway from inhalation by food and secretions. The aryepiglottic folds and the false and true vocal cords offer a three-layered defence. Apart from its action in swallowing, the larynx may close the airways instantly in a reflex response to olfactory and other stimuli and it also plays a part in the cough reflex.

Cough

The cough comprises the following actions: (i) sometimes a preliminary inspiration; (ii) closure of the glottis (vocal cords); (iii) contraction of the abdominal musculature and bracing by intercostal musculature; (iv) sudden release of the glottis.

The reflex is provoked by physical or chemical stimulation of irritant receptors in the larynx, trachea or bronchial tree (particularly near bifurcations), or by inflammation in these sites.

The result is a forceful expiratory blast which may remove inadvertently inhaled solid or fluid material. The force of expiration in a vigorous cough is accompanied by a large pressure drop from the alveoli to the trachea and major bronchi which causes compression with invagination of the posterior non-cartilaginous part of the wall. This narrows the airway down to a U-shaped slit resulting in very high flow rates very close to the surface of the mucous membrane, which imparts a shearing force promoting upward movement or actual expulsion of inhaled material or collections of abundant mucus.

Mucociliary escalator

Ciliated cells are present from the terminal bronchiole to the larynx. They are very sparse peripherally and become the predominant cell proximally. The upward movement of a 'raft' of mucus (the gel layer) on the surface of thinner fluid (the sol layer) (Fig. 1.5) propelled by the forward movement of the tips of cilia beating in organized waves is a wonderful clearance mechanism which is crucial to pulmonary health. Regulation of the composition of the airway secretion is probably complex. Alveolar fluid containing lipid surfactant together with material contributed by Clara cells forms the layer peripherally. The quantity and composition of the sol layer seems to be regulated by the brush border of ciliated cells (overall considerable reabsorbtion of fluid is needed as branching airways come together). Goblet cells and mucus glands provide mucus itself. Mucus glycoprotein, the main component, is responsible for the visco-elastic properties of sputum and is composed of a central polypeptide core from which come long chains of sugars. Bonds between these chains give mucus its stability. Viscosity and elasticity of the mucus layer are probably important to ciliary effectiveness; both are complex and difficult to study. A certain elasticity (or recoverable stretching) of mucus by each cilial beat is essential if the mucus is to move forward whilst the cilia recover for the next beat. A degree of viscosity to retard the recovery of the deformed mucus sheet is also important for movement. Excessive viscosity, however, impedes the movement of the cilia. Mucus secretion by goblet cells appears to be increased by local inflammation; mucus gland secretion is under vagal control. Increased mucus production has a protective function, limiting penetration of noxious soluble substances and increasing the likelihood of impaction of particulate matter, but excessive quantities of mucus produced, for example, in chronic bronchitis lead to less effective clearance.

Performance of cilia is affected by smoke, acidosis and toxins; viral infection causes widespread shedding of ciliated cells. The rate of movement of the mucus blanket seems to be faster peripherally than centrally where it is about 1 mm per minute. Material deposited in the airways is normally completely cleared within 24 hours.

Proteins in respiratory secretions

Apart from mucus glycoprotein, respiratory secretions contain proteins derived from plasma which are represented in proportions determined by their intravascular concentration and molecular size. Albumin is present but of more importance are α_1-antitrypsin (the major anti-protease; see p. 224) and immunoglobulins. IgG seems to be present in quantities explained by passive transudation but IgA may be actively transported after binding to the secretory piece on epithelial cells. IgA is an important part of surface defence against inhaled micro-organisms. Resistance in populations is proportional to IgA concentrations. IgA production is defective in malnourishment; it is lower in smokers and may be congenitally absent. Animal work has shown that parenteral immunization leads to IgG production which diffuses into secretions, whereas surface immunization leads to IgA production as well and this may be concentrated at the site of immunization. Bronchial associated lymphoid tissue (BALT) could play a role in this process.

All respiratory secretions contain lysosomal enzyme and interferon.

Alveolar macrophages

Macrophages are normally present within alveoli and within the inter-stitium of the lung parenchyma. They are ultimately of bone marrow origin although they appear able to reproduce locally. Recruitment to the lung is increased by inflammation and products of tissue necrosis. Macrophages are actively phagocytic and largely responsible for dis-posing of particulate matter that reaches alveolar level. Some macro-phages are drawn up on the mucociliary escalator; some appear able to pass through cell junctions peripherally with their burden of ingested matter eventually reaching the lymphatics. Prior opsonization of micro-organisms may be required before the macrophage is able to ingest them. Phagocytic function of macrophages may be impaired by factors such as air pollutants (for example, smoke and ozone), viral infection, alcohol ingestion and malnutrition. In addition to their phagocytic role, macrophages are able to secrete enzymes. They can kill ingested micro-organisms by intracellular production of peroxidase. Macrophages are activated by immune complexes and produce lysosomal enzyme and neutrophil chemotactic factor. The lung can of course recruit large numbers of neutrophils in response to infection and this can be con-sidered a further component of defence. Neutrophils release lysosomal enzyme which may kill micro-organisms and also proteolytic enzymes (especially elastase which may damage lung tissue; see p. 225). The role of lymphocytes within the airways is uncertain. The full range of humoral and cellular immunological, inflammatory and some healing reactions are available within lung tissue itself, constituting a further range of defences which will not be considered here.

Pulmonary lymphatics

Increased lymphatic drainage controls the effects of increased capillary permeability which accompanies alveolar insult. The intrapulmonary and hilar lymph nodes form further defences against general infection by organisms entering the lung.

Particle penetrance

Penetration of airborne particles into the respiratory tract is largely dependent upon their size. In practice, aerodynamic shape also plays a part and the relevant index is referred to as mass mean diameter (MMD). Particles more than about 10 μm in diameter are largely removed by the nose; those of 5–10 μm penetrate the tracheobronchial tree and particles smaller than about 3 μm may reach alveoli. Some particles actually change size as they enter the respiratory tract through hygroscopic attraction.

Particle deposition

Impaction

Heavier particles tend to be flung outwards where there is a change in direction of airflow. A high proportion thus make contact with the wall in the turbulent upper airways and others reaching lower down become impacted where bronchi divide. In particles of intermediate size which

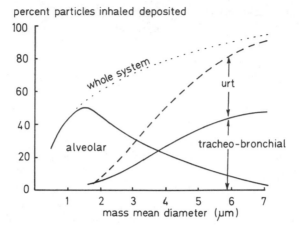

Fig. 4.1. *Deposition of inhaled particles.* Graph showing percentage of particles inhaled which is deposited in the airways—divided into tracheobronchial section and upper respiratory tract (urt)—and the percentage deposited at alveolar level. Particles with a diameter of less than about 3 μm are more likely to be retained at alveolar level than to be removed at a higher level. (After Hatch, 1966.)

reach the bronchi, deposition may to a large extent be determined by slow gravitational settling. Even though the airstream is moving more or less continuously, particles tend to move downwards in the airstream and a proportion make contact with the wall. Very small particles forming a perfect aerosol may impact by chance brownian movement, though this is not thought to be very important; particles of this size are largely exhaled without deposition. Fig. 2.2 shows the relationship between size of particle and deposition in the upper respiratory tract, tracheobronchial tree and alveoli. Patterns of deposition have most immediate relevance in the context of occupational lung disease: some impressively dusty occupations may not be threatening if particles are relatively large and not harmful to clearance mechanisms; other occupations with less impressive dust which penetrates deeply and impedes clearance may result in serious disease. Virus particles when excreted in droplet form dry to a very small desiccated nucleus of less than 0.5 μm. On being inhaled by the host they may behave as very small particles, but they may rehydrate very rapidly during inhalation and impact like larger particles. Consideration of particle size and deposition are obviously of importance in the administration of therapeutic aerosols (see p. 177).

CHAPTER 5 / THE HISTORY—
SYMPTOMS OF RESPIRATORY
DISEASE

Assessment of the patient with respiratory disease hinges on thorough, unhurried history-taking and not upon tests of pulmonary function or the chest X-ray. The aim, as in all history-taking, is to obtain a clear impression of particular symptoms and combinations of symptoms and most importantly to build up a clear picture of their progress or variation with time. The following notes are not intended to be exhaustive but they may be helpful in suggesting ways in which enquiry may be extended.

Dyspnoca (see p. 31)

CHARACTER

What words does the patient use? 'Tightness' may indicate airways obstruction or angina; 'gasping' and 'panting' suggest hyperpnoea—excessive but not necessarily laboured or obstructed breathing. The patient may liken the dyspnoea to the sensation which normally follows running. Is there accompanying noise? A wheezing sound is suggestive of airways narrowing (which may accompany disease not primarily affecting the airways such as pulmonary embolism or incipient pulmonary oedema). A frothy bubbling may accompany frank pulmonary oedema. It is often helpful when in doubt to mimic the sounds in question (wheezing can be reproduced by first breathing quietly right out almost to residual volume and then giving a further sharp forced expiration).

CIRCUMSTANCES

Is it related to time of day, exercise, meals, posture, etc.? Patients with long-standing overinflation dislike bending intensely; asthma has a characteristic diurnal variation (p. 163) and so on.

HOW SEVERE IS IT?

The effect upon a patient's activities is the best guide to severity.

41

Exercise tolerance may be crudely but usefully graded as follows:

	Grade
Short of breath at rest.	4
Short of breath walking about the house and undertaking light activity such as washing.	3
Has to stop even when walking at own reduced pace on the level.	2
Asks friends of own age to slow down but keeps going at own reduced pace on level.	1
Able to walk with friends at normal pace on level but unable to keep going on hills or when hurrying.	0

Inexperienced clinicians are peculiarly prone to preoccupation with the detailed assessment of the nature and severity of current disability and may fail to make a penetrating assessment of its duration and rate of progress—both of which may contain information of critical diagnostic importance. Useful insight may sometimes be gained into the rate and progress of disability by noting change in a patient's *range*. When was he last shopping in a distant centre, when last shopping locally or visiting park or pub? When was the patient last beyond the street in which he lives, the garden gate, the front door, one floor of the house, one room, chair or bed?

Cough and sputum

The duration and annual or daily pattern of cough and sputum production should be clearly established. Nocturnal cough is particularly likely to be associated with asthma or left heart failure. The approximate volume, texture and colour of sputum should be recorded. Black particles usually only reflect local atmospheric pollution, yellow sputum usually indicates a high cellular content due to bacterial infection but in asthma eosinophil clumps can produce similar appearances. Regular production of green sputum may indicate bronchiectasis, as may long-standing day-long production of large volumes of sputum. Enquiry should be made regarding previous *haemoptysis*, its quantity and possible association with epistaxis, fever, chest pain or other respiratory symptoms.

Chest pain

The association of chest pain with respiratory movement, coughing or turning over will suggest a pleural origin. It is sometimes helpful to mimic the wince and grunt which an inspiration evokes in the presence of pleural pain—this is generally recognized immediately by patients who have experienced the symptom. Normal individuals may experience occasional pleural pain which is transient and relieved by gradually taking a deep breath in small steps and this phenomenon is referred to as the 'Catch syndrome'. Sometimes localized anterior chest pain of this sort is accompanied by tenderness of one costochondral junction and this is referred to as Tietze's syndrome or costochondritis: a benign condition. Obese individuals are sometimes troubled by brief costal-margin pain interrupting a breath related to a rib (usually the ninth) rolling over the rib above (clicking rib). Shoulder-tip pain suggests irritation of diaphragmatic pleura and radiation of precordial pain to the neck and arms suggests a myocardial origin. Precordial pain may also accompany mediastinal enlargement, pericarditis and oesophagitis all of which may have special additional features. Pain in the epigastrium and around the costal margin is common in severe airways obstruction and may be related to peptic ulceration, oesophagitis and extreme muscular effort.

Previous respiratory illness

If a patient reports previous episodes of 'bronchitis', 'influenza', 'pneumonia', etc. it is important to obtain a clear account of the nature of the illness and not merely to accept the offered diagnosis at face value. Careful enquiry may reveal that a reported episode of 'bronchitis' had features very suggestive of asthma or that 'pneumonia' might in fact have been pulmonary embolism. The extent of previous investigations and the response to treatment may provide valuable clues. Enquiry should always be made regarding previous X-ray examinations; a surprising proportion of the adult population in the UK has had a chest X-ray at some time or other and, if previous films can be located, they may sometimes provide invaluable information.

Associated allergies

Allergic lung disorders, particularly asthma, are so common that enquiry should always be made about previous skin disorders (eczema, 'dermatitis'), hay fever, recurrent or persistent colds, nasal obstruction, nasal operations, etc.

Family history

A similar enquiry should be made regarding allergic disorders in the family and this should be extended to include 'bronchitis' wheezing and excessive cough and breathlessness as well as tuberculosis. It is worthwhile pausing whilst the patient reviews each generation in turn; if enquiry is hurried it is very likely to be negative.

Occupational history

A clear sequential account of a patient's previous occupations including descriptions of the actual tasks and names of materials encountered may be vital (see especially Asthma, Allergic Extrinsic Alveolitis, Asbestos, Pneumoconiosis).

Smoking history

It is important to obtain a clear account of total smoking exposure and not to be misled by patients who may have recently reduced their consumption or stopped smoking.

CHAPTER 6 / EXAMINATION OF THE CHEST

Some important clues relating to the respiratory system may be evident from the moment the patient is first seen, and these signs should be noted carefully lest they be overlooked during formal examination of the chest. They include the character of the breathing and its relationship to activity and speech, the shape of the shoulders (Fig. 6.1) and spine and the character of the cough. The presence of partial nasal obstruction may be apparent when the patient first speaks but is likely to be overlooked later.

Inspection

Cyanosis

Cyanosis is generally apparent when about 5 g/100 ml of haemoglobin is present in the reduced state within the blood vessels of the skin.

PERIPHERAL CYANOSIS

This is commonly due to local circulatory slowing resulting in more complete extraction of oxygen from the blood. The regions in question are commonly cool.

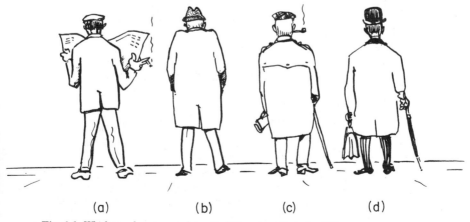

(a)   (b)   (c)   (d)

Fig. 6.1. *Which man has airways obstruction?* (Answer at foot of p. 59.)

CENTRAL CYANOSIS

This is said to exist when the bluish coloration involves areas not normally prone to local circulatory changes. The best site to examine is the tip of the tongue. The lips may sometimes appear blue due to local pigmentation or local circulatory change but the tip of the tongue always has adequate blood supply. Central cyanosis indicates that there is desaturation of arterial blood. When using tissue colour to assess arterial oxygenation note should obviously be taken of the pinkest area visible. Arterial oxygenation cannot be worse than the level suggested by this area. When there is frank central cyanosis arterial P_{O_2} will almost always be below 6 kPa (45 mmHg) depending on haemoglobin content and arterial pH.

Clubbing

Clubbing is easier to recognize than to define rigidly. There is increased curvature of the nail and the nail-bed is raised so that the normal angle between the proximal part of the nail and the skin over the dorsum of the terminal phalanx is lost (Fig. 6.2). The base of the nail may be palpable

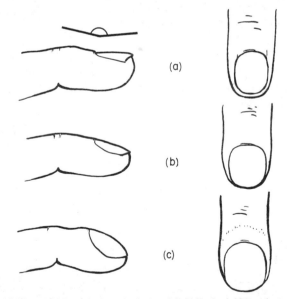

(a)

(b)

(c)

Fig. 6.2. *Clubbing.* (a) Normal, showing the 'angle'. (b) Early clubbing; the angle is absent. (c) Advanced clubbing. The nail shows increased curvature in all directions, the angle is absent, the base of the nail is raised up by spongy tissue and the end of the digit is expanded.

through the skin and an abnormal sponginess may be apparent when pressure is applied over it. Clubbing is associated with:

1 bronchial carcinoma
2 bronchiectasis and other forms of chronic suppurative lung disease
3 pulmonary fibrosis
4 pleural and mediastinal tumours
5 subacute bacterial endocarditis
6 cyanotic congenital heart disease
7 cirrhosis and coeliac disease.

Breathing pattern

From the beginning of the encounter with the patient there will be the opportunity to observe whether he appears to be breathless or distressed, grunting or in pain, wheezing or panting, etc. and these important features should be carefully noted. If it is suspected that the **respiratory rate** may be increased it should be counted over a whole minute as the error inherent in counting for a shorter period such as 15 seconds is large and reduces the value of the observation, particularly if the rate is being counted serially.

The character of the cough

The sound produced by a cough is a most valuable (and widely ignored) physical sign. The patient should be requested to give several sharp coughs (not merely clearing the throat). A rattling sound may give clear indication of the presence of abundant bronchial secretions. A 'bovine cough' lacking the usual explosive onset may suggest vocal cord paralysis. Most importantly, a muffled wheezy cough may provide a very vivid indication of the presence of otherwise quite unsuspected airways obstruction.

Stridor

This (often sinister) sign is likely to be noticed early in the interview as the patient draws breath whilst talking rather than during formal examination of the chest. It can be imitated by breathing in and out with the vocal cords held in the position of the whispered word 'air'. It indicates localized obstruction of the larynx, trachea or large bronchi.

Jugular veins

Examination of the jugular veins should never be omitted. The patient should be examined in a semi-reclining position with the trunk between 30 and 45 degrees from the horizontal. It is very important that the head should be in line with the trunk and fully supported so that the sterno-mastoid muscles are relaxed and soft (if not in use as accessory muscles of respiration). The jugular veins reflect intrathoracic pressure changes and assessment of the level and character of the jugular venous pulse can be difficult when breathing is laboured, but useful information can still be obtained if the patient is asked to take one or two extremely slow, shallow breaths. If he is requested to stop breathing briefly then the glottis is generally closed and the venous pressure is spuriously raised.

Inspection of the chest

Inspection of the chest should begin with an overall view of the shape of the chest and thoracic spine to note any obvious kyphosis, asymmetry, scars, prominent veins, etc. It is then helpful for the patient to adopt the semi-reclining position described above. Flattening, overinflation or other asymmetry may then be assessed by viewing from the front.

Respiratory movements

Regional asymmetry. Despite its semi-rigid nature the chest reflects filling of the underlying lung remarkably well in its movements. The diseased side always moves least. Movement of the upper part of the chest may be more easily appreciated by placing the hands exactly symmetrically on either side of the upper sternum. Contraction of pectoralis major sometimes complicates this observation. Expansion of the lower zones may be appreciated by spreading the hands with the fingers directed backwards and the thumbs close to the mid-line. The relative movement of the two hands and the separation of the thumbs is then observed closely.

Movement of the costal margin. Observation of the movement of the costal margin may reveal a lateralized abnormality; it may also provide a very valuable clue to the presence of airways obstruction. The observation is made in the semi-recumbent position described and movement is best appreciated by placing the fingertips on the costal margin just lateral to the outer edge of rectus abdominis in the position of the circles shown in Fig. 6.3. As the patient breathes, the fingertips should follow

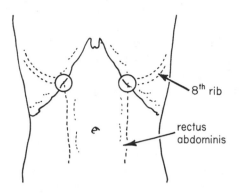

Fig. 6.3. *Movement of the costal margin.* The position for observing costal margin movement with the fingertips is indicated by the circles (see text p. 48).

the costal margin and the distance separating the fingertips of the two hands is closely observed (Fig. 6.4).

(a) In normal quiet breathing the hands move apart on inspiration and towards each other on expiration.

(b) In severe airways obstruction the hands may move towards each other on inspiration and apart again on expiration.

(c) Sometimes in severe airways obstruction the main abnormality is in expiration when there is an outward and then an inward movement.

Patterns (b) and (c) are referred to here as costal margin paradox. The sign is associated with a high inspiratory impedence at a high lung volume. Clinical observation supports the following conclusions.

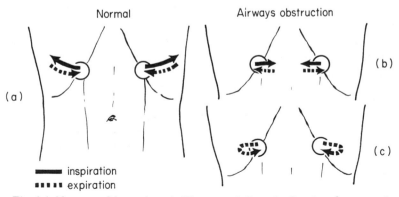

Fig. 6.4. *Movement of the costal margin.* The arrows indicate the direction of movement in normal individuals and in those with severe airways obstruction (see text p. 48).

1   When costal margin paradox is observed there is substantial airways obstruction present.

2   Where severe airways obstruction is already known to be present (by use of a spirometer) but costal margin movement is in the *normal* direction then there is almost always either:

(i)   some factor limiting the volume of the lungs (diffuse fibrosis, infiltration, kyphosis, etc.) or

(ii)   severe emphysema is present (see p. 226).

Costal margin paradox is most commonly seen in association with severe chronic obstructive lung disease (p. 227). It is also seen in infants with bronchiolitis and in subjects of all ages with severe asthma. A change from paradoxical costal margin movement to normal outward movement is a reassuring sign of improvement in an asthmatic crisis, which is particularly useful in those unable to perform simple ventilatory tests. The sign is not present in other causes of dyspnoea such as pulmonary fibrosis or heart failure—with the occasional exception of those cases of pulmonary oedema in which wheezing and airways obstruction are prominent.

Movement of the sternum. In patients with laboured breathing the movement of the sternum should be observed carefully either by viewing from the side or by placing the fingertips of one hand lightly over the lower third of the sternum. Attention is paid to the *anteroposterior* movement of this point. Normally the whole sternum moves forwards during inspiration and backwards during expiration. If the reverse is observed (i.e. indrawing of the lower sternum during inspiration) it generally indicates a high inspiratory impedence at a low lung volume. The sign is referred to here as lower sternal paradox and it is seen in very severe pulmonary fibrosis in which the lungs are contracted and stiff and in localized upper airways obstruction (for example, tracheal narrowing or a blocked endotracheal tube). The sign may help in distinguishing between severe upper airways obstruction causing stridor and severe diffuse airways obstruction.

Summary:

> Costal margin paradox = high volume impeded breathing
>
> Lower sternal paradox = low volume impeded breathing
>   without costal margin paradox

Palpation

Cervical and axillary lymph nodes

These nodes should always be carefully palpated.

Position of the mediastinum

This is assessed by localization of the trachea above and the cardiac apex below.

Ribs

Particularly where there is chest pain the ribs should be palpated carefully, seeking localized tenderness suggesting fracture or swelling suggesting bony metastasis. It may help to compress the chest gently but firmly, laterally and anteroposteriorly; localized pain suggests rib fracture.

Percussion

All areas should be percussed paying particular attention to compare the note obtained with the finger placed exactly symmetrically on the two sides. The presence or absence of hepatic and cardiac dullnesses should be noted—they disappear when the lungs are overinflated (for example, during a deep breath). The position of the tympanitic gastric resonance on the left may provide a clue to the position of the diaphragm. When percussing the back it may be helpful to ask the patient to place one elbow on top of the other in front of him—this has the effect of bringing the scapulae forwards out of the way.

Auscultation

The effect of lung tissue on the transmission of sound gives important information to the clinician (Fig. 6.5).

Source of sound

With the exception of abnormal added sounds (crackles, wheezes, etc. dealt with later), the source of audible sound in the lungs is (i) turbulent air flow in the larynx and central airways and (ii) the voice. Both have high and low pitched components and these are transmitted differently by normal and abnormal lung.

Normal breath sounds

These amount to a faint, low-pitched rushing sound with a gentle

Chapter 6

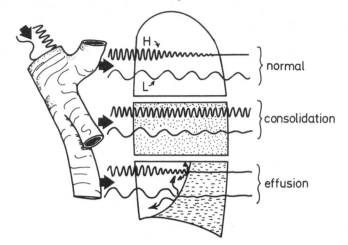

Fig. 6.5. *Summary of sound transmission in the lung.* Sound is generated either by turbulence in the larynx and large airways or by the voice. Both sources are a mixture of high (H) and low (L) pitched components. *Normal aerated lung* filters off the high-pitched component but transmits the low-pitched component quite well. This results in soft low-pitched breath sounds, well conducted vocal resonance and easily palpable very low-pitched sound (vocal fremitus). *Consolidated lung* transmits high-pitched sound well and filters off some of the lower-pitched sound. This results in loud high-pitched breath sounds (bronchial breathing), high-pitched bleating vocal resonance (aegophony) and easy transmission of the high-pitched consonants of speech (whispering pectoriloquy). *Pleural effusion* causes reduction in the transmission of all sound—probably because of reflection of sound waves at the air–fluid interface. Breath sounds are absent, vocal resonance much reduced and vocal fremitus is absent.

beginning and end during inspiration and again rather briefly during expiration. The source of the sound is the larynx and upper airway; normal lung attenuates the higher frequencies leaving the small amount of medium- and low-pitched sound typical of normal breathing. There is some variation in the intensity and character of normal breath sounds consequent upon the thickness of the chest wall, breathing pattern, body size, etc. Breath sounds are normally harsher anteriorly in the upper zones particularly on the right. Two further terms are still occasionally used to describe breath sounds. 'Vesicular breathing' is synonymous with 'normal breath sounds' and derives from an age when it was believed that the entry of air into alveoli generated the sound. 'Air entry' is a loose term used to indicate that breath sounds have been heard with greater or lesser ease. Both of these terms are redundant.

Bronchial breathing

This can be heard over consolidated areas of lung. These areas conduct the high-frequency 'hiss' component from the larger airways quite well. Bronchial breathing is characteristically rather similar in inspiration and expiration and there is a momentary silent pause between the two. The sound can be imitated by listening with a stethoscope over the larynx whilst the subject breathes in and out with the vocal cords held in the position of a whispered 'ee'.

Vocal resonance

The character of vocal resonance—observed by auscultation over the chest during speech—provides further evidence of the lung's ability to transmit or filter different sound frequencies. Normal aerated lung transmits the booming low-pitched components of speech and attenuates the high frequencies. Consolidated lung on the other hand filters off the low frequencies and transmits the higher frequencies so that speech takes on a telephonic or bleating quality (aegophony). The facilitated transmission of high frequencies can be demonstrated by the clear transmission of whispering over consolidated lung (whispering pectoriloquy). Pleural fluid reduces the intensity of all frequencies, most specially low frequencies.

Vocal fremitus

(Included here because it concerns sound transmission.) Normal aerated lung transmits *low* frequencies well and a sonorous voice produces easily palpable fremitus (a buzzing vibration) over the chest wall. Consolidated lung transmits fremitus less well and pleural fluid very severely dampens it and may obliterate the vibrations altogether.

Added sounds (adventitiae)

Semantic difficulties arise here. The term râle is taken by some to mean any added sound and by others as synonymous with crackle and for this reason it is perhaps best avoided.

WHEEZING (RHONCHI)
Wheezes or rhonchi are sustained musical sounds of varying length and pitch. They may be heard during inspiration or expiration (more

commonly the latter) and they are then produced by a flow-limiting mechanism (see p. 15). They tend to be heard in the presence of airways obstruction but they are not inevitably present in this situation and are generally a poor indication of the severity of the obstruction.

CRACKLES (FORMERLY CALLED CREPITATIONS)
A series of very brief clicking sounds which may be loud and coarse or fine and high-pitched. Fine high-pitched crackles can be imitated by rolling a few hairs together close to the ear. The sounds are probably produced by the opening of previously closed bronchioles. The timing of crackles is of some significance.

Early inspiratory crackles
These are associated with diffuse airways obstruction. A series of clicks are commonly heard very close together at the beginning of inspiration with relative silence afterwards. These sounds do *not* indicate pulmonary oedema, left ventricular failure, etc.

Pan-inspiratory or late inspiratory crackles
These are associated with diffuse fibrosis, pulmonary oedema (actual or incipient), bronchiectasis and partial consolidation (Fig. 6.6).

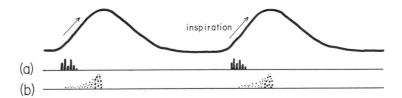

Fig. 6.6. *Timing of crackles.* Diagramatic representation of: (a) early inspiratory crackles—commonly associated with airways obstruction; (b) paninspiratory or late inspiratory crackles—commonly associated with early pulmonary oedema, lung fibrosis, etc.

Probable explanation. During inspiration areas of lung open up in sequence according to their compliance (distensibility). Compliant areas open up first and then, as the retractive forces in the lung increase, increasingly stiff areas participate in receiving inspired air.

In the case of airways obstruction there may be widespread terminal airways closure during expiration particularly in relatively compliant (floppy) parts of the lung. During inspiration these areas accept air most readily and the clicks are probably produced by the opening of their airways early in inspiration.

The disorders associated with late inspiratory crackles cause reduced lung compliance (increased stiffness) which is to some extent patchily distributed. During inspiration air passes first to the more compliant (distensible) parts—that is to the more normal parts—and only begins to enter the stiffer abnormal areas later in inspiration as lung recoil forces build up in the stretching lung.

PLEURAL RUB

Pleural rubs are commonly creaking or groaning sounds and sometimes take the form of an interrupted dry scuffing sound. They are often quite localized and indicate roughening of the normally slippery pleural surfaces.

The sputum

The sputum should *always* be inspected. Truly clear sputum is unusual in city dwellers and if it is thin, slimy and bubbly the specimen is probably saliva. Greyish mottled fragments are usually present in the true mucoid sputum. In asthma, mucoid sputum may be so tenacious that it is impossible to tip it out of a container and it frequently has a glary refractile appearance. If the sputum is creamy or yellow it is referred to as purulent and this appearance commonly reflects active bronchial bacterial infection. Green or khaki coloured sputum indicates delay in production of sputum and suggests bronchiectasis or chronic lung abscess. Brown sputum may be produced by intra-alveolar haemorrhage or a resolving haemoptysis. Solid chunks of sputum are seen in asthma and small bronchial casts may sometimes be seen hanging like fronds below the surface if sputum is suspended in water. A transparent container is an advantage when inspecting sputum, particularly if there is a large amount of saliva and an ordinary universal container is useful in this context.

SIGNS OF LOCAL LUNG DISEASE

Warning

Certain distinctive combinations of physical signs have for generations been recognized as allowing some crude but useful assessment of the type of gross pathological change within the chest. The correlation between the signs and the underlying changes is, however, much looser than is the case in cardiological examination and it is as well to be aware of the limitations of physical examination. In developed countries it is realistic to regard the chest X-ray as a normal extension of physical examination where there is good reason to suspect localized lung disease. The appearances of the chest X-ray frequently modify the interpretation of the physical signs.

Signs of consolidation (airless but not collapsed lung)

Movement of the affected side may be less.
Percussion note is dull—not usually profoundly so.
Vocal fremitus may be somewhat reduced.
Bronchial breathing may be heard.
Crackles may be heard (pan-inspiratory or late inspiratory).
Vocal resonance may have a bleating quality (aegophony).
Whispering pectoriloquy may be heard.

SUMMARY
Moderate dullness, often crepitations and characteristically well conducted high-pitched sound.

Signs of collapse

Reduction in lung volume may be apparent from movement of the *trachea* towards the collapsed side. The chest wall may appear flattened on the affected side. The apex may be displaced towards the collapse. Movement of the affected side may be reduced. The gastric resonance may be exceptionally high in left-sided collapse.

Breath sounds are usually diminished over the collapsed lobe. In addition to these signs there may be signs of consolidation as outlined above—collapse and consolidation commonly occur together.

Note. These signs may be present in massive collapse but sometimes negligible signs accompany collapse, particularly of a lower lobe.

SUMMARY
Perhaps evidence of localized loss of lung volume with reduction in movement, breath sounds and moderate dullness on percussion.

Signs of pleural effusion

Trachea and apex may be displaced away from the effusion if it is massive.

Movement of the affected side may be reduced.

Dullness on percussion. This is the most important sign of pleural fluid and is maximal at the base and in the axilla. At least 500 ml of fluid seem to be necessary before dullness becomes detectable.

Vocal fremitus is reduced or absent over pleural fluid.

Breath sounds are reduced or absent. Towards the upper part of an effusion there may be signs of consolidation.

SUMMARY

Striking dullness on percussion with reduction of breath sounds and vocal fremitus.

Signs of pneumothorax

WITHOUT TENSION

In a small pneumothorax there may be *no* signs at all.

Percussion is usually unremarkable ('hyperrcsonance' is usually unconvincing).

Breath sounds arc absent or much reduced and this may be the only sign. A clicking sound in time with the heart is sometimes heard in small left-sided pneumothoraces due to intermittent contact of the two pleural surfaces over the heart. Othcr signs are generally lacking.

TENSION PNEUMOTHORAX

Trachea and apcx are displaced away from the affected side (important).

Movement of the side may be reduced and the chest may appear fuller on that side.

Percussion may yield a hyperresonant note.

Breath sounds are absent over the pneumothorax.

Vocal resonance and fremitus are somewhat reduced. Tachypnoea and respiratory distress are usual and there may be hypotension, sweating and congestion of neck veins.

SUMMARY

Absent or reduced breath sounds without dullness or signs of consolidation. In tension pneumothorax: displacement of the mediastinum, reduced movement, overdistension and signs of circulatory embarrassment.

Signs of pleural thickening

This is difficult to diagnose with certainty from signs alone.
Movement of the side may be reduced if thickening is extensive.
Dullness on percussion is usual but may not be striking.
Breath sounds are reduced.
Vocal resonance and fremitus are impaired.
Other signs: a pleural rub may be audible but other signs are generally lacking.

SUMMARY
Signs suggestive of a small pleural effusion with sometimes reduced movement of the side in question.

Signs of local pulmonary fibrosis

This is difficult to distinguish from collapse. Upper lobe fibrosis (usually related to old tuberculosis) may produce deviation of the trachea towards the affected side with flattening and reduced movement of the upper chest. Slight dullness, bronchial breathing and crepitations may be evident over the upper lobe.

SIGNS OF DIFFUSE LUNG DISEASE

Diffuse pulmonary fibrosis (p. 203)

Pulmonary oedema (p. 282)

Bronchiectasis (p. 138)

Signs of diffuse airways obstruction

Note: The only really important signs of airways obstruction are provided by a spirometer or a peak flow meter (see p. 64 and p. 63). There are a number of signs which are regularly associated with airways obstruction (described below and see p. 221) but they are not particularly reliable as indicators of its presence or severity, and it is quite easy for experienced observers to overlook severe airways obstruction. The assessment of airways obstruction does NOT hinge merely upon the amount of wheezing audible on auscultation.

The character of the cough is wheezy or muffled—a convenient and very valuable sign.

Signs of overinflation. These can be mimicked by taking in a full breath when it will be found that:

1 The shoulders are high (Fig. 6.1).
2 The antero-posterior diameter of the chest is increased.
3 Accessory muscles of respiration are in operation.
4 Further expansion is limited and accompanied by *inward* movement of the costal margin (Fig. 6.4) and sometimes by descent of the larynx.
5 Percussion reveals absent hepatic and cardiac dullness.

Movement of the costal margin. Inward movement of the costal margin on inspiration is an important sign of severe airways obstruction. An outward movement of the costal margin early in expiration has similar significance. Absence of these signs does not exclude severe airways obstruction (see Figs 6.3 and 6.4 and accompanying text).

Breathing pattern. In severe airways obstruction the patient appears to snatch at inspiration and to have a (relatively) prolonged expiration. In less severe obstruction prolonged expiration is not very obvious. Pursed-lip breathing may be noted.

Wheezes (rhonchi). These may be of high or low pitch and tend to be more marked towards the end of expiration. Very severe airways obstruction can exist without rhonchi. The loudness of rhonchi is related to breathing pattern and is a very poor indicator of severity of obstruction. Prominent inspiratory rhonchi are suggestive of asthma.

Crackles. Early inspiratory crackles and clicks may be heard (p. 54, Fig. 6.5).

Prolonged forced expiratory time. A maximum forced expiration from a position of full inspiration can normally be completed within about 5 seconds. Prolongation beyond this time generally indicates airways obstruction. The end of expiration can be determined by auscultation over the trachea.

From Fig. 6.1. (b) has airways obstruction: note high position of the shoulders.

CHAPTER 7 / PULMONARY FUNCTION TESTS AND BLOOD GASES

Despite the bewildering profusion of sophisticated investigations now employed in testing pulmonary function it (happily) remains possible to obtain most of the information relevant to clinical practice with the aid of a few fairly simple tests. In this section the emphasis will be on simplicity and practicality.

SIMPLE TESTS OF VENTILATORY FUNCTION

Ventilation refers to the process of moving air into and out of the lungs.

Normal values

Ventilatory performance varies widely with body size, age and sex (Fig. 7.1). Tables and nomograms are available which take these variables

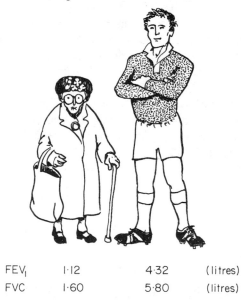

FEV$_1$	1·12	4·32	(litres)
FVC	1·60	5·80	(litres)

Fig. 7.1. *Normal values.*

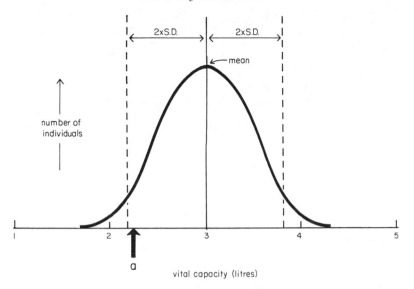

Fig. 7.2. *Distribution of vital capacity in normal individuals of one particular age, height and sex (see text).*

into account and display 'predicted normal values' for individuals of particular age and height. These 'predicted' values are the *mean* values derived from study of a normal population and it should be understood that there is considerable variation about this mean (Fig. 7.2). For example, the standard deviation of the mean predicted value for vital capacity is about 500 ml. In effect this means that if a medium-sized adult has a vital capacity which is 1 litre below the predicted normal value, the low result *may* be the result of respiratory disease but, on the other hand, the value is only 2 standard deviations from the mean and perhaps 5% of normal individuals of the same age and size will be found to have a lower vital capacity than this. The practice of expressing results as a 'percentage of predicted normal' is thus potentially misleading: the finding of a vital capacity of 75% of the predicted value does not indicate a 25% disability and is still compatible with normality.

Vital capacity

The vital capacity is the volume of air expelled by a maximal expiration from a position of full inspiration and this can be measured with any spirometer (Fig. 7.3).

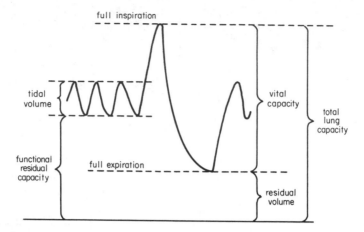

Fig. 7.3. *The more commonly used subdivisions of total lung capacity.*

Vital capacity is reduced in the following circumstances.
1   Reduced lung compliance (lung fibrosis, infiltration, loss of lung volume, pulmonary oedema, etc.).
2   Deformity of the chest (kyphoscoliosis, ankylosing spondylitis, etc.).
3   Muscular weakness (myopathy, myasthenia gravis, etc.).
4   Airways obstruction. (Although the main defect is a limitation in rate of airflow, reduction in vital capacity is almost inevitable.)

Peak expiratory flow rate (PEFR or PEF)

This is measured with a peak flow meter or a peak flow gauge (Fig. 7.4). It is the maximum *rate* of airflow which can be achieved during a sudden forced expiration from a position of full inspiration. The best of three attempts is usually accepted as the PEFR. The value achieved is a little dependent on effort but is mainly determined by the calibre of the airways. The importance of lung volume in determining maximal expiratory airflow has already been mentioned (p. 15) and it follows from this that it is essential that the forced expiration should be performed from the full inspiratory position. The results must be related to body size. PEFR is particularly impaired in the presence of diffuse airways obstruction, but it is also somewhat impaired in conditions which reduce lung volume.

The importance of measurement of peak flow rate stems from its reproducibility, speed, simplicity and convenience. It is particularly

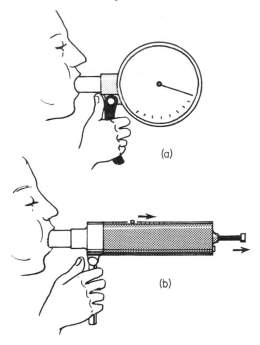

Fig. 7.4. *Measurement of peak expiratory flow rate (PEFR).* (a) Wright peak flow meter (distributed by Air Med, Clement Clarke International); (b) peak flow gauge (Ferraris Development Engineering Ltd.).

The subject takes a *full inspiration*, applies the lips to the mouthpiece and delivers a *sudden* maximal expiratory blast. In (a) a spring-loaded vane is pushed by the expired air uncovering a slot through which air escapes. A ratchet retains the vane at its furthest excursion and PEFR is read from the dial which is calibrated in litres per minute. In (b) the vane is replaced by a piston which uncovers a slot at the top of the cylinder. A ratchet retains the piston at its point of maximum excursion and PEFR is read from a scale on the top of the cylinder. Good agreement is obtained between results obtained with the two instruments.

Another peak flow device which is widely available—the mini Wright peak flow meter—is very similar to the peak flow gauge and is available in two forms, standard and low-reading (Air Med. Clement Clarke International).

important in asthma in which airways obstruction varies considerably (Chapter 15). Occasional measurements of pulmonary function made in the laboratory or clinic are of limited relevance in this condition and much more information about severity, provoking factors and response to treatment (and even about the diagnosis of asthma itself) can be obtained from frequently repeated measurements made by the patient in his or her own home or work environment. This illustrates the fact that sophisticated sensitive tests of pulmonary function do not necessarily yield more discriminatory or relevant information.

The forced expiratory volume in one second (FEV_1) and the forced vital capacity (FVC)

The FEV_1 is the volume of air expelled in the first second of a maximal forced expiration from a position of full inspiration. The forced vital capacity is obtained by continuing the forced expiration until no further air can be expelled.

The FEV_1 is reduced in any condition which reduces vital capacity but it is particularly reduced when there is diffuse airways obstruction. The relationship between FEV_1 and FVC is clinically very useful as it is to a large extent independent of body size and age.

In a forced expiration about 75% of the air is expelled in the first second (FEV_1/FVC = 0.75, this is sometimes referred to as the forced expiratory ratio). In the presence of diffuse airways obstruction a smaller proportion of the air is expelled in the first second (the forced expiratory ratio is reduced).

'Restrictive' and 'obstructive' patterns of ventilatory impairment

When lung volume is restricted by pulmonary fibrosis or infiltration or by rigidity of the chest wall the VC is reduced and the FEV_1 is also reduced in proportion and the forced expiratory ratio is normal or even higher than normal. This pattern of ventilatory impairment is described as a **restrictive defect**.

In the presence of airways obstruction, VC and FEV_1 are again reduced but the FEV_1 is proportionately greater affected than the VC. The forced expiratory ratio is reduced and this pattern is referred to as an **obstructive defect**.

The division of ventilatory defects into obstructive and restrictive patterns is clinically useful but it should be noted that, although diffuse pulmonary fibrosis and parenchymal infiltrations generally produce a restrictive defect, sometimes an obstructive pattern is seen. Pulmonary function tests always require to be interpreted in the light of all additional available information concerning the individual patient.

The forced expiratory spirogram

Any spirometer equipped with a fast-moving recording chart may be used to record the forced expiratory spirogram from which the FEV_1

and FVC may be read. It is important that a true maximum forced expiration is achieved. This can be checked by observing the striking reproducibility of the true forced expiratory spirogram. The FEV_1 and FVC are generally taken as the best of three closely reproducible attempts. Comparison of successive attempts and other useful features of the spirogram can be observed most readily with spirometers which are equipped to start the expired tracing at the same point at each attempt. A widely available self-triggering bellows-type spirometer (Vitalograph) possesses this important facility as well as a number of other features of practical importance (Fig. 7.5). Some commonly-encountered patterns of forced expiratory spirogram are shown in Fig. 7.6.

In addition to FEV_1 and forced VC (FVC) a number of other indices may be calculated from a forced expiratory spirogram. Probably the most useful additional measurement is the maximal mid-expiratory flow rate measured over the middle half of the forced expiration ($FEF_{25-75\%}$). $FEF_{25-75\%}$ is dependent upon age and height, normal values lying between 1.5 and 3.5 litres per second in women and 1.5 and 5.5 litres per second in men.

A further important point to be noted from the spirographic tracing is the forced expiratory time. Normally this is less than 4 seconds and the expiratory curve should be virtually flat at this time. If a substantial proportion of forced expiration is exhaled after 4 seconds then airways

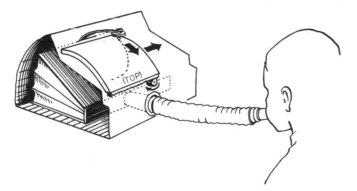

Fig. 7.5. *Schematic view of Vitalograph dry spirometer.* The main components are a bellows and a moving record chart. An arm attached to the bellows carries a writing point which moves forwards across the chart as air enters the bellows. As soon as the bellows moves a microswitch is triggered and a motor causes the record chart to move steadily from left to right. The combination of lateral movement of the chart and forward movement of the writing point causes an oblique line to be inscribed upon the chart (see Fig. 7.6).

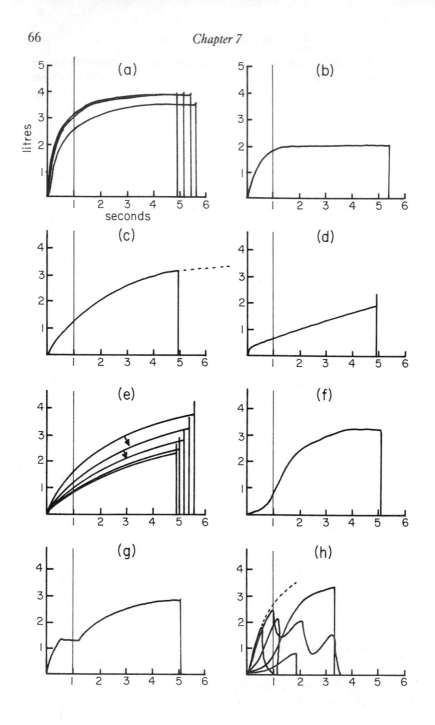

obstruction can be assumed to be present. Although the chart of the Vitalograph spirometer moves only for the first 6 seconds (later models 12 seconds) this is sufficient to observe whether the curve is flat or continuing (Fig. 7.6c,d,e).

$FEF_{25-75\%}$ and observation of forced expiratory time are helpful in borderline cases of airways obstruction and where there appears to be a

Fig. 7.6. *Forced expiratory spirogram tracing obtained with a Vitalograph spirometer.*
(a) *Normal.* Four expirations have been made. Three of these were true maximal forced expirations as indicated by their *reproducibility.* The FEV_1 is 3.2 litres and the VC is 3.8 litres. The forced expiratory ratio (FEV_1/VC) is 84%.
(b) *Restrictive ventilatory defect.* Patient with pulmonary fibrosis. The VC in this case was 2 litres less than the predicted value for the subject. The FEV_1 is also reduced below the predicted value but it represents a large part of the VC. Forced expiratory ratio is greater than 90%.
(c) *Obstructive ventilatory defect.* The FEV_1 is much reduced. The rate of airflow is severely reduced as indicated by the reduced slope of the curve. Note that the forced expiratory time is increased—the patient is still blowing out at 5 seconds. The vital capacity has not been adequately recorded in this case because the patient did not continue the expiration after the chart stopped moving; he could have expired further (this is a common technical error).
(d) *Severe airways obstruction.* The FEV_1 is about 0.5 litres. VC is also reduced but not so strikingly as FEV_1. Forced expiratory ratio 23%. Very low expiratory flow rate. This pattern of a very brief initial rapid phase followed by a straight line indicating little change in maximal flow rate with change in lung volume is sometimes associated with severe emphysema.
(e) *Airways obstruction and bronchial hyperreactivity.* Five expirations have been made, FEV_1 and VC become lower with each expiration. Patient with asthma. This feature suggests poor control of asthma and liability to severe attacks.
(f) *A non-maximal expiration.* Compare with (a). In a true forced expiration the steepest part of the curve always occurs at the beginning of expiration which is not the case in (f). A falsely low FEV_1 and forced expiratory ratio are obtained. Usually the patient has not understood what is required or is unable to co-ordinate his actions. Occasional patients wish to appear worse than they really are. This pattern is unlikely to be mistaken for a true forced expiration because of its shape and because it cannot be reproduced repeatedly.
(g) *Escape of air* from the nose or lips during expiration.
(h) *Inability to perform the manoeuvre.* Five attempts have been made. In some the patient has breathed in and out. Other attempts are either not maximal forced expirations or are unfinished. Bizarre patterns such as this are often seen in patients with psychogenic breathlessness and in the elderly and demented. Even with poor co-operation it is often possible to obtain useful information. In the example shown (h) significant airways obstruction can be excluded because of the steep slope of at least two of the expirations which follow an identical course and show appropriate curvature (dotted line) and the VC can be estimated as not less than 3.2 litres.
    Note: VC in this section is actually *forced* vital capacity (or FVC). Especially in airways obstruction VC performed slowly is rather larger than forced VC.

mixed ventilatory defect. Amongst elderly women in particular airways obstruction (sometimes due to asthma) may be reflected by reduction in VC with the FEV_1 being reduced more or less in proportion so that the forced expiratory ratio is close to 0.75. Inspection of $FEF_{25-75\%}$ and forced expiratory time reveals the true nature of the defect.

The flow–volume loop

In recent years there has been greater interest in another method of displaying maximum (or forced) ventilatory manoeuvres—the flow–volume loop. This is at first a little harder to interpret than the familiar spirometer trace (which represents a plot of volume against time) but it is helpful to bear in mind that the flow–volume loop is merely another way of looking at the same information. There are a number of ways of obtaining an instantaneous record of air **flow**. One way is to use a pneumotachograph which is a transducer comprising a small resistance to air flow through which the subject breathes. Pressure drop across this specially designed laminar-flow resistance is directly proportional to air flow. The pressure is converted to an electrical signal and displayed on an oscilloscope or plotter. The **volume** of air moved can be derived from electrical integration of the flow signal or it can be obtained independently using a spirometer. The flow–volume relationship is usually displayed as in Fig. 7.7, with lung volume on the horizontal axis and flow on the vertical axis. Conventionally full inspiration is to the left and expiration to the right. The horizontal line (Z–Z in Fig. 7.7) itself

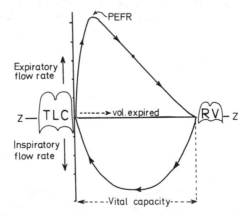

Fig. 7.7. *The flow–volume loop.* Air flow is represented on the vertical axis and lung volume on the horizontal axis. The line Z–Z represents zero flow. Expiratory flow appears above the line; inspiratory flow below. PEFR, peak expiratory flow rate; TLC, total lung capacity; RV, residual volume.

represents no flow. Expiratory flow is represented above the line and inspiratory flow below. The combined expiratory and inspiratory limbs form a loop—the **flow–volume loop**. The shape of the normal loop is as shown and it is quite distinctive. Peak expiratory flow rate (PEFR) is

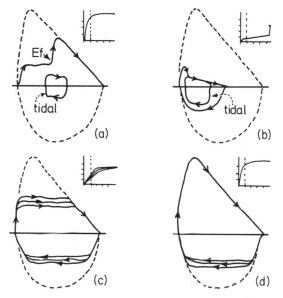

Fig. 7.8. *Further flow–volume loops.* The dotted outline represents a typical normal loop. The small graphs show the appearances of a forced expiration on a Vitalograph spirometer (as in Fig. 7.6). (a) *Demonstration of maximum flow.* A normal individual makes an unhurried expiration from full inspiration and then about half way through the vital capacity a maximal expiratory effort (Ef) is made. The flow–volume tracing rejoins the maximum flow–volume curve which describes the highest flow which can be achieved at that lung volume. Also shown in (a) is the flow–volume loop of typical tidal breathing. At the resting lung volume there is an abundant reserve of both inspiratory and expiratory flow available. (b) *Very severe airways obstruction* in an individual with emphysema. Maximum expiratory flow is very severely reduced. There is a brief peak (probably caused by airways collapse) after which flow falls very slowly. Also shown in (b) is a loop representing quiet tidal breathing. It is clear that every expiration is limited by maximum flow. Expiratory wheezing or purse lip breathing would be expected. There is some inspiratory reserve of flow but hardly any expiratory reserve. Ventilation could be increased slightly by adopting an even higher lung volume and by speeding up inspiration. (c) *Fixed intrathoracic large airways obstruction:* for example, tracheal compression by a mediastinal tumour. Here the peak inspiratory and expiratory flows have been truncated in a characteristic pattern. (d) *Variable extrathoracic obstruction.* Severe extrathoracic obstruction results in inspiratory collapse of the airway below the obstruction (but still outside the thorax). In this example expiration is normal, and this suggests a variable check-valve mechanism such as might be caused by bilateral vocal cord paralysis.

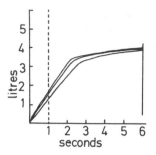

Fig. 7.9. *Large (central) airways obstruction.* Typical tracing obtained with a vitalograph spirometer. The subject has made three maximal forced expirations. Each shows a striking straight section which then changes relatively abruptly at about the same volume to the expected curve of the forced expiratory spirogram. The straight section is not as reproducible as a normal spirogram. A 'family' of similar tracings is thus obtained, each with straight and curved sections. *Explanation:* Over the straight section flow is limited by the fixed intrathoracic localized obstruction. Above a particular expiratory effort there is collapse of the large airway above the obstruction—a flow-limiting mechanism (p. 15)—this is little influenced by lung recoil so the critical flow is similar during expiration and the spirogram appears straight. A lung volume is eventually reached where maximum flow is even lower than that permitted by the central obstruction. The ordinary forced expiratory spirogram is described after this point. In the example shown there must be an element of diffuse airways obstruction as forced expiratory time is somewhat prolonged (see also Fig. 7.8c).

reached early in expiration from total lung capacity (TLC) and it is somewhat faster than peak inspiratory flow. There is a steady fall in the maximum expiratory flow that can be achieved as expiration progresses. The expiratory limb is highly reproducible: the subject finds it impossible to break out of the boundary of the loop (Fig. 7.8a). The line describes the maximum flow that can be achieved at each particular lung volume. Inspiration is rather less reproducible; maximum inspiratory flow is achieved in mid inspiration.

The flow–volume curve may be used to derive indices of maximum flow towards the middle or end of expiration (for example, the maximum flow after 50% or 75% of the vital capacity has been expired ($FEF_{50\%}$ or $\dot{V}_{max50}$; $FEF_{75\%}$ or $\dot{V}_{max75}$). These indices may be more sensitive to increased resistance in the small airways (in contrast to PEFR and FEV which are predominantly influenced by diffuse changes affecting medium-sized and larger airways) and they have found some applications in research. A further application of the flow–volume loop is in the elucidation of localized narrowing of the large airways (Fig. 7.8). In practice there is quite often difficulty in diagnosing obstruction of the large airways: usually because the possibility is not considered in the first place. It is therefore of some importance to be able to recognize the pattern produced by fixed intrathoracic large airway obstruction using an ordinary spirometer (Fig. 7.9).

BLOOD GAS MEASUREMENT

Alveolar ventilation

Measurement of P_{CO_2}

The only satisfactory means of assessing the adequacy of ventilation is measurement of alveolar or arterial P_{CO_2} (see p. 21).

MEASUREMENT OF P_{CO_2} BY REBREATHING TECHNIQUE
Changes in arterial P_{CO_2} are mirrored by changes in mixed venous P_{CO_2} (provided CO_2 production and cardiac output are not grossly disturbed). The rebreathing technique first described by Campbell and Howell permits mixed venous P_{CO_2} to be measured quickly and conveniently at the bedside or in the consulting room by non-invasive means (Fig. 6.10).

Procedure (abbreviated version of the method)
1   A rubber bag is filled with about 2 litres of oxygen.
2   The patient breathes quietly in and out of the bag for 90 seconds.
3   The CO_2 concentration of the mixture in the bag is measured using a modified Haldane apparatus.

During the period of rebreathing the concentration of CO_2 in the bag rises sharply to start with but only very slowly towards the end of 90 seconds (Fig. 7.10). By this time there is equilibrium (with respect to CO_2) between the blood in the pulmonary capillaries (mixed venous blood) and the air going back and forth between bag and lungs. Mixed venous P_{CO_2} is then the same as the P_{CO_2} of the contents of the bag. The latter is obtained by multiplying the percentage concentration of CO_2 in the bag by the available barometric pressure (barometric pressure less water vapour pressure at 37°C).

The mixed venous P_{CO_2} measured by this means is about 1.2 kPa (9 mmHg) higher than the arterial P_{CO_2}. For most clinical purposes it is justifiable and convenient to subtract this amount and to quote the result as an 'arterial' P_{CO_2} (rebreathe method).

Arterial P_{CO_2} is normally between 4.8 and 6.1 kPa (36 and 46 mmHg).

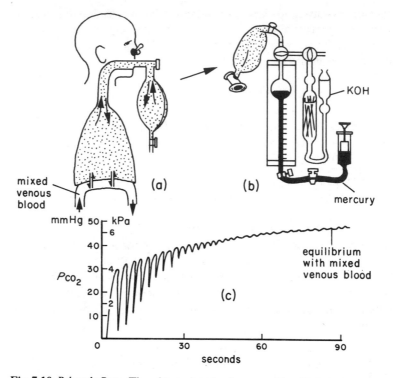

Fig. 7.10. *Rebreathe* P_{CO_2}. The subject rebreathes from a small bag filled with oxygen until equilibrium between the bag, lungs and venous blood is achieved (a). The CO_2 concentration of the contents of the bag is then measured with modified Haldane gas analysis apparatus (b). (c) shows the result of rapid CO_2 analysis of the bag contents during the procedure. Equilibrium is achieved after about 90 seconds. After this there is a very slow rise in CO_2 concentration of the bag (and the subject's arterial blood). The value for P_{CO_2} obtained at 90 seconds approximates to that of mixed venous blood.

MEASUREMENT OF ARTERIAL P_{CO_2} BY ELECTRODE

Arterial P_{CO_2} is almost always measured with an electrode of the Severinghaus type. It is now common for this to be miniaturized and incorporated within an automated system together with electrodes measuring pH and P_{CO_2} enabling small samples to be handled in a standardized manner. The CO_2 electrode comprises a pH electrode with a thin film of bicarbonate kept in position over its tip by a polypropylene membrane and fitted into a small sample chamber. When blood comes into contact with the membrane, CO_2 diffuses rapidly across into the bicarbonate solution and the pH in the solution stabilizes at a value related to the sample P_{CO_2}. The meter is calibrated to read

P_{CO_2} directly and the electrode is calibrated using gases of solutions of known P_{CO_2}

MEASUREMENT OF P_{CO_2} BY CALCULATION FROM PH
AND BICARBONATE LEVEL
It is now quite common for pH, P_{CO_2} and plasma bicarbonate all to be measured directly in the laboratory. If any two of these are known the third may be calculated or read from a graphical representation of the Henderson–Hasselbalch equation such as that shown in Fig. 7.15.

MEASUREMENT OF P_{O_2}
See p. 82.

ACID–BASE BALANCE

Background

RELATIONSHIP BETWEEN [H⁺] AND P_{CO_2}
If a solution of bicarbonate is brought into equilibrium with several gas mixtures in turn, each with a different P_{CO_2}, and if hydrogen ion concentration, [H⁺], is measured after each equilibrium it will be found that there is a direct relationship between P_{CO_2} and [H⁺] (Fig. 7.11). This relationship between P_{CO_2} and [H⁺] is a representation in graphic terms of the Henderson–Hasselbalch equation.

Dissolved CO_2 forms carbonic acid which dissociates into H_2O and CO_2 in a constant relationship:

$$K = \frac{[H^+][HCO_3^-]}{[H_2CO_3]}$$

The [H⁺] can be expressed thus:

$$[H^+] \propto \frac{[H_2CO_3]}{HCO_3^-}$$

The concentration of H_2CO_3 is directly related to the prevailing partial pressure of CO_2 so the formula can be written:

$$[H^+] \propto \frac{P_{CO_2}}{[HCO_3^-]}$$

In other words there is a direct linear relationship between P_{CO_2} and [H⁺] of the sort shown in Fig. 7.11.

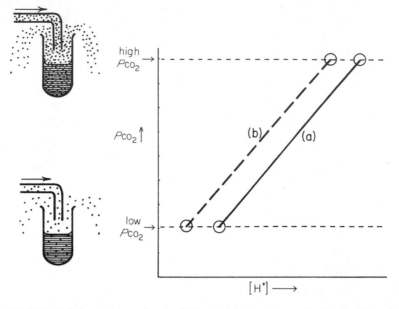

Fig. 7.11. *Relationship between* $P\text{CO}_2$ *and hydrogen ion concentration in a bicarbonate solution.* A solution of bircarbonate is equilibrated with two gases of known $P\text{CO}_2$. H^+ is measured. (a) shows the relationship between $P\text{CO}_2$ and H^+ for that solution (the buffer line). (b) shows the relationship for a solution with a higher bicarbonate concentration.

If in this model some bicarbonate is added to the solution and the same procedure repeated it will again be found that there is a direct relationship between $P\text{CO}_2$ and $[H^+]$ but at each level of $P\text{CO}_2$ the $[H^+]$ will be lower than previously (b in Fig. 7.11).

$[H^+]$ is generally expressed as pH, which is the negative logarithm of $[H^+]$ but this does not prevent a convenient linear plot of pH against $P\text{CO}_2$ if the latter is given a logarithmic scale (Fig. 7.12). For any particular bicarbonate solution a line may be plotted which describes the relationship between pH and $P\text{CO}_2$ in that solution. Interpretation of acid–base status requires knowledge of pH, $P\text{CO}_2$ and bicarbonate concentration.

BICARBONATE CONCENTRATION

Bicarbonate concentration can be calculated if $P\text{CO}_2$ and pH are known (see Fig. 7.15) and it can also be measured directly: the *Actual*

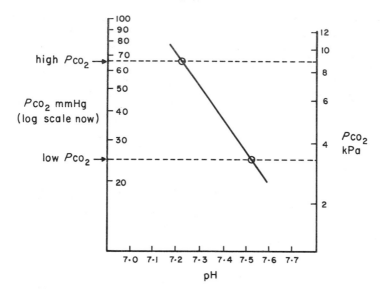

Fig. 7.12. *Plot of PCO₂ and pH.* This figure shows the same relationship as in Fig. 6.8. The [H⁺] scale has been converted into the more widely used pH. pH is the negative logarithm of [H⁺]. High [H⁺] is now on the left and low [H⁺] on the right and the buffer line now slopes the other way. Because pH is a logarithmic term, PCO₂ has been given a logarithmic scale so that the straightline relationship between the two is retained.

bicarbonate concentration. *Standard bicarbonate* is a calculated value indicating what the bicarbonate concentration would be at a standard PCO_2 (of 5.3 kPa or 40 mmHg). Two other expressions can also be obtained by calculation if haemoglobin is known; they are *base excess* and *buffer base.* These expressions recognize the fact that there are other buffers apart from bicarbonate in the blood. There is little to choose between these parameters of the buffering capacity of blood—actual or standard bicarbonate, buffer base and base excess—it is a matter of individual preference which is employed. They all behave in a similar fashion in disturbances of acid-base homeostasis.

Review of patterns of disturbance of acid–base balance

Although there are other buffering systems in the body, the $CO_2/$ bicarbonate system is the most accessible and the most responsive and, for clinical purposes, disturbances of acid–base balance are usually discussed in terms of the changes observed in it. pH is determined by the ratio of P_{CO_2} to bicarbonate concentration. Changes in pH which are caused primarily by an alteration in P_{CO_2} are termed **respiratory**; P_{CO_2} is determined by alveolar ventilation. Changes in pH which are brought about by changes in bicarbonate concentration are termed 'non-respiratory' or, by convention, **metabolic**. The renal tubule modulates bicarbonate concentration in response to the prevailing P_{CO_2} but this is very slow. (The kidney has other important functions in acid–base regulations which will not be reviewed here).

Acid–base diagrams

It is usual to employ a diagram to assist discussion of this topic. The three variables pH, P_{CO_2} and bicarbonate can be displayed by several graphical means, all based upon the Henderson–Hasselbalch equation and all having about equal merit. The format already described with axes comprising log P_{CO_2} and pH is a convenient base from which to

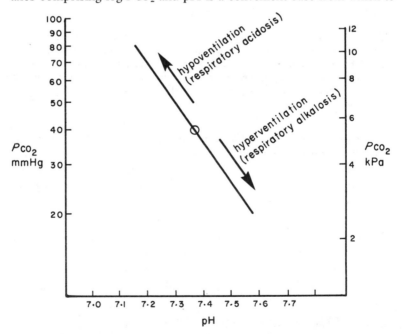

Fig. 7.13. *'Respiratory' acidosis and alkalosis.* If the bicarbonate concentration remains unaltered then changes in pH of the blood must be due to changes in P_{CO_2}. P_{CO_2} is determined by alveolar ventilation. Hyperventilation causes fall in P_{CO_2} and a rise in pH and movement of the arterial point downwards along the buffer line as shown above. Hypoventilation causes increase in P_{CO_2} and an upward movement of the arterial point.

start. In the following section outlining the principal types of disturbance the reader should refer frequently firstly to Fig. 7.13 which allows the three components to be related to each other and secondly to Fig. 7.16 which shows the direction in which disturbances from the normal are observed to occur in well-defined experimental or clinical situations where there is an uncomplicated 'pure' disturbance of either ventilation (respiratory) or bicarbonate (metabolic) compounds.

RESPIRATORY ACIDOSIS (ACUTE)

Reduction in alveolar ventilation causes an increase in arterial P_{CO_2}. In the short term there is insufficient time for renal compensation by reabsorbtion of bicarbonate so that the bicarbonate concentration remains almost unchanged. The change in pH is entirely due to change in P_{CO_2} and the arterial blood point is plotted in the direction indicated in Fig. 6.10.

Note: In practice the changes *in vivo* are slightly different from the expected changes because of the operation of other buffering systems apart from bicarbonate (see Fig. 7.16).

There is *some* increase in the bicarbonate level because increase in P_{CO_2} leads to increase in dissolved CO_2. Dissolved CO_2 is a small part of the total and the change in bicarbonate in pure respiratory disturbances is small (Fig. 7.15).

Causes. An acute underventilation–obstruction of the airway, opiate overdosage, massive neurological damage, paralysis etc.

Pattern. pH reduced, P_{CO_2} raised, bicarbonate normal.

RESPIRATORY ALKALOSIS

Alveolar hyperventilation causes a fall in P_{CO_2} and the arterial point is plotted in the direction indicated (Fig. 7.16). Bicarbonate concentration is virtually unchanged and the change in pH is due principally to the change in P_{CO_2}. In long-sustained respiratory alkalosis there is some renal adaption with reduction in plasma bicarbonate (restoring pH towards normal) but this compensation is slow and partial.

Causes. Any form of acute hyperventilation—pulmonary embolism, acute asthma, salicylate poisoning, anxiety and hysteria etc.

Pattern. pH raised, P_{CO_2}, reduced, bicarbonate normal.

METABOLIC ACIDOSIS

The primary disturbance is generally an increase in acid. This has an effect on the equilibrium $H^+ . HCO_3' \rightleftharpoons H_2O + CO_2$ pushing it to the right. The CO_2 produced is removed by increased ventilation and the nett result is a lowering of plasma bicarbonate. An acute fall in bicarbonate results in an acute shift of the 'buffer line' to the left (Fig. 7.14). In practice the resulting fall in pH causes further respiratory stimulation so that the P_{CO_2} is reduced promptly and the arterial point moves in the direction indicated in Fig. 7.16—the lowering of P_{CO_2} ensures that the change in pH is much less dramatic than would otherwise have been the case. This respiratory compensation is an inevitable accompaniment in metabolic acidosis—acute and chronic—unless there is some other factor limiting ventilatory function or responsiveness.

Causes. Diabetic ketoacidosis, acute circulatory failure and other forms of lactic acidosis, renal tubular acidosis, etc.

Pattern. pH reduced, P_{CO_2} reduced, bicarbonate reduced.

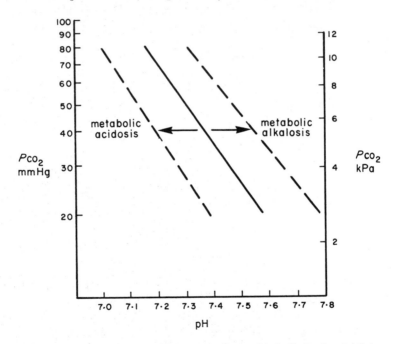

Fig. 7.14. *'Metabolic' acidosis and alkalosis.* The position of the buffer line has already been noted to be dependent upon the bicarbonate concentration of the solution. Changes in the level of plasma bicarbonate are the result of non-respiratory metabolic changes. pH change which is largely the result of altered bicarbonate buffering is loosely referred to as 'metabolic'. The buffer line moves to the left with fall in bicarbonate (metabolic acidosis) and to the right with increase in bicarbonate (metabolic alkalosis). In the Siggard–Andersen plot of P_{CO_2} and pH various indices which reflect bicarbonate content and buffering capacity of the blood can be read directly from the intersection of the line with special nomograms.

METABOLIC ALKALOSIS

Increase in bicarbonate concentration has the effect of moving the 'buffer line' to the right (Fig. 7.14). In practice the P_{CO_2} usually increases a little so that the change in pH is a little less than would otherwise have occurred. This compensatory fall in alveolar ventilation is usually slight and the correction partial.

Causes. Administration of excessive alkali, loss of acid through vomiting, reabsorbtion of bicarbonate, e.g. in hypokalaemia.

Pattern. pH raised, P_{CO_2} normal or slightly raised, bicarbonate raised.

CHRONIC RESPIRATORY ACIDOSIS

(Sometimes called chronic compensated respiratory acidosis.) If underventilation from whatever cause is sustained for some days renal tubular reabsorption of bicarbonate will achieve significant elevation of plasma bicarbonate level and this has the effect of correcting the acidosis. The arterial point moves on the diagram toward the right (Fig. 7.16). The correction is usually not complete so that the pH remains a little low.

Causes. Any cause of sustained hypoventilation—most commonly chronic obstructive pulmonary disease.

Pattern. pH normal or slightly reduced, P_{CO_2} elevated, bicarbonate elevated.

MIXED DISTURBANCES

These are quite common. Mixed disturbances are represented in Fig. 7.16 by the spaces between the limbs of the shaded area; the nature of the mixed disturbance is indicated by the adjacent limbs. For example, point (a) in Fig. 7.16 (low pH, normal P_{CO_2}, low bicarbonate) indicates a mixed metabolic and respiratory acidosis. Note that an element of respiratory acidosis can be deduced even though the P_{CO_2} is not significantly raised. This is because the P_{CO_2} is higher than would have been expected in an individual with a 'pure' metabolic disturbance.

Interpretation of mixed disturbances

In mixed disturbances there are usually a number of possible interpretations. For example point (a) (Fig. 7.16) is equally compatible with the following totally different clinical situations.

1 A patient with acute pulmonary oedema who is severely hypoxic and also in low-output cardiac failure. The metabolic acidosis reflects probable lactic acidosis from critically low peripheral oxygen delivery (Chapter 26) and the P_{CO_2} suggests that, despite the ventilatory stimuli

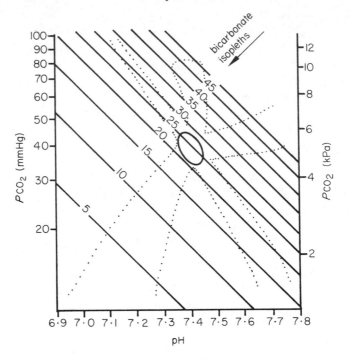

Fig. 7.15. *Relationship between P_{CO_2}, pH and actual bicarbonate ion concentration* (compare with Figs 7.13 and 7.14). If two of the indices are known the third may be estimated from the diagram. The oval indicates normal values. The dotted areas indicate the direction of the main patterns of acid-base disturbance; these are shown in Fig. 7.16.

stemming from the acidosis, hypoxia and the pulmonary oedema the patient's ability to hyperventilate is compromised.

2 A patient in renal failure with accompanying acidosis who has been given a narcotic agent which has suppressed the ventilatory response to the acidosis.

Unless the clinical situation is known beforehand, it is generally not possible to interpret the acid–base data beyond describing the components of the mixed disturbance.

Further examples of mixed disturbances (Fig. 7.16)

Point (b). This could represent the situation soon after a cardiac arrest where a severe lactic acidosis exists and the emergency artificial ventilation or the patient's spontaneous ventilation has been insufficient.

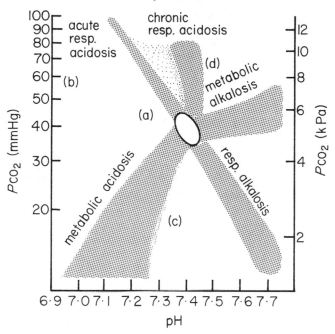

Fig. 7.16. *Acid–base disturbances.* The oval indicates the normal position. The shaded areas indicate the direction of observed 'pure' or uncomplicated disturbances of acid–base balance. Bicarbonate levels are omitted for clarity but are shown in Fig. 7.11. Letters a–d are referred to in the text (see Interpretation of mixed disturbances).

Point (c). This could represent the situation in severe aspirin poisoning where aspirin-induced hyperventilation has been complicated by aspirin-induced metabolic acidosis.

Point (d). This could represent the situation of an individual with chronic ventilatory failure due to chronic obstructive lung disease (e.g. previously with P_{CO_2} 75 mmHg, 10 kPa and pH 7.4) who is stimulated to increase ventilation shortly before the sample was taken by physiotherapy, pulmonary embolism, IPPV, etc.

SCOPE AND LIMITATIONS OF ACUTE ACID–BASE DATA
1 Has limited diagnostic potential considered on its own.
2 May help by indicating that a disturbance is mixed rather than simple.
3 May provide a useful indication of the severity of a disturbance.

4   May provide useful information concerning the trend of a disturbance.
5   Only rarely requires direct treatment. Almost always the disturbance is managed by taking measures to reverse the primary process giving rise to the abnormality rather than by giving acid or alkali.

ARTERIAL OXYGENATION

A note on arterial blood sampling

Sampling from the radial artery at the wrist has advantages over other sites such as the femoral or brachial arteries.
1   The artery is readily palpable.
2   There is no big vein accompanying it.
3   It is easily compressed against the radius after puncture.
4   If a haematoma does develop it is soon detected and not hidden beneath clothes.
5   In the unlikely event of the artery becoming damaged there is an excellent collateral circulation via the palmar arch.

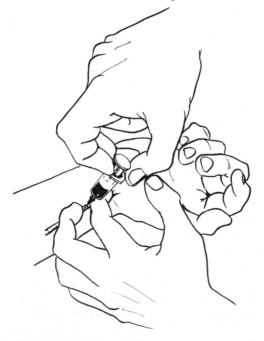

Fig. 7.17. *Sampling arterial blood from radial artery.*

There is no need to transfix the artery by a vertical stab; it may easily be entered by an angled approach along the line of the vessel (Fig. 7.17). For clinical purposes it is perfectly acceptable to use a small plastic syringe and a fine needle provided only light suction is applied and the specimen is analysed promptly. Use of a fine needle followed by good compression causes minimal trauma to the artery and repeated sampling from the same site is possible.

Capillary blood sampling

Capillary blood sampled from a warmed ear-lobe or finger yields blood gas values very close to those of arterial blood. The samples are collected into heparinized capillary tubes which are sealed. The method is not suitable when the peripheral circulation is impaired.

Arterial oxygenation can be assessed by measurement of either oxygen tension or saturation.

Oxygen tension Pco_2

This is measured using a Clark-type platinum polarigraphic electrode which comprises a platinum cathode and a silver anode in a tiny electrolytic cell biased by a small voltage and separated from the blood sample by a thin membrane. The current output of the cell is proportional to the availability of oxygen molecules at the platinum surface and hence to Po_2. Transcutaneous oxygen electrodes are now available but they require expert handling and have limited clinical uses.

Oxygen saturation

Saturation is generally measured using spectrophotometric methods based on the different absorption of light of particular wavelengths by reduced and oxygenated haemoglobin—a difference which is apparent from the difference in colour. In some intruments the intensity of the light transmitted through the specimen is measured and in others the reflected light is measured. The Kipp haemoreflectometer is a robust and practical example of the latter type. It is possible to monitor arterial saturation continuously using an ear oximeter. A small clip containing a light source and photocell with appropriate filters is attached to the ear which is transilluminated.

Saturation or tension?

There is little to choose between the two forms of oxygen measurement up to a Po_2 of about 9.3 kPa (70 mmHg) and one may be obtained from the other if the pH of the blood is known. Oxygen tension is more widely used, perhaps because it is also useful in the higher range above a Po_2 of 70 mmHg where saturation hardly changes at all.

Interpretation

The normal range in healthy young adults is from about 10.5 to 14 kPa (80–105 mmHg). In older or immobile individuals lower values would be expected even in the absence of notable lung disease. Cyanosis in individuals with normal haemoglobin concentration and pH begins to be evident at an arterial Po_2 below about 6.4 kPa (48 mmHg) at which level saturation is about 80%. It is very obvious below 5.3 kPa (40 mmHg) when saturation is below 75%.

Arterial oxygen Po_2 falls reciprocally with the increase in Pco_2 when there is overall (alveolar) underventilation (see Fig. 2.7). Hypoxaemia is also caused by regional underventilation. One form of this is represented by a widened spread of ventilation/perfusion ratios—a common disturbance in lung disease (see Fig. 2.10). Sometimes hypoxaemia during exercise reveals impairment of pulmonary function. Faster transit of blood through the alveolar capillaries and greater desaturation of the venous blood returned to the lungs exaggerates the effects of impaired gas transfer and of ventilation/perfusion disturbance respectively. For a discussion of hypoxia see Chapter 26.

SI units—pressure

The unit of pressure employed is the kilopascal (kPa) which is equivalent to 7.5 mmHg.

To convert kPa to mmHg multiply by 7.5

To convert mmHg to kPa multiply by 0.13 (add a third and divide by 10)

A nomogram relating kPa and mmHg appears as an Appendix (p. 374).

TRANSFER FACTOR

Transfer factor (TLCO) is also known as diffusing capacity (DLCO). It expresses the overall ability of the lungs to transfer carbon monoxide from the alveoli to the blood. Another term, K_{CO} (transfer coefficient), is an expression of this ability corrected for the volume of lung (see below).

Background

The important influence of ventilation–perfusion relationships upon gas exchange has already been noted. At one time the ability of gases to diffuse across the alveolar–capillary membrane was thought to be the principal factor limiting gas exchange in disease. This led to the concept of 'diffusing capacity'—a measurement of the rate at which gas passes from the alveoli to the bloodstream.

Diffusing capacity = quantity of gas transported across in each minute for every unit of pressure gradient.

The measurement was found to be clinically useful. Later when it was realized that many factors apart from diffusion affected gas transfer in the lungs the expression was renamed 'transfer factor'. Oxygen transport is obviously of most interest to clinicians, but special difficulties are encountered in studying this gas because transport stops when haemoglobin becomes saturated. The difficulties can be partly overcome by using very low concentrations of oxygen which do not permit saturation of the blood, but other problems are then encountered. Carbon monoxide is usually employed in the measurement of transfer factor. Very low concentrations are used so that the blood remains avid for the gas during its passage through the pulmonary capillary.

Outline of measurement

Two pieces of information are required:
1   the quantity of CO transferred per minute;
2   the pressure gradient across the alveolar membrane (this is in effect the alveolar partial pressure of CO as blood CO tension can be ignored).

Steady-state method

The patient breathes air containing a known low concentration of CO from a Douglas bag and expired air is collected in another Douglas bag over a timed period of some minutes. The rate of CO transfer (i) can be calculated from the difference between inspired and expired concentrations. The alveolar CO level (ii) is more difficult to establish because it varies during each breath as CO is lost into the blood. A mean alveolar level can be calculated by estimating deadspace ventilation for CO_2 and assuming that this same volume was filled with unchanged inspired CO mixture. The short-fall in expired CO must then be entirely due to a lower concentration in the alveolar fraction which can be calculated.

Single-breath method

This is more widely used. The patient takes a measured breath containing small amounts of both helium and CO, holds the breath for 10 seconds and then breathes out. A sample of expired air is obtained (after the initial deadspace air has escaped) and the concentration of CO is measured.

The expired concentration of helium is lower than the inspired because it has been diluted by mixture with air already in the lungs at the beginning of the breath (but, being insoluble, no actual absorption has occurred). The volume of air in the lungs during the breath-hold can be calculated. The expired concentration of CO is also lower than the inspired level but the fall is proportionately greater than in the case of helium because some CO has been absorbed into the bloodstream.

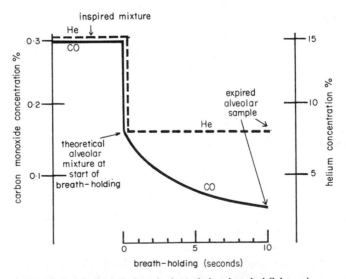

Fig. 7.18. *Measurement of transfer factor by the single-breath method.* Schematic representation of the helium and carbon monoxide concentrations in the inspired mixture and in alveolar air during breath-holding.

The calculation of the rate of CO transfer (i) and alveolar CO tension (ii) is based on the assumption that the CO is instantly diluted in the same proportion as He at the beginning of the breath-hold and that the alveolar CO concentration then falls exponentially towards the expired level (Fig. 7.18). Integration yields an expression of the relationship between rate of fall of concentration of CO and alveolar concentration of CO. When account is taken of the volume of air involved the rate of CO transfer in ml per minute per mmHg partial pressure of CO can readily be calculated.

Transfer factor is normally of the order of 20 ml min^{-1} mmHg^{-1} and is related to age, sex and body size. Transfer factor in SI units is expressed as mmol min^{-1} kPa^{-1} and is normally of the order of 6.7 mmol min^{-1} kPa^{-1} (to convert from SI units to 'old' units multiply by 3).

Factors influencing transfer factor

Transfer factor is influenced by many considerations which include:
1 Ventilation/perfusion imbalance—in disease much of the inspired gas may not reach perfused alveoli.
2 The thickness of the alveolar–capillary membrane.
3 The area of the membrane.
4 The pulmonary capillary blood volume.
5 The haemoglobin concentration.
6 The rate of reaction of CO with haemoglobin.

Impairment of transfer factor does not necessarily mean impairment of diffusion. Despite the number of factors which perturb it, transfer factor remains an extremely useful measurement (the same could be said of the ESR).

Transfer coefficient (K$_{CO}$)

This is obtained by dividing transfer factor by the alveolar volume (the volume in which the helium became diluted is usually used for this purpose). It is an expression of gas transferring ability per unit volume of lung. It assists interpretation when a reduced transfer factor is encountered. For example, an individual who has had one lung removed will have a reduced transfer factor but a normal K$_{CO}$ and diseases which cause lung shrinkage produce the same effect. Where, however, the lung parenchyma becomes damaged by disease (for example in fibrosing alveolitis or in emphysema), lowered transfer factor is accompanied by lowering of the K$_{CO}$. Normal values for K$_{CO}$ depend on age and sex. Fit young adults have values around 1.5 (SI units are mmol min^{-1} kPa^{-1} l^{-1}); the very elderly may have normal values as low as 1.0.

Interpretation

In the presence of normal ventilatory function the finding of a significantly reduced transfer factor is a strong indication of the presence of a parenchymal lung disorder involving the alveoli or their blood supply.

In the presence of a restrictive ventilatory defect an impairment of transfer factor suggests fibrosis, oedema or infiltration if the reduction is more severe than would be expected from simple reduction in lung volume—that is to say, if K_{CO} is also reduced to about the same extent. In diffuse parenchymal disease measurement of transfer factor may provide a crude index of severity and progress.

The significance of impairment of transfer factor in the presence of an obstructive ventilatory defect is more difficult to assess and depends to some extent on the relative severity of the two defects and upon clinical circumstances. Persistent impairment of transfer factor and K_{CO} provides support for a diagnosis of emphysema.

EXERCISE TESTS

Exercise tests may provide valuable insight into the performance of the cardio-respiratory apparatus as a whole. Often very useful information may be obtained by merely walking with a patient on the level or up stairs. More precise information is obtained if pulse, minute ventilation and oxygen uptake are measured during graded exercise using an ergometer. Measurement of maximum exercise tolerance is useful but not without hazard in the elderly and those with cardiac disease. It is sometimes helpful to measure arterial blood gas tensions or steady-state transfer factor during exercise, particularly when the cause of dyspnoea is obscure.

SUMMARY OF THE BASIC TESTS
OF PULMONARY FUNCTION

PEFR	Wright peak flow meter	Allows detection of major degrees of airways obstruction. Its major role is in recording patterns of *change* in severity of obstruction by means of frequent recordings in the home and at work. This helps both diagnosis and assessment of treatment.
FVC FEV$_1$	Spirometer, e.g. Vitalograph	Permits recognition of defects of ventilation and provides information about their nature, e.g. obstructive or restrictive.
P_{CO_2}	Rebreathing method, arterial blood/CO_2 electrode	Allows assessment of alveolar ventilation. Together with pH and/or bicarbonate concentration gives information relating to acid–base status.
P_{O_2}	arterial blood/O_2 electrode	Allows assessment of ventilation/perfusion mis-match.
Transfer factor	Steady-state or single-breath methods	Provides useful non-specific information relating to gas-transfer function of the lungs which may not be readily gained by other means.
Exercise testing		Assessment of global cardio-pulmonary performance.

CHAPTER 8 / ELEMENTS OF
RADIOLOGY OF THE CHEST

The interpretation of physical signs particularly of local disease is a valuable skill but far from infallible, and the ready availability of chest radiography in developed countries makes it important that the clinician should be familiar with the elements of interpreting chest radiographs almost as an extension of physical examination.

The normal chest X-ray

Some of the more useful landmarks of the normal chest X-ray are indicated in Fig. 8.1. It is desirable that the film should be examined systematically to avoid missing useful information. The centring and penetration of the film should be quickly noted as these factors have considerable influence on the shape of the heart and mediastinum and upon the character of the vascular markings in the lung fields. The shape and bony structures of the chest wall should be surveyed and the position of the diaphragms and trachea noted. The heart's shape and size and the appearance of the mediastinum and hilar shadows are examined. On the right side the horizontal fissure is a particularly useful landmark and should be carefully identified. The size, shape and disposition of the vascular shadows are next noted and the pattern of the lung markings in different zones carefully compared. Whenever a localized abnormality of any sort is evident or suspected a lateral film becomes essential for accurate localization. The main features of the lateral film are indicated in Fig. 8.2.

Collapse

Collapse of a lobe is usually evident from shift of landmarks (fissures, mediastinum, blood vessels) and the collapsed lobe itself *may* cast a characteristic shadow (Fig. 8.3). However, the changes are often very difficult to see on a postero-anterior (PA) chest film and lateral or even oblique or lordotic views may be required to identify the collapsed lobe. Note that in right middle lobe collapse there may be little to see on the PA film apart from lack of definition of the right border of the heart. This is a useful sign which helps to distinguish it from lower lobe collapse where the right border of the heart remains clearly defined. In left lower lobe collapse there may be a triangular area of increased density visible behind the heart shadow but this may not be evident and lateral or oblique views may be required. In complete collapse of the left lower lobe some small upward-curving linear shadows often appear in the left lower zone just outside the apex of the heart on the PA film.

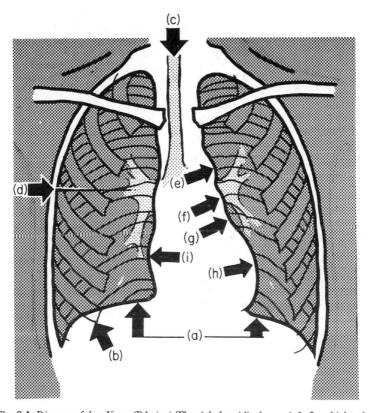

Fig. 8.1. *Diagram of chest X-ray (PA view).* The right hemidiaphragm is 1–3 cm higher than the left (a) and on full inspiration it is intersected by the shadow of the anterior part of the sixth rib (b). The trachea (c) is vertical and central or very slightly to the right. The horizontal fissure (d) is found in the position shown or slightly lower and should be truly horizontal. It is a very valuable marker of change in volume of any part of the right lung. The left border of the cardiac shadow comprises: (e) aorta; (f) pulmonary artery; (g) concavity overlying the left atrial appendage; (h) left ventricle. The right border of the cardiac shadow normally overlies the right atrium (i) and above that the superior vena cava.

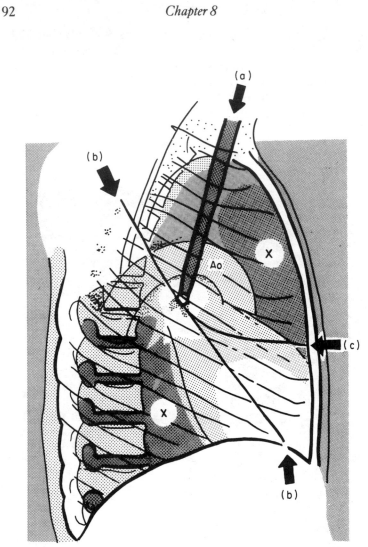

Fig. 8.2. *Diagram of chest X-ray (lateral view).* (a) Trachea. Ao: aorta. (b) Oblique fissure. (c) Horizontal fissure. It is useful to note that in a normal lateral view the radiodensity of the lung field above and in front of the cardiac shadow is about the same as that below and behind (x).

Consolidation

Consolidated ares of lung appear as uniform areas of opacification which conform to the outline of a lobe or segment; there is often a variable amount of collapse present.

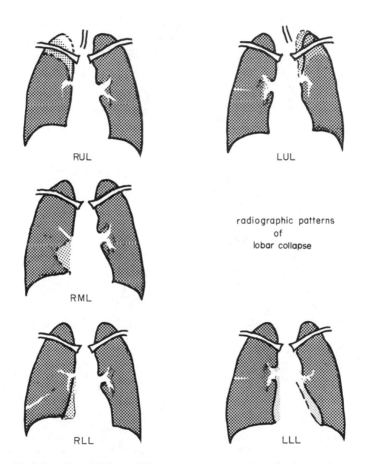

Fig. 8.3. *Lobar collapse.* Collapsed lobes occupy a surprisingly small volume and are commonly overlooked on the chest X-ray. In the above diagram note the position of the diaphragms in each case. Helpful information may be provided by the position of the trachea, the hilar vascular shadows and the horizontal fissure. RUL, right upper lobe; RML, right middle lobe; RLL, right lower lobe; LUL, left upper lobe; LLL, left lower lobe.

The silhouette sign (Fig. 8.4)

The sharp edge of structures such as heart, mediastinum and diaphragm is due to the contrast between aerated lung and the pleural
surface. When there is abnormal shadowing overlying such a border in a
postero-anterior X-ray the silhouette sign may enable the observer to
decide where exactly the abnormal area is in the chest. If the sharp
outline, for example that of the heart border, is lost then the abnormal
pulmonary shadowing must be adjacent to the structure rather than
merely projected so as to overly it. If the sharp outline, or silhouette, is
visible through the pulmonary shadowing then the reverse is true and
the shadowing does not abut against the structure at that point.

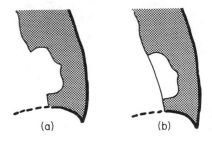

(a)   (b)

Fig. 8.4. *The silhouette sign.* Diagram showing abnormal lung shadowing in the left lower
zone. Where the sharp outline of mediastinal structures or diaphragm is lost because of
abnormal lung opacification it can be concluded that the shadowing is immediately
adjacent to the structure (and vice versa). In example (a) the shadowing must be anterior
and next to the heart as the sharp outline of the heart is lost. In (b) it must be posterior as
the heart outline is preserved.

Pleural effusion

Small pleural effusions (of 300–500 ml) cause no more than blunting of
a costophrenic angle; larger effusions cast a characteristic shadow with a
curved upped edge rising into the axilla (even though the upper level in
fact runs horizontally round the chest wall). Very often effusions cause
uniform opacification of one side of the chest and there may be shift of
the mediastinum towards the opposite side.

Fibrosis

Localized fibrosis causes streaky shadows with evidence of traction
upon neighbouring structures. Upper lobe fibrosis causes traction upon

the trachea and also elevation of the hilar vascular shadows. Generalized interstitial fibrosis produces a hazy shadowing, sometimes with a fine reticular (net-like) or nodular pattern. Advanced interstitial fibrosis results in a honeycomb change which is apparent on the chest X-ray as diffuse opacification containing multiple circular translucencies a few millimetres in diameter.

Rounded shadows

Carcinoma of the lung is by far the commonest cause of rounded shadows of the lung; other causes include:

    Metastatic tumour (? multiple)
    Tuberculoma (? calcification)
    Lung abscess (usually cavitates in time)
    Pulmonary infarct (not usually round; tends to disappear)
    Rare primary benign tumours (hamartoma, adenoma, etc.)
    Encysted interlobar effusion
    Hydatid cyst (rare, ? hair-like outline)
    Arteriovenous malformation (? adjacent vascular shadow).

Early thoracotomy is indicated in the case of rounded shadows without obvious cause as they are so often due to surgically curable carcinoma and diagnosis is commonly impossible by other means.

Miliary mottling

This term is used to describe the appearance produced by numerous minute opacities in the lung fields 1–3 mm in diameter (which may resemble millet seeds)—an appearance which may be caused by a very large number of pathological processes, some of the commoner causes being:

    Miliary tuberculosis (p. 126)
    Pneumoconiosis (p. 304)
    Sarcoidosis (p. 216)
    Fibrosing alveolitis (p. 205)
    Lymphangitis carcinomatosa (p. 250)
    Pulmonary oedema (usually perihilar, transient and accompanied by larger fluffy shadows).

Mediastinal masses

Metastatic tumour or lymphomatous involvement of the mediastinal lymph nodes is the commonest cause of an abnormal mediastinal shadow but other masses may cast shadows and the particular site of the mass may give a clue to its cause (Fig. 8.5).

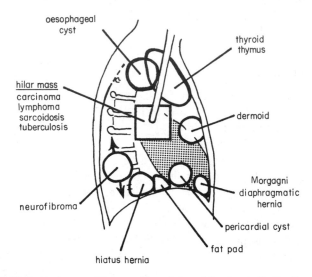

Fig. 8.5. *Mediastinal masses.* Diagram of lateral view of the chest indicating the sites favoured by some of the commoner mediastinal masses.

Special techniques

Tomography

In this technique the film and the X-ray tube move in opposite directions along parallel axes pivoting about a point situated at the level of particular interest within the chest. The movement causes blurring of shadows except those situated in the plane of the pivotal point which remain fairly sharply defined giving the effect of a cross-section at this level. Adjustment of the apparatus allows several 'cuts' to be made in the region under scrutiny. The technique may yield useful information in the investigation of pulmonary opacities, particularly those situated near the hilum which may be difficult to distinguish from vascular shadows. Tomography may give a clearer outline of a pulmonary shadow, reveal the presence of calcification or cavitation not evident on a plain film and may demonstrate the relationship between a shadow and adjacent bronchi and blood vessels.

Bronchography

A variety of techniques are employed for the introduction of an iodized oily contrast medium into the trachea, generally under local anaesthesia. It is an uncomfortable procedure. Immediately after instillation of about 20 ml (for one side) of the medium the patient is rolled and tipped into lateral, supine, prone and head-down positions to fill the main broncho-pulmonary segments. Oblique, postero-anterior and lateral views are taken. Bronchography may be useful where it is important to confirm the presence or extent of bronchiectasis or in the investigation of bronchial obstruction especially where this is beyond the range of the bronchoscope. Bronchography should not be undertaken lightly—particularly in the presence of asthma or severe respiratory disability.

Fluroscopy ('screening')

This is generally carried out with the aid of image-intensifying equipment. It permits movement of the lungs and diaphragms to be observed which may be important in the investigation of suspected diaphragmatic paralysis. Movement of the paralysed side is defective and if the patient sniffs the paralysed diaphragm will show paradoxical upward movement. Screening may also permit air-trapping in large localized areas of lung to be observed.

Computerized axial tomography (CAT)

This revolutionary imaging technique has had rather less impact on the diagnosis of pulmonary disease than it has had on disease elsewhere, probably because the presence of air in the lungs has always offered excellent contrast for plain X-ray investigation. Nevertheless, computerized tomography is able to reveal fine detail of abnormal lung structure. It is for example able to detect small nodular lesions of 3 mm or so in diameter whereas such lesions are commonly not detected on a plain chest radiograph.

It has revealed some points of interest in diffuse lung disease; for example, fibrosing alveolitis is shown to involve the periphery of the lung rather more than the more central zones and this distribution is particularly evident posteriorly in the lower lobes. In pleural thickening due to asbestos exposure the technique has revealed the presence of fibrosis strands extending inwards from the pleural surface in some cases indicating that more than merely pleura is involved. Computerized tomography may also allow earlier non-invasive diagnosis of meso-thelioma particularly where appearances are obscured by pleural effusion or pleural adhesions following repeated pleural aspiration.

Computerized tomography has found some application in the staging of lung cancer but decisions on the question of operability are not usually based on the results of the investigation alone. The technique finds its most important thoracic application in the diagnosis of mediastinal masses and their differentiation from normal structures and in particular in distinguishing deposits of fat from other structures.

Pulmonary arteriography

Radio-opaque contrast material is injected into the pulmonary artery through a catheter which has been passed from a peripheral vein through the right side of the heart. The usual indications are (i) confirmation of pulmonary embolism and (ii) identification of arteriovenous mal-formations.

Radioisotope lung scanning

The major application of isotope scanning is in the diagnosis of pulmonary embolism (see p. 267 for description).

PERFUSION SCANNING

Isotope-tagged macroaggregated albumin particles are injected intra-venously and lodge in the lungs in proportion to local blood flow. The distribution of the isotope is displayed using a scanning gamma counter or a gamma camera. Dissolved Xenon-133 may be injected as an alternative (this is rapidly evolved into perfused alveoli which can provide additional information but also leads to practical difficulties).

VENTILATION SCANNING

The patient breathes a mixture containing radioactive Xenon-133 in a closed-circuit spirometer. Krypton 81 is easier to use and has a very short half-life enabling general images to be undertaken at one examin-ation. A gamma camera is used to demonstrate the distribution of the gas. Insight into regional ventilation is gained by observing the rate of 'washing in' and later 'washing out' of the isotope after the patient has begun and ended the period of closed-circuit breathing. The technique may be helpful in providing additional information about lungs involved by bullae, carcinoma or other disease where extensive surgical resection is being considered. It has also proved useful in small children and babies with wheezing dyspnoea where localized bronchial obstruction—for example by a foreign body—may be difficult to distinguish from generalized airways obstruction.

CHAPTER 9 / ACUTE RESPIRATORY INFECTION

Most acute respiratory infections are of viral origin. A variety of different viruses are responsible. Some viruses are regularly associated with a particular clinical pattern, most are capable of producing differing respiratory illnesses depending upon such factors as severity of infection, age of the patient and the presence of pre-existing disease.

Diagnosis in acute respiratory infections goes only so far as identification of the clinical pattern or the level of the respiratory tract which is principally affected. Pursuit of the actual organism is usually only carried out in severe disease in special centres or in the study of epidemiology.

Principal patterns

Common cold

Rhinorrhoea, nasal obstruction and variable conjunctivitis and epiphora are the main features sometimes associated with a scratchy mild pharyngitis.

Acute pharyngitis

The common 'sore throat' is more usually associated with fever and a variable degree of malaise. The throat and soft palate are reddened and the tonsils may be inflamed and swollen. After a day or two the tonsillar lymph nodes may be enlarged. In young people about 25–33% of sore throats are due to infection by a haemolytic streptococcus; the proportion appears to be falling. Sore throat due to haemolytic streptococcus is indistinguishable from sore throat due to a virus.

Acute tracheo-bronchitis

Cough is the principal symptom. In the early stages it is irresistible, repetitive and unproductive. A barking sound is often produced by flapping vibrations of the inflamed posterior tracheal wall.

Audible wheezing and rhonchi are sometimes present. Reflex laryngeal spasm or actual oedema of the larynx may cause stridor. In young children inspiratory distress and croaking stridor may be prominent and the illness is termed *croup*. Occasionally this produces dangerous acute respiratory failure.

Acute bronchiolitis

This term is used to describe lower airways inflammation occurring in babies mainly between 1 and 6 months of age. Initial upper respiratory tract symptoms, irritability and difficulty in feeding are followed by cough, wheezing and grunting respiratory distress with inspiratory rib recession accompanied by evidence of overinflation and, in severe cases, signs of respiratory failure. The baby is not usually pyrexial. The illness normally lasts 3–4 days and a rattly cough may last for 2–3 weeks. In severe cases respiratory distress may persist longer and it may be complicated by respiratory failure and exhaustion requiring artificial ventilation. Bronchopneumonia is a rare complication!

Pneumonia

The term pneumonia infers inflammation of the lung parenchyma. Fever, tachypnoea sometimes with pleural pain and cyanosis together with clinical and radiological signs of consolidation are the main features. There may be profound systemic upset with delirium and circulatory collapse. (Pneumonia is discussed in more detail on p. 106.)

Influenza

The term influenza may be used by the lay public to describe almost any pyrexial illness but is generally used to describe an acute illness in which symptoms of malaise and particularly myalgia may be out of proportion to the upper respiratory tract symptoms and accompanying fever.

The patient is commonly prostrate and pyrexial for 3–4 days and may feel unwell and easily tired for a fortnight or so. Sometimes lethargy and depression develop and may persist over many weeks. The term influenza naturally acquires greater precision during the course of epidemics.

Principal respiratory viruses

Rhinoviruses

There are more than ninety different serotypes of this class of virus; identification and study are difficult. The incubation period is short and the commonest pattern of illness is the common cold. It is believed that rhinovirus may precipitate acute exacerbations of chronic bronchitis and may occasionally cause pneumonia in infancy.

Adenoviruses

There are about thirty different serotypes of adenovirus which may cause pharyngitis and conjunctivitis in adults, severe bronchitis in childhood and, rarely, severe pneumonia in infancy.

Respiratory syncytial virus

Respiratory syncytial virus is so called because it induces syncytial formation in tissue culture. This organism is the principal cause of bronchiolitis in infancy and is probably responsible for a proportion of cases of 'cot death'. Infection is commonest at about 3 months and is unusual before 1 month or later than 6 months, generally occuring in winter epidemics. Maternal IgG antibody does not confer immunity. Resistance to infection requires the development of specific IgA in the respiratory secretions. The virus may be identified by an immuno-fluorescent technique from naso-pharyngeal or tracheal aspirates, by its isolation or by later serological changes. The organism may be associated with mild apyrexial upper respiratory tract infections in older individuals.

Influenza virus

Two main serological types are found, A and B. Influenza B causes mild recurrent outbreaks of influenza. There are several serological types but spontaneous antigenic variety is slight. Influenza A causes pandemic influenza. Spontaneous antigenic variation occurs from time to time resulting in rapid spread of the organism. Minor epidemics occur every winter and pandemics occur every 4–5 years or so. In epidemics patients with persisting chronic respiratory disease and the elderly are particularly at risk but occasional young adults may also suffer over-

whelming infections sometimes complicated by influenzal or staphylococcal pneumonia, myocarditis and encephalitis.

Parainfluenza virus

There are four serotypes, types 1 and 3 being most frequently encountered. Epidemics occur which in the case of type 1 may show an
alternate-year pattern. In adults this virus is associated with pharyngitis,
laryngitis and tracheitis; hoarseness is a common feature. Fever is
unusual. In children it causes croup (especially type 3). It may cause
lower respiratory tract infections and a few cases of bronchiolitis are
caused by it.

Coxsackie and ECHO viruses

These enteroviruses play a relatively minor role in acute respiratory
infection. Well documented outbreaks of acute mild respiratory illness
due to Coxsackie A have been reported in closed communities amongst
army recruits, students, etc. Coxsackie B may cause pleurodynia
(epidemic myalgia, Bornholm disease) characterized by fever and
frighteningly severe lateralized chest pain on movement. This agent also
causes pericarditis and rarely overwhelming myocarditis. Coxsackie A is
known to cause herpangina-pharyngitis with vesicle formation.

Measles virus

Pneumonia and tracheobronchitis may complicate severe measles. It is
difficult to distinguish the effects of virus infection from those of later
bacterial invasion which may be protracted and lead to permanent
bronchial damage. Measles may cause overwhelming pneumonia in
children receiving treatment for leukaemia.

Epstein–Barr (EB) virus

This agent is known to cause infectious mononucleosis which
commonly produces upper respiratory symptoms, principally pharyngitis and tonsilitis in addition to the other well known features of the
illness.

Other viruses

Herpes simplex virus may occasionally affect the respiratory tract but is not commonly responsible for common syndromes of acute respiratory infection. Rarely it may cause pneumonia but almost always this is during the course of another illness or treatment which impairs immunological competence (leukaemia, immunosuppressive treatment). Cytomegalovirus may cause severe interstitial pneumonia under similar circumstances. During the course of chicken-pox the varicella-herpes zoster virus may cause pneumonia which may leave specks of calcification which remain visible after chest X-ray. Chest pain due to pre-eruptive herpes zoster may cause diagnostic problems and sometimes herpes zoster is accompanied by diaphragmatic palsy.

Mycoplasma pneumoniae; Psittacosis/ornithosis (see p. 116).

Treatment

Antibiotics have no effect upon the viruses described above but may occasionally be called for where bacteriological complications have developed.

Common cold

No treatment is generally required. Disabling epiphora, rhinorrhoea and nasal congestion may be ameliorated by an oral preparation containing pseudoephidrine.

Special risk cases

Patients who are thought to have had acute rheumatic fever or acute glomerulonephritis must receive penicillin for sore throats. Individuals with rheumatic fever should have continuous penicillin prophylaxis until they are aged at least 20. Penicillin may be given orally but prophylaxis may be more secure with monthly injections of a long-acting preparation.

Tracheo-bronchitis

Uncontrollable unproductive cough causing sleeplessness may merit treatment with a mild cough suppressant such as codeine linctus.

Mixtures containing antihistamines are commonly found useful in children probably because of their sedative effects. If the sputum is frankly purulent and improvement is delayed an antibiotic such as amoxycillin, septrin or tetracycline may shorten recovery. Tetracycline should not be given in pregnancy or under the age of about 9 years because of effects on teeth and bone. Croup in infants may be helped by maintaining a warm humid environment.

Bronchiolitis

Antibiotics have no effect. Treatment is directed towards presenting adequate hydration, oxygenation and feeding until spontaneous improvement occurs. Very occasionally progressive respiratory failure and exhaustion require the use of artificial ventilation—a specialist procedure not lightly undertaken. In severe deteriorating cases suspicion of staphylococcal superinfection may lead to administration of flucloxacillin.

Pneumonia (see p. 106)

Prophylaxis

Highly vulnerable individuals with advanced cardiac or respiratory disease may reduce the incidence of infection if they limit their contact with others by avoiding large gatherings, etc. The common respiratory viruses are transmitted by droplet spread and it is almost impossible completely to prevent infection by isolation. Some protection against epidemic strains of influenza A is now possible with the use of attenuated live vaccines. Their use is normally limited to particularly susceptible individuals and injections given 2–3 months before the expected epidemic. The large number of antigenic varieties among the other common respiratory viruses has prevented wider application of vaccination in this field. During an epidemic, amelioration of an influenzal infection may be possible with the use of amantadine (used in the treatment of Parkinson's disease) if treatment is started very promptly.

CHAPTER 10 / PNEUMONIA

Definition

Pneumonia is a general term used to denote inflammation of the gas-exchange region of the lung. Usually pneumonia is due to an infective agent but the term is also used to cover inflammation due to physical, chemical or allergic processes.

Bronchopneumonia/Lobar pneumonia

These terms have little clinical relevance but are nevertheless in widespread use. Bronchopneumonia is the name given to the most common pattern of pneumonia where there is patchy involvement of lung parenchyma, particularly in the lower zones. The term lobar pneumonia merely indicates that one or more lobes are uniformly affected by inflammation and consolidation with relative sparing of the remainder of the lungs. At one time lobar pneumonia was a common form and almost always due to the pneumococcus. Nowadays classical lobar pneumonia is rather uncommon and it is frequently not due to the pneumococcus.

Causative factors

In practice the clinical features of pneumonia give little guidance as to the nature of the agent responsible but the circumstances of the illness may give some clue (Fig. 10.1) (e.g. severe pneumonia in an epidemic of influenza A is commonly staphylococcal).

Host factors

Pneumonia may develop secondary to a breakdown of the normal defence processes of the respiratory tract: for example, from failure to clear bronchial secretions due to impaired consciousness, age and weakness, overwhelming bronchial infection, or lack of tissue resistance due to severe illness, malnutrition, alcoholism or immunosuppression due to disease or drugs, etc. Localized pneumonia may be related to bronchial obstruction by foreign body or carcinoma, or to infection of a

106

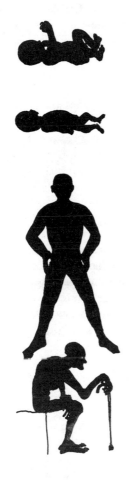

Previously well infant
1. RSV
2. Adenovirus and other viruses
3. Bacterial

Previously ill infant
1. Staphylococcus
2. *E. coli* and gram-negative bacteria
3. Viruses and opportunistic organisms

Children and previously fit adults
1. Viral
2. Pneumococcal
3. Mycoplasmal, psittacosis
4. Legionella
Post-influenzal: Staphylococcal,
    streptococcal

Previous respiratory illness. Elderly and
    debilitated
1. Pneumococcal
2. *Haemophilus influenza*
3. Staphylococcal
4. Klebsiella
If no response to antibiotic treatment
    think of:
Tuberculosis
Mycoplasma pneumoniae
Carcinoma

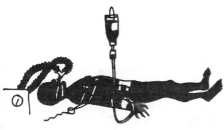

In the course of major illness or during
    immunosuppression
1. Staphylococcal
2. *Ps. aeruginosa* and other gram-
    negative organisms
2. Opportunistic organisms—
    Pneumocystis carinii. cytomegalovirus,
    tuberculosis
4. Non-infective forms of pneumonia

Fig. 10.1. *Some organisms associated with pneumonia.* Age and previous health are important in assessing cause of pneumonia.

pulmonary infarct, persistent bronchiectasis, etc. On the other hand, some agents appear to be able to produce pneumonia in previously normal individuals without obvious impairment of defence mechanisms.

Organisms responsible

Some of the more important organisms are indicated in Fig. 10.1 and short notes on individual forms of pneumonia appear at the end of this chapter.

Pathology

The common feature of pneumonias is the presence of a cellular exudate in the alveolar spaces. In secondary bacterial pneumonia suppuration may cause necrosis and damage to the lung architecture producing abscesses, cysts or damage to the respiratory bronchioles resulting in centrilobular emphysema. In lobar pneumonia due to pneumococcus and in some viral pneumonias resolution of the inflammatory intracellular exudates occurs, largely through the action of macrophages, and the lung tissue may return to its former state.

Clinical features

The severity of the illness and precise manner of presentation vary considerably. There is almost always malaise, fever and cough. There is commonly pleural pain and sometimes dyspnoea. Examination may reveal tachypnoea, tachycardia and sometimes cyanosis. There may be signs of consolidation (p. 56), sometimes associated with a degree of collapse or evidence of accompanying airways obstruction.

In severe pneumonia there may be severe prostration, delirium, jaundice, oliguria and peripheral circulatory failure.

Management

Not all patients with pneumonia require admission to hospital; in fact, the majority of cases is now managed at home. Hospitalization is generally necessary in the very young, the very ill and in cases where domestic circumstances do not permit the necessary level of elementary nursing care.

Investigation

1 Chest radiology

A chest X-ray is important at some stage in the illness and as early as possible in the case of the severely-ill patient requiring hospital admission. The extent and pattern of the changes on the chest X-ray is very variable but shadowing in at least one section of the lung field is virtually always seen. The best X-ray may reveal important evidence of related disease (e.g. bronchial carcinoma, pulmonary tuberculosis, heart disease or signs suggesting pulmonary embolism, etc.).

2 Sputum examination

Early examination of a gram-stained smear of sputum is important in seriously-ill patients. This will usually distinguish pneumococcal and staphylococcal pneumonia from that due to gram-negative organisms such as *E. coli, Ps. aeruginosa* or *Klebsiella pneumoniae* which require different antibiotics. Interpretation is difficult if antibiotic treatment has already been given. A Ziehl-Neelsen smear should not be omitted in case of tuberculosis.

3 Sputum culture

Culture of the sputum is always desirable and is very important in those critically ill, but treatment cannot be withheld until the results of culture are available. Interpretation of the results of sputum culture demands some caution—the organism retrieved may not be the causative agent, particularly if antibiotics have already been given. Where there is good access to an interested laboratory specimens may be despatched for virological culture or immunofluorescence diagnosis. Sputum should be examined for tuberculosis in every patient with pneumonia.

4 Blood culture

In severely-ill patients it is often very helpful to carry out blood culture. Treatment appropriate to pathogenic organisms isolated by this means is imperative.

5   Pleural aspiration and lung aspiration

Culture of pleural fluid may provide helpful corroboration of the significance of sputum findings and lung aspiration with a fine needle may occasionally be justified in cases causing difficulty and grave concern.

6   Serological tests

Serological tests may allow a retrospective diagnosis of pneumonia if a rising antibody titre to one of the commoner viral agents or the organism of legionnaires' disease (*Legionella pneumophilia*) can be demonstrated. This is rarely very helpful.

Treatment
General

Mild pneumonia in a robust individual with a capable family member to provide domestic nursing can be managed in the home. Where there is cyanosis, hypotension and altered consciousness hospital admission is desirable. The following measures are frequently necessary.
1   Encouragement of oral fluid intake to avoid dehydration.
2   Aspirin or paracetamol for severe fever, malaise and aching.
3   Stronger analgesics such as codeine, or morphine for pleural pain. (Beware patients with previous airways obstruction if opiates are used, as respiratory failure may be precipitated.)

Severe illness

More severely-ill patients may require:

OXYGEN
If cyanosis is present and respiratory drive is good, oxygen should be given by nasal catheter or whatever method is best tolerated and in sufficient concentration to relieve cyanosis. Care is again required if there is associated airways obstruction as the patient may have unsuspected chronic respiratory failure (p. 237).

INTRAVENOUS FLUIDS
Severely-ill patients with tachycardia, hypotension and a cool periphery may have low plasma volumes reflected by a low central venous pres-

sure. Large volumes of saline or dextran may be required before central venous pressure rises and adequate circulatory filling is restored.

CORTICOSTEROIDS

In very severely-ill patients intravenous hydrocortisone is generally felt to be beneficial although clear evidence in support of this is lacking.

Antibiotic and chemotherapy

PNEUMONIA IN PREVIOUSLY HEALTHY INDIVIDUALS

The first choice of treatment will depend on the organisms most prevalent in the environment. In some parts of the world almost all of the acute pneumonia is due to pneumococcus and the prevalent strain is fully penicillin sensitive. Under these circumstances penicillin used alone is highly satisfactory. Intramuscular or intravenous benzyl penicillin should be given until there is obvious improvement when oral treatment with phenoxymethyl penicillin may be substituted.

In the UK, however, the increased incidence of legionella pneumonia and occasional resistance of the pneumococcus has led to the suggestion that the initial treatment in acute pneumonia occurring outside hospital should be erythromycin together with either penicillin in high dosage or ampicillin. In influenza epidemics severe staphylococcal pneumonia may develop and at these times flucloxacillin should be included from the start together with benzyl penicillin as the organism is now commonly a penicillinase producer.

PNEUMONIA COMPLICATING PRE-EXISTING DISEASE

Where a patient is alcoholic, debilitated or immunosuppressed or has bronchiectasis, the possibility of a gram-negative organism should be borne in mind. *Klebsiella pneumoniae* demands treatment with streptomycin 1 g twice daily in young adults (less in the aged) together with cotrimoxazole. If *Ps. aeruginosa* is isolated and if the patient's condition gives cause for concern or the blood culture is positive, gentamycin and carbenicillin should be given. This organism is often present in the sputum of debilitated patients and its significance is then difficult to assess.

OVERWHELMING PNEUMONIA

In critically-ill patients it may be necessary to treat blindly for possible pneumococcal, staphylococcal, klebsiella, legionella or pseudomonas infection.

Chapter 10

Failure to respond

Successful treatment is usually accompanied by obvious improvement within 24 or 48 hours. If the patient fails to respond to treatment the clinician should be alert to the possibility of underlying malignant disease, gram-negative infection, tuberculosis, mycoplasmal infection, or legionnaires' disease.

Complications

Pneumonia due to staphylococcus may produce cavitation and abscess formation fairly early in the course. Klebsiella pneumonia may be very slow to respond and commonly leads to abscess formation and to empyema (p. 296).

Lobar collapse may complicate any pneumonia and bronchoscopy may be felt necessary if it persists in order to exclude intraluminal obstruction by carcinoma, foreign body or secretions. Bronchiectasis and localized pulmonary fibrosis may follow severe pneumonia.

Prognosis

The outlook in pneumococcal pneumonia occurring in previously well individuals is good and the mortality is of the order of 5%. Severe pneumococcal pneumonia in which more than one lobe is involved and where there is hypotension carries a more serious prognosis and hospital series have recorded mortalities of over 20%. Much the same applies to legionella pneumonia. Klebsiella pneumonia still carries a mortality of about 45%. Staphylococcal pneumonia is always serious, even in previously well patients, and the mortality is about 20%. The most important factors affecting prognosis relate to host resistance. Factors such as advanced chronic cardiac or pulmonary disease, diabetes, alcoholism, malnutrition and immune incompetence secondary to disease or drugs all weigh heavily against a successful outcome.

NOTES ON SOME INDIVIDUAL FORMS OF PNEUMONIA

Pneumococcal pneumonia

The pneumococcus (*Streptococcus pneumoniae*) is a paired, capsulated gram-positive organism. There are numerous serotypes and those causing pneumonia are generally not those found as common upper respiratory commensals. The organism is still the commonest cause of acute pneumonia. The involvement of the lungs is commonly, but not always, lobar in distribution. The affected lobe usually maintains its normal shape and size when it becomes consolidated. Early in untreated pneumonia the alveolar exudate contains abundant red cells and the term 'red hepatization' was used by pathologists to describe the liver-like change in the lung in those dying soon after the onset. Later the exudate contains abundant white cells and alveolar macrophages and the term 'grey hepatization' was employed to describe the naked-eye appearance. These labels are of little more than historical significance.

The clinical features are those of an acute pneumonia (see above) and vary greatly in severity. Sometimes recovery is protracted and radiological improvement delayed but the outcome is usually satisfactory. Pneumococcal meningitis is a rare but serious complication.

TREATMENT
Intramuscular benzyl penicillin, 600 mg twice daily until improvement is seen followed by oral phenoxymethyl penicillin is the usual recommendation. Amoxycillin orally from the beginning is probably just as effective and is more convenient and comfortable.

Staphylococcal pneumonia

The organism may be evident in gram-stained smears of sputum as a gram-positive clustered coccus. About 1% of pneumonias occurring outside hospital are due to the staphylococcus. The proportion is higher in pneumonia occurring in those already ill in hospital. Hospital organisms are usually penicillin resistant and 'domestic' organisms penicillin-sensitive. Staphylococcal pneumonia has no early special features but tends to be severe and is common as a sequel to Influenza A infection in epidemics. Even very fit young adults may be victims of overwhelming pneumonia. Shock may be present early in the illness and after a few days cavitation, overdistended air-cysts and localized lung abscesses may occur. Staphylococcal pneumonia may be complicated by remote septic systemic emboli.

TREATMENT
Penicillin resistance must be assumed until sensitivity tests are eventually available and flucloxacillin 500 mg four times daily by mouth or intravenously should be given until improvement occurs. Two or three

times this dose together with large doses of benzyl penicillin may be employed in the very ill, even if penicillinase-producing organisms are responsible (resistance to penicillin is relative rather than absolute).

Klebsiella pneumonia

This condition is also referred to as Friedlander's pneumonia. The organism responsible, *Klebsiella pneumoniae* is a gram-negative capsulated rod-shaped organism. It generally presents as an acute severe pneumonia in patients who either have pre-existing lung disease (e.g. bronchiectasis) or impaired resistance to infection (alcoholism, malnutrition, diabetes and other underlying diseases). It may present with lobar or multilobar involvement of the lung and causes profound illness. Rapid destruction of lung tissue occurs with cavitation. The course is usually stormy and protracted despite appropriate antibiotic therapy.

TREATMENT
Opinion is divided on the most suitable regimen. Some favour streptomycin and cotrimoxazole given together; gentamycin and chloramphenicol are also potentially effective.

Haemophilus influenzae pneumonia

Pneumonia attributed to this gram-negative bacillus usually arises in a severe exacerbation of chronic bronchitis and chronic obstructive lung disease. As well as the features of the pre-existing lung disease there may be fever, pleural pain, a pleural rub, localized crepitations and irregular radiological shadowing which lead to the diagnosis of pneumonia. A lobar pattern is uncommon. *Haemophilus influenzae* is frequently recovered from the sputum in this situation and presumed to be the cause of the pneumonia. The pneumococcus is commonly recovered at the same time.

TREATMENT
Either amoxycillin or cotrimoxazole is appropriate. Resistance to amoxycillin is uncommon but probably increasing. It is in part a consequence of β-lactamase production by the organism.

Pseudomonas aeruginosa pneumonia

Infection with this organism almost always arises in debilitated individuals with pre-existing lung disease or recently acquired bronchial obstruction, aspiration pneumonia, etc. It is particularly likely to occur in desperately-ill patients who are elderly, who have had antibiotic therapy in hospital, who are undernourished, who are receiving intra-venous therapy over a long period, who are being artificially ventilated and who have a tracheostomy (all of these factors individually and together predispose to pseudomonas pneumonia). Diagnosis can be difficult because the organism can very often be cultured from such individuals whether or not they have pneumonia. Blood culture may be helpful. The condition is always serious.

TREATMENT
A combination of intravenous azlocillin with gentamycin or tobramycin is often used. Alternatively, intravenous ceftazidime or cefotaxime may be given.

Legionnaires' disease

This is a severe form of pneumonia caused by a recently discovered bacterium (*Legionella pneumophilia*) and it takes its name from an Ameri-can Legion Convention in 1976 where the first recognized outbreak occurred. Most cases in Britain have developed the illness on holiday in Spain but sporadic local cases are now being reported in some cities. The infection appears to be air-borne and in some instances suspicion has centred on air-conditioning systems as a possible vehicle. The incubation period is short and pneumonia may be evident after 3 or 4 days of malaise, myalgia and fever and is accompanied by the usual symptoms and signs. The illness is usually severe with marked confusion and sometimes acute renal failure. It is not unusual for artificial ven-tilation to be necessary. The mortality is about 15–20%. Spontaneous recovery may be protracted. The diagnosis may be confirmed by a fourfold rise in serum antibody titre; it is difficult to culture or to identify the organism antemortem.

TREATMENT
Erythromycin is the drug of choice and may bring about dramatic sudden improvement. Complete or near-complete resolution of pul-monary changes is usual. Tetracycline may be almost as effective.

Pneumonia caused by *Mycoplasma pneumoniae*
(Primary atypical pneumonia)

Mycoplasma pneumoniae (Eaton agent) belongs to a group of the smallest organisms capable of replication outside living cells. It may cause fever, sore throat, myringitis or pneumonia. It tends to attack in winter and occasionally causes local epidemics within families and closed communities. Children and young adults are the usual sufferers.

The pneumonia may be characterized by dramatic radiological shadowing usually in both lower lobes which may contrast with rather mild illness. Sometimes fever and symptoms of pneumonia may be very protracted if the cause is not recognized. Permanent damage or serious complications are rare.

The diagnosis is usually suspected on clinical and radiological grounds, supported by a prompt response to tetracycline and confirmed by a rising titre of complement fixing antibody over 10 days. Cold agglutinins to type O human red cells are usually demonstrable in mycoplasma pneumonia.

TREATMENT
The organism is sensitive to tetracyclines and erythromycin.

Psittacosis/ornithosis

These names refer to the illness in man produced by *Chlamydia psittaci* which is a rickettsial type of organism transmitted from infected birds either of the psittacine type (parrots, parakeets, budgerigars) or others (e.g. pigeons).

The illness begins with a high swinging fever and dramatic prostration with headache, photophobia and sometimes delirium. There may be widespread myalgia and severe neck stiffness. This may lead to an initial diagnosis of meningitis. Splenomegaly may sometimes be detected. Attention is often not drawn to the chest until a chest X-ray is carried out although a persistent cough may be present. A few fine crepitations localized to one or more areas of the lungs are usually the only pulmonary signs. Enquiry usually reveals obvious contact with birds and occasionally the recent acquisition of a sick bird.

The chest X-ray reveals some pulmonary shadowing which is usually rather undramatic and may be limited to one segment. Confirmation of the diagnosis is provided by demonstration of a rising titre of complement-fixing antibody.

TREATMENT

Tetracyclines produce prompt subsidence of fever and recovery is usually uneventful and complete.

Virus pneumonias

The main respiratory viruses are reviewed briefly on p. 102.

Influenza A pneumonia

Influenza A causes epidemic infections and may produce severe pneumonia sometimes resembling pulmonary oedema.

Adenovirus pneumonia

A few of the serotypes of adenovirus which produce respiratory infection may cause pneumonia but upper respiratory infection is much more common. Pneumonia is confined to children and young adults. There is a tendency for pneumonia due to adenovirus to develop in individuals convalescing from infectious mononucleosis. The adenovirus may be recognized by electron microscopy of lung aspirate or lung biopsy and can be grown in tissue culture. Bacterial infection may follow adenovirus pneumonia.

Varicella pneumonia

Acute widespread patchy pneumonia may accompany severe chicken pox, especially when it occurs in an adult or in the course of immuno-suppressive therapy. The diagnosis is generally obvious from the associated severe skin eruption but it is sometimes necessary to exclude tuberculosis and other treatable causes of widespread infiltration. After recovery, the chest X-ray may reveal the development of small calcific nodules of uniform size (about 2–3 mm) which are permanent markers of the earlier infection.

Opportunistic pneumonias

A number of agents may produce pneumonia in circumstances in which there is severe depression of immunological responsiveness, although some are otherwise incapable of causing it. These organisms are loosely termed 'opportunistic'. Groups of patients particularly at risk are those undergoing combination chemotherapy for leukaemia or lymphoma, those receiving immunosuppression for renal, cardiac or marrow transplantation and patients with AIDS (Acquired ImmunoDeficiency Syndrome).

Pneumocystis carinii

This organism appears as minute oval bodies or cysts $5-10\ \mu$m in length and is probably related to the protozoa. It causes pneumonia in babies of a few months of age and in adults who are immunosuppressed. Breathlessness and tachypnoea are the main features, other physical signs are rarely helpful. Gas exchange becomes progressively impaired with progressive fall in transfer factor and ultimately cyanosis. The chest X-ray shows widespread mottling which is slowly progressive.

The diagnosis may be confirmed by lung biopsy (usually by peripheral transbronchial biopsy p. 255) or by bronchoalveolar lavage. Typical minute cysts are revealed with a special silver staining technique. *Pneumocystis carinii* and cytomegalovirus infections sometimes co-exist. The disease carries a high mortality partly related to the circumstances in which it arises. It may respond to treatment with cotrimoxazole (in approximately twice the standard dosage) or pentamidine.

Cytomegalovirus

This infection is most often seen in patients receiving large doses of corticosteroids and immunosuppressive drugs in the course of transplantation or during intensive treatment of leukaemia and lymphomas.

The presentation is as pneumonia, which is frequently severe and sometimes protracted, lasting many weeks. The chest X-ray tends to show nodular shadowing irregularly distributed in the lung fields. The diagnosis may be confirmed by rising antibody titres (immunosuppressives permitting), or by isolation of the organism from lung aspirate, blood or urine. Lung biopsy may reveal typical inclusion bodies in the inflammatory intra-alveolar cells. There is no effective treatment.

Other opportunists

These include:

Measles, which may cause severe overwhelming pneumonia in treated leukaemia (giant cell pneumonia).

Varicella, see above
Adenovirus, see above
Pseudomonas, see p. 111
Tuberculosis see p. 121

The differential diagnosis of widespread pneumonic shadowing during treatment with immunosuppressive and antineoplastic drugs can be difficult. Many of the drugs are themselves capable of producing a pulmonary reaction resembling pneumonia due to an opportunist infection (see Chapter 25). Furthermore, pulmonary shadowing may be due to neoplastic infiltration by the disease under treatment.

Aspiration pneumonia

Aspiration of acid stomach contents into the lungs can cause a very severe pneumonia accompanied by bronchial irritation and bronchoconstriction. Sometimes the picture is that of extensive pulmonary oedema which may develop after aspiration of quite small quantities of gastric contents (Mendelsohn's syndrome). Acute aspiration pneumonia usually occurs as a complication of states of impaired consciousness of whatever cause in which the normal protective reflexes are in abeyance.

Recurrent episodes of less severe aspiration pneumonia may occur in association with hiatus hernia, oesophageal stricture and diverticulae, weakness of the bulbar muscles, epilepsy, etc. The episodes tend most frequently to affect the posterior segment of the right lung. Abscess formation is common. There may be very little to indicate the cause of the episodes of pneumonia. Organisms isolated may include *Ps. aeruginosa, E. coli* and anaerobic species.

Lipoid pneumonia

This is a special form of aspiration pneumonia due to the repeated unwitting inhalation of animal or mineral oils medicinally (usually as laxatives or nose-drops; liquid paraffin is the commonest culprit). The inhaled oil causes patchy areas of pneumonia and collapse which may be widespread or localized, varying or relatively constant. Granulomatous lesions may develop which can mimic carcinoma. Cough is almost always present but there may be few other clues to suggest pulmonary disease. The diagnosis may be suspected when a chest X-ray reveals bizarre opacities in a moderately-ill elderly individual who is found to be using an oily preparation. Microscopic examination of the sputum (or

sometimes of biopsy material) shows 'foamy' macrophages which contain abundant globules of oil.

NOTE

The term lipoid pneumonia is also used to describe cholesterol and fat
deposition in incompletely resolved pneumonic areas accompanying a
variety of pulmonary diseases. The lipid here is of endogenous origin.

CHAPTER 11 / TUBERCULOSIS

Tuberculosis is an infection due to *Mycobacterium tuberculosis* characterized by necrosis and granuloma formation. It most commonly affects the lungs but may involve other isolated organs or be widespread.

Prevalence and mortality

A hundred years ago more than 30 000 persons died from tuberculosis in the UK annually (about the same mortality rate as for bronchial carcinoma today). A steady fall in mortality has occurred since that time due initially to improved nutrition and living conditions, later to improved public health measures such as early identification and isolation and in the last 30 years to the development of effective chemotherapy. Death from tuberculosis is now rare in the UK, occurring mainly in the elderly and sometimes being unrecognized in life. Despite the dramatic fall in mortality, tuberculosis remains an important disease and the annual notification rate for new cases is of the order of 20 per 100 000. The average age of newly-notified cases is increasing steadily. In undeveloped countries the disease is still responsible for a large mortality and the pattern of the disease resembles that prevalent in developed countries some 50 years or so ago.

Pathology

The typical appearances comprise the tuberculosis granuloma with central necrosis which has a macroscopic 'cheesy' appearance (caseation) and which in time commonly contains calcium salts (Fig. 11.1). Healing lesions are generally accompanied by extensive fibrosis. The extent to which proliferative changes, fibrosis or caseation predominate is probably determined by the immunological status of the individual.

Evolution of the disease (Fig. 11.2)

Knowledge of the time-course of tuberculous infection comes from before the days of effective chemotherapy; the disease is no longer seen to evolve in the characteristic fashion in the UK.

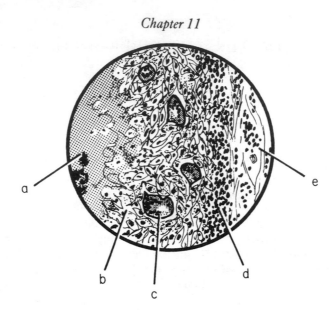

Fig. 11.1. *Diagram of main histological features of tuberculous lesion.* The centre of the lesion is to the left of the diagram. (a) Caseating central portion containing calcium deposits; (b) epitheloid cells; (c) giant cells of Langhans type; (d) lymphocytic infiltration of the outer layers; (e) fibrous tissue. The appearances vary considerably depending upon the age of the lesion, its situation and the degree of immunoreactivity of the host.

Primary tuberculosis

Source of infection

The disease is always acquired from an infected individual who is excreting bacteria; usually the contact is close and the exposure heavy. Less than 1% of tuberculosis is bovine in origin in developed countries and this source will not be considered further here.

The primary complex

The primary complex comprises the reaction at the site of the initial infection together with that which develops in the regional lymph nodes. The commonest example is the primary pulmonary focus accompanied by tuberculous hilar adenopathy (Fig. 11.2). This develops within 4 weeks of first infection and usually its progress is limited and there are few, if any, symptoms. Occasionally erythema nodosum develops at this stage. Healing then takes place, the tuberculin test becomes positive, a degree of immunity to the tubercle bacillus is developed and the lymph nodes subside. The peripheral lung lesion becomes reduced to a small nodule which may calcify and be evident on the chest X-ray indefinitely (Gohn focus).

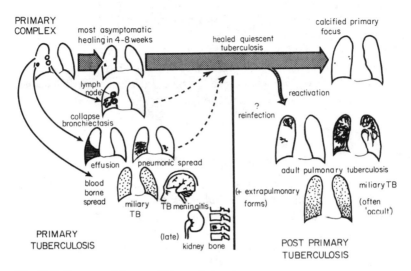

Fig. 11.2. *Summary of the natural history of tuberculosis.*

Progression of pulmonary primary complex

In children the lymph nodes may become much enlarged and cause pulmonary collapse by compressing lobar bronchi. Occasionally air-trapping causes overinflation of an obstructed lobe. Diffuse areas of radiological hazy opacification may be associated with lymph-node enlargement. This phenomenon is referred to as epituberculosis; it may be due to a parenchymal hypersensitivity reaction and it usually gradually subsides. In young adults the parenchymal pulmonary reaction may enlarge and cavitate with progressive pulmonary spread. Small parenchymal lesions may present with a pleural effusion identifiable by pleural biopsy.

SPREAD OF INFECTION

At any time in the course of tuberculous infection, spread may occur by several routes:

Bronchial tree
This leads to spread to other areas of lung or, via the sputum, to the
larynx (causing ulceration) and gastrointestinal tract.

Lymphatic system
This leads to regional lymphadenopathy or ultimately indirectly to blood
spread via the lymphatic duct causing miliary spread.

Bloodstream
Pulmonary veins draining pulmonary lesions may carry infective
material leading to remote spread of the disease particularly to bone,
kidney, adrenal gland, brain and meninges.

Post-primary infection

This term refers to any development of tuberculosis beyond the first few
weeks of a primary infection and after the development of hypersensitivity. It includes cases of reinfection and reactivated primary
infection even when this occurs years later. Reactivation tends to occur
in old age and in the course of illness or drug treatment which impairs
immunological competence. The lungs are the most usual site of post-
primary disease and the apices of the lungs are the commonest pulmonary site.

Clinical presentation

In developed countries the diagnosis is usually suggested by the finding
of compatible changes on chest X-ray during investigation of patients
with:
1   *Persistent cough and purulent sputum.*
2   *Haemoptysis.*
3   *Unresolved pneumonia.*
4   *Non-specific symptoms.* Investigation of patients of beyond middle age
with fever, malaise and weight-loss may reveal tuberculosis. Immigrants
from Asia and Africa may present unusual forms of tuberculosis with
fever, malaise and splenomegaly associated with hilar or cervical gland
enlargement.
5   *No symptoms.* Tuberculosis may be revealed during the course of
routine examinations or by mass miniature radiography (MMR).

Physical signs

Almost any combination of physical signs may be found (e.g. consolidation, effusion, fibrosis, collapse). Quite often the signs are rather slight even in the presence of advanced pulmonary tuberculosis.

Radiological features (Fig. 11.3)

These override the physical signs of importance. A great variety of appearances is encountered including:

1 *Patchy solid lesions* or irregular shape tending to be localized to one lung or part of a lung or to the upper lobes.

2 *Cavitated solid lesions.*

3 *Streaky fibrosis.*

4 *Flecks of calcification.* Calcification is always suggestive of tuberculosis but occurs in other conditions. All of these changes may be present together.

Other patterns which may be encountered include:

5 *Solitary round shadows.* Less than a quarter of these shadows are tuberculous and the majority of the remainder are of neoplastic origin.

6 *Hilar gland enlargement.* The combination of hilar enlargement and a solid lesion which may be cavitated tends to resemble bronchial carcinoma.

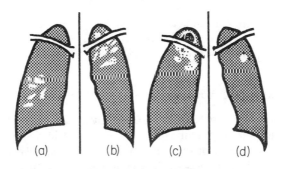

(a)   (b)   (c)   (d)

Fig. 11.3. *Radiographic appearances in pulmonary tuberculosis.* Tuberculosis can produce almost any form of pulmonary shadowing. Some common forms are indicated above. (a) Irregular mottled shadowing of any part of the lung especially (b) one or both apices. (c) Cavitation of an apical lesion is particularly suggestive but cavitation also occurs in carcinoma. (d) Solitary tuberculoma presenting as a 'coin' shadow. Calcification suggests tuberculosis but the diagnosis is generally only established at thoracotomy; the majority of such shadows is caused by carcinoma.

7   *Pleural effusion.*
8   *Pneumothorax.*
9   *Miliary mottling* (see below).

Miliary tuberculosis

This term refers to the widespread dissemination of tuberculosis usually with multiple (millet-seed size) nodules evident in the lung fields on the chest X-ray which is generally believed to follow entry of a large amount of infective material into the circulation either via the lymphatic system or the veins draining a local lesion. Formerly this variety of the disease was most usually seen following primary infection in children but it is now encountered more frequently in the older age groups. Usually the patient is ill, pyrexial and anorexic but occasionally individuals appear to be active and fairly well. A low-grade fever is the most constant of the non-specific features. Sometimes anaemia is the most obvious clinical feature and the blood picture may show abnormal cells suggesting a diagnosis of leukaemia. Occasionally these non-specific features are present without any miliary changes on the chest X-ray and the diagnosis may then be exceedingly difficult. Persisting fever in an elderly individual who is deteriorating may call for a therapeutic trial of specific antituberculous therapy even if attempts to isolate the tubercle bacillus have failed.

Diagnosis of tuberculosis

The combinations of clinical and radiological features described will often make a diagnosis of tuberculosis virtually certain but definitive diagnosis requires identification of the tubercle bacillus.

Sputum smear examination

Examination of a sputum smear stained by the Ziehl-Neelsen method by adequately-trained individuals is a vital step in diagnosis. Identification of acid and alcohol-fast bacilli is presumptive evidence of tuberculosis and of infectivity (in an untreated case). Repeated sputum examinations are indicated where suspicion of tuberculosis is high.

Sputum culture

The tubercle bacillus can be cultured *in vitro* on Dover's medium. This takes between 4 and 7 weeks. Assessment of *in vitro* sensitivity to antituberculous drugs may take a further 3 weeks after positive identification.

Guinea-pig inoculation

This technique permits isolation of tubercle bacilli when they are present in very small numbers in the material. It is expensive and rarely required.

Biopsy

The diagnosis can sometimes be made from biopsy material and this is particularly the case with isolated pulmonary nodules which require thoracotomy, pleural effusion and tuberculous cervical adenopathy.

Tuberculin testing

After 3 weeks or so from the time of the initial infection hypersensitivity to a protein part of the tubercle bacillus is developed. Hypersensitivity can be detected by intradermal injection of a purified protein derivative (PPD) of cultured tubercle bacilli. The response is of the Type IV cell-mediated variety and takes the form of a raised area of induration and reddening of the skin. In the Mantoux test 0.1 ml of tuberculin solution is injected intradermally (not subcutaneously). The test is read at 48–72 hours. A positive result is indicated by redness and induration at least 10 mm in diameter (the lesion is slightly oedematous and can be located by palpation with the eyes shut). If active tuberculous infection is very likely 1 TU should be used, otherwise 10 TU is normally employed and the test repeated with 100 TU if the result is negative.

HEAF TEST AND TINE TEST
The Heaf test and Tine test are widely used and convenient (Fig. 11.4). Positive Mantoux 1:100 (10 TU) or less, Grade III Heaf test and a positive Tine test are roughly equivalent.

Significance
A positive tuberculin test merely indicates previous tuberculous infection. A negative test virtually excludes active tuberculosis (except in rare cases of overwhelming disease or severe immunosuppression). A weak reaction to tuberculin (less than 10-mm induration; Heaf Grades I

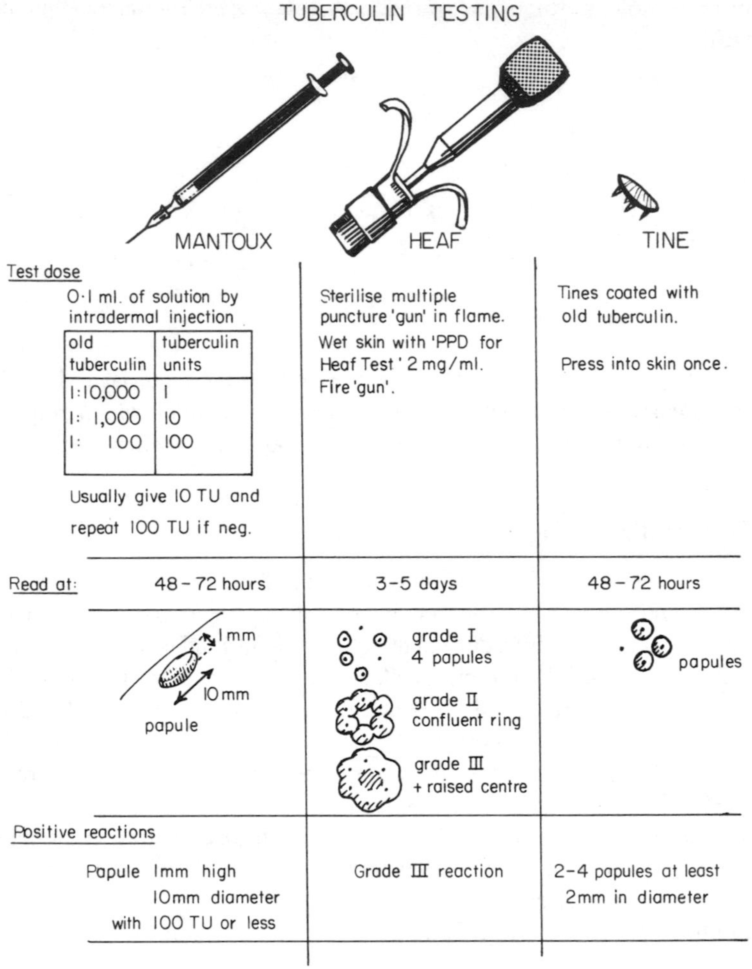

TUBERCULIN TESTING

	MANTOUX	HEAF	TINE
Test dose	0·1 ml. of solution by intradermal injection	Sterilise multiple puncture 'gun' in flame.	Tines coated with old tuberculin.
	old tuberculin / tuberculin units	Wet skin with 'PPD for Heaf Test' 2 mg/ml.	Press into skin once.
	1:10,000 / 1 1: 1,000 / 10 1: 100 / 100	Fire 'gun'.	
	Usually give 10 TU and repeat 100 TU if neg.		
Read at:	48 – 72 hours	3–5 days	48 – 72 hours
	 1mm 10mm papule	 grade I 4 papules grade II confluent ring grade III + raised centre	 papules
Positive reactions	Papule 1mm high 10mm diameter with 100 TU or less	Grade III reaction	2–4 papules at least 2mm in diameter

Fig. 11.4. *Tuberculin testing.*

to II) may be non-specific and indicate hypersensitivity to other myco-bacteria. Weaker responses tend to be seen in the elderly. Exceptionally vigorous reactions suggest currently active disease. The principal role of tuberculin testing is epidemiological. Spontaneous conversion in child-hood is presumed to indicate primary infection and treatment is usually advised. A source amongst adult contacts must be carefully sought. In the UK the policy of BCG vaccination of tuberculin-negative children at about 14 years reduces the usefulness of the tuberculin test above this age.

Case detection

The great majority of new cases of tuberculosis are detected by chest X-ray examination of individuals in the high-risk groups already mentioned. Mass miniature radiography is important where the prevalence of tuberculosis is high. In the UK the yield of new cases from this source is now extremely small (less than 1 in 2000 X-rays) and the service is being contracted.

MANAGEMENT OF TUBERCULOSIS

The management of tuberculosis may be summarized as follows.

Curative chemotherapy. Achieved by ensuring that the patient receives:
1   at least two drugs to which his organism is sensitive
2   in appropriate dosage
3   for long enough.

Prevention of spread of infection. Achieved by:
1   rapidly sterilizing antituberculous chemotherapy
2   isolation of infective cases (now rarely necessary)
3   identification of close contacts who have become infected or who may be the source of the infection. This remains very important
4   chemoprophylaxis (may be recommended in certain high-risk susceptible contacts).

Curative chemotherapy

The aims stated above are simple but treatment nevertheless demands expertise and attention to detail, and it should be supervised by doctors working as part of a health team with special experience of the problems involved.

Refinement of antituberculous treatment

Effective treatment for tuberculosis really began in 1947 with the introduction of streptomycin given by daily intramuscular injection. This was given together with oral para-aminosalicylic acid (PAS) and isoniazid (INH) to discourage the development of mycobacterial resistance. For about 25 years this remained the standard combination of drugs; all three being given together for 3 months and PAS and INH being continued for a further 9 months. Some regimens were substantially longer. Treatment with these drugs revolutionized the outlook in tuberculosis which had previously had a very high mortality indeed. There were, however, difficulties with the treatment which included (i) hypersensitivity reactions and other unwanted side-effects of the treatment (including the need to give streptomycin by injection); (ii) the development of resistant organisms; (iii) imperfect compliance because of long treatment duration; (iv) a significant relapse rate requiring long follow-up and (v) the need to isolate cases still excreting organisms because of uncertain persisting infectivity. Over the past 10 years or so the introduction of rifampicin to replace streptomycin, and ethambutol to replace PAS has led to significant improvements on all of these counts. Until recently the standard regimen in the UK has been to give rifampicin, INH and ethambutol together for 2 months and to continue with two of these until a total of 9 months of treatment have been completed. These treatments are all oral, well tolerated, rapidly sterilizing and virtually 100% effective if compliance is perfect. In practice a relapse rate of about 2–3% is encountered. Antituberculosis treatment has undergone a continuous process of refinement accompanied by scrupulous continuous assessment of its effectiveness; much of this work has been undertaken in Africa and Asia. Even shorter treatment using a 6 month regimen with four drugs in the initial phase has now been shown to be extremely effective and well tolerated, and this is being adopted as the standard regimen in many developed countries.

Modern short course treatment

INITIAL TREATMENT
For 2 months the patient takes orally: rifampicin, INH, ethambutol and pyrazinamide daily in the morning.

CONTINUATION TREATMENT
For a further 4 months rifampicin and INH are taken orally daily in the morning.

To this simple schedule it is usual to add a small daily dose of pyridoxine to prevent the development of peripheral neuropathy due to INH. Tolerance is good, compliance is assisted by the relatively short duration. Results are excellent so that continued follow-up is not necessary where there have been no irregularities with treatment. Resistance is a great rarity. Although treatment is now very simple attention must be paid to encouraging perfect cooperation on the part of the patient and to some relevant points of detail. It is particularly important to ensure that patients, members of their families and all health workers involved understand that the treatment is all taken together in the morning—not as divided doses.

There are a number of other proved and effective regimens available for the treatment of tuberculosis but these will not be detailed here. It is worth noting that these include regimens in which treatment is given three times weekly. This allows supervision of each dose where there would otherwise be inadequate compliance with treatment.

Review of principal antituberculous drugs

RIFAMPICIN

Rifampicin is a broad spectrum antibiotic which is outstandingly effective against *Mycobacterium tuberculosis*. It is taken by mouth in a single daily dose of 600 mg by individuals weighing 50 kg or more and in a dose of 450 mg by those who are lighter.

Adverse effects are uncommon. Itching of the skin and an erythematous rash may develop early. Withdrawal and re-introduction of treatment usually resolves the problem. Jaundice may appear early in treatment and a rise in serum transaminase is fairly common. If jaundice is evident, rifampicin is temporarily withdrawn until bilirubin levels are normal once more. The drug can then be re-introduced without further jaundice developing. Thrombocytopaenia and haemolytic anaemia are rare adverse effects. Rifampicin is largely excreted by the liver but enough appears in the urine to colour it red and suitable testing is easily carried out to confirm patient compliance.

ISONIAZID (INH)

Isoniazid is an effective, well tolerated antituberculous drug given orally in a single daily dose of 300 mg (for normal sized adults).

The acetylator status of the individual affects the rate of disposal of INH but the above doses are sufficient to allow for rapid disposal by fast acetylators, and concurrent treatment with pyridoxine affords adequate protection against neuropathy in slow acetylators so that it is not essential to establish acetylator status in all patients.

Apart from peripheral neuropathy, side-effects are rare. Skin rashes and hepatitis are occasionally attributable to INH and it is one of the drugs known to cause a form of systemic lupus erythematosus.

ETHAMBUTOL

Ethambutol is a bacteriostatic antituberculous compound given in a once daily oral dose of 25 mg per kg in the initial part of short course treatment—otherwise 15 mg per kg.

Its main importance appears to lie in the deterrence of bacterial resistance since it has an individual action on the tubercle bacillis and it is very rare for resistance to other antituberculous agents to be shared. The most important adverse effect is optic neuritis. If treatment is stopped as soon as the patient is aware of any visual impairment there is usually gradual recovery of visual acuity; severe visual loss may not be fully reversible. The incidence of the effect appears to be related to the total dose. Pretreatment screening and regular checking of vision during treatment does not permit prediction or early warning of the development of the side-effect.

PYRAZINAMIDE

Pyrazinamide is an effective bactericidal antituberculous agent given in a single oral daily dose of 2 g in patients weighing 50 kg or more than 1.5 g in those who are lighter.

It appears able to kill mycobacteria inside cells and it penetrates the cerebrospinal fluid well. Together with rifampicin it ensures rapid reduction in infectivity of sputum-positive patients. Pyrazinamide may cause arthralgia or even frank gout. Hepatotoxicity is also seen. This is occasionally severe and pyrazinamide is not reintroduced if jaundice seems attributable to it.

OTHER DRUGS

Streptomycin

Streptomycin is a bactericidal antituberculous aminoglycoside antibiotic given by intramuscular injection once daily in a dose of 1 g in normal sized adults with normal renal function. Beyond middle age the daily dose is reduced by 0.75 g or 0.5 daily.

The principal side-effect is vestibular damage which may cause permanent disabling ataxia. Generalized rashes and fever may also occur.

Para-aminosalicylic acid (PAS)
This is now little used as it is unpleasant to take and has a high incidence of adverse effects and relatively low effectiveness. It is cheap and finds application in undeveloped countries.

Thiacetazone
This is cheap, variably tolerated and only moderately effective. It is not used in developed countries.

Cycloserine, prothionamide, capreomycin, viomycin and kanamycin
These are expensive little-used 'reserve' antituberculous drugs. Their main application is in the treatment of drug-resistant disease. Drug resistance is now largely confined to patients treated with older regimens which do not include rifampicin and to those individuals who, for psychosocial reasons, have not proved able to take treatment properly. Rifampicin is the drug of choice in 'resistant' disease where it has not already been used.

Prevention of the spread of infection

INFECTIVITY
1   For practical purposes, only persons with acid- and alcohol-fast bacilli (AAFBs) in the sputum on direct examination are infectious. In sputum-negative patients, even if a culture is subsequently positive, the numbers of bacteria must be so small as to make infection of others very unlikely.
2   Patients with sputum positive for AAFBs may be considered technically non-infectious after they have completed 2 weeks of a modern three or four drug regimen which includes rifampicin.
3   Admission to hospital is unnecessary except (a) in the gravely ill, (b) in a few degenerated alcoholic patients, vagrants and others in whom it might otherwise prove impossible to initiate proper treatment. The patient's own family will already have been exposed to the risk of infection for some considerable time before diagnosis so that segregation at the time of diagnosis is irrelevant: the infectivity of the patient will diminish very rapidly indeed once treatment is started.
4   In the case of patients who require to be in hospital for some reason, those with sputum negative for AAFBs may be managed in the same way as any other patients. Patients with sputum positive for AAFBs should be nursed in a single room until at least 2 weeks of chemotherapy have been completed. Patients should not cough over other individuals and

the sputum should be regarded as highly infectious. Staff should wash the hands on leaving the cubicle. More elaborate measures—masks, gowns, gloves, separate crockery and afterwards fumigation of the room—are all unnecessary.

5   At home, patients with sputum positive for AAFBs should remain in their homes until at least 2 weeks of short course treatment containing rifampicin have been completed. Young children from other families should not visit the house during this time.

6   Patients may continue to produce AAFBs in the sputum for many weeks despite taking effective chemotherapy. If treatment is being taken correctly these organisms may be regarded as killed after 2 weeks and cultures should prove negative.

CONTACT TRACING

This is important. About 10% of all tuberculosis diagnosed in the UK is detected by examination of contacts of known cases. Persons living in the same household are those most at risk. About 10% develop active disease where the index case is sputum-positive. It is usual to limit contact tracing to household contacts, but the search is generally widened to include close family members who visit frequently and also to include any young children who visit. Close friends and sexual partners are contacts. Other casual contacts including those encountered at work are only rarely sufficiently close to merit tracing, and examination. Particularly high rates of tuberculosis are found in the contacts of Asian immigrants with the disease.

Adult non-immigrant contacts

Adults should have a chest X-ray performed immediately. In contacts of sputum-negative patients this is all that is required. Contacts of patients with sputum positive for AAFBs should have a repeat chest X-ray 3 and 12 months after the patient starts treatment. In most UK communities tuberculin testing of non-immigrant adults is unrewarding as a high proportion of the normal population give positive results.

Adult Asian immigrant contacts and all children under 16 who have not had BCG

Contacts should be Heaf-tested and those with a reaction of Grade III or more should be treated. Where there is no evidence of the disease process, treatment may amount to prophylaxis using INH alone for 6 months. Those who are Heaf-negative should be offered BCG vaccination. Those who are Heaf-positive should have a chest X-ray which should be repeated at 3 and 12 months. Asian contacts and ideally all household contacts of sputum-positive patients should have a further chest X-ray at 24 months.

Children who have definitely had BCG vaccination
These contacts require a chest X-ray which should be repeated at 3, 12 and, in the case of sputum-positive index cases, at 24 months.

Note
Heaf-testing of contacts is best deferred until 6 weeks after a sputum-positive index case has started effective treatment. Otherwise testing could take place before the development of skin hypersensitivity to tuberculin in a very recently infected individual (leading to a false negative Heaf test).

Prophylaxis

BCG VACCINATION
(Bacillus Calmette-Guérin) is a live-attenuated strain of tuberculosis which confers a useful degree of immunity in some communities. It is still offered to all tuberculin-negative children at about 14 years in the UK. It is given by intradermal injection. A local skin reaction is produced at about 4 weeks and there may be regional lymphadenopathy. The tuberculin test is positive after this time in successful 'takes'. Its continued use as a universal prophylactic is being questioned in countries where the risk of tuberculosis is low.

BCG is given to babies and children in contact with known cases of tuberculosis.

CHEMOPROPHYLAXIS
Treatment is normally advised when positive tuberculin tests are encountered in children who have not received BCG. This is particularly important in adolescent girls because of the possibility of occult genital tuberculosis and subsequent sterility. A modified regimen may be adopted using INH alone in a single daily dose of 100–300 mg for a year. Prophylactic treatment may also be indicated in particular high-risk groups: for example, patients with evidence of 'healed' tuberculosis who undergo treatment with steroid or other immunosuppressive drugs.

Atypical mycobacteria

About 1.5% of pulmonary tuberculosis is due to opportunistic myco-bacteria, the commonest of which is *M. kansasii.* Others include *M. xenopii* and *M. avium intracellulare.* The disease presents as indolent pulmonary tuberculosis and is identified in the laboratory. These bacteria are relatively resistant to antituberculous therapy. Where progress is unsatisfactory surgery may assist in controlling the disease. The degree of infectivity is low. A substantial proportion of patients with 'tuberculosis' cervical lymphadenopathy harbour these organisms.

CHAPTER 12 / BRONCHIECTASIS

Definition

Bronchiectasis is a state of dilatation of at least some of the bronchi. The bronchial wall is irreversibly damaged as a consequence of earlier inflammation and infection of the bronchus or neighbouring lung tissue, and the normal transport of mucus is impaired. In severe cases there is chronic local suppuration. The condition is characterized by cough and the regular production of large amounts of purulent sputum.

Prevalence

Most cases of bronchiectasis arise in childhood as a consequence of severe lower respiratory infection. As the population becomes replaced by individuals who have grown up in the antibiotic era the prevalence is falling and the mean age of those with established disease is increasing. The relative importance of bronchiectasis due to congenitally acquired defects of mucociliary clearance or to immunodeficiency is increasing as these varieties become more widely recognized and as childhood suppurative lung disease becomes rarer.

Pathological features

There is great variation in the extent and severity of bronchiectasis. The gross anatomical appearances are sometimes described as saccular, varicose or cylindrical but the actual form has little significance in terms of aetiology, course or management. The mucosal surface is always abnormal showing loss of ciliated epithelium, squamous metaplasia and heavy inflammatory cell infiltration. During infective exacerbations there may be sloughing, ulceration and abscess formation. The neighbouring lung is generally reduced in volume with patchy scarring and consolidation and may have been the site of earlier pneumonia. In severe cases the distal lung is replaced by fibrous tissue containing pus-filled cystic spaces.

Pathogenesis

The essential elements in bronchiectasis are firstly impaired mucociliary clearance and, secondly, structural change in the wall of the
bronchi. In some cases the structural changes in the bronchi are the
consequence of impaired clearance and associated infective complications: for example, in those cases due to defects in ciliary motility. In
others damage to the ciliated mucosa and to the bronchial wall may
occur together: for example, in the course of an acute severe lower
respiratory infection or as a result of chronic low grade infection in
individuals with immunodeficiency syndromes.

The majority of current adult cases still have their origin in severe
bronchial and pneumonic infection in childhood. Severe whooping
cough and measles are particularly prone to be followed by bronchiectasis. Bronchial obstruction by tuberculous lymph nodes was formerly a
common childhood cause of later bronchiectasis. Bronchial obstruction
due to other causes such as carcinoma or foreign body may lead to
bronchiectasis in the collapsed lung distal to the block. Proximal
bronchiectasis may accompany allergic aspergillosis (p. 196).
Bronchiectasis is generally present in congenitally atelectatic lobes.

In some cases of bronchiectasis there is an underlying genetically
determined defect of ciliary function. In Kartagener's syndrome,
dextrocardia occurs in association with bronchiectasis. There is
impaired ciliary function and a structural abnormality of the cilia
involving the dyenin rods. The 'immotile cilia syndrome' is a term used
to describe cases in which the cilial abnormality occurs without dextrocardia. It is now evident that there are a number of different types of
primary ciliary dyskinesia, only some of which are associated with
structural abnormality of the cilia detectable by electron microscope.
Techniques now exist for assessing ciliary beating (usually from samples
obtained through the nose) but to date there seems to be no close
relationship between the severity of functional abnormality of cilia
examined outside the body and the severity of clinical disease. In
primary ciliary dyskinesia symptoms are invariably present from birth.

Clinical features

The cardinal clinical features of bronchiectasis is the frequent coughing
up of green sputum. There is considerable variation in severity:

Mild

Rattly cough and green sputum after colds only.
Changing position may produce sputum.
Occasionally small haemoptysis.
Patient generally very well; normal pulmonary function.
Normal chest X-ray.

Moderate

Rattly cough all the time.
Able to produce a specimen of sputum at any time—usually green, rarely mucoid. Occasional haemoptysis.
Patient or relatives may notice hallitosis.
Patient usually generally well, pulmonary function usually normal.
Rarely clubbing. Crackles commonly audible.
Chest X-ray usually near normal.

Severe

Very large volumes of khaki-coloured sputum.
Occasional pneumonic illness with haemoptysis and pleural pain.
Clubbing very common.
Particularly if associated with airways obstruction, dyspnoea, cyanosis and respiratory failure may develop.
Patient often generally unwell, off work frequently, may vomit during expectoration.
Pyogenic skin and ocular infections common.
Gram-negative bacteria commonly present in sputum.
At risk from pneumonia, septicaemia, remote abscess formation and (rarely) amyloidosis.
Widespread crepitations audible.
Chest X-ray may show increased bronchovascular markings and sometimes multiple cysts containing fluid levels.

Investigation

1 Sputum examination

Naked-eye inspection of the sputum is essential to confirm the patient's account. Direct smear examination and culture for tuberculosis should be included in the initial assessment. Bacteriological examination is often unhelpful despite the obvious purulence of the sputum. *Haemophilus influenzae* and staphylococci are commonly isolated but more often no pathogens are recovered. More advanced cases tend to harbour *Ps. aeruginosa* or klebsiella species. Anaerobic culture techniques carried out in specialist laboratories have shown that there are usually very many different saprophytic organisms present in sputum which appears sterile on standard culture.

2 Chest X-ray

This is necessary in order to exclude obvious localized lung disease but the appearances are often normal. Peribronchial thickening and visible cysts may be evident in severe disease.

3 Bronchography (see p. 97)

This investigation is expensive and uncomfortable and need not be carried out where the diagnosis is clear and management is satisfactory. It may be necessary where the diagnosis is in doubt: for example, in the investigation of haemoptysis or recurrent regional collapse. It may also be necessary where management is unsatisfactory and there are grounds to suspect that the condition might be localized and treatable by resection.

Occasionally major saccular or varicose bronchiectasis is revealed but more usually the appearances are less dramatic and comprise: disturbance of the normal tapering pattern of part of the bronchial tree, abrupt failure to fill small bronchi in these areas and crowding of bronchi reflecting a degree of collapse in the part of the lung supplied (Fig. 12.1). The condition is generally patchy, basal and bilateral. Occasionally only one lobe is involved; left lower lobe and lingula are the commonest sites for localized disease. Allergic bronchopulmonary aspergillosis has been shown to be accompanied sometimes by proximal bronchiectasis (see p. 197). In general, however, the pattern of the bronchial abnormality is not helpful in suggesting aetiology.

Management

The most important elements in the management of the patient with bronchiectasis are generally explanation and reassurance. The patient is

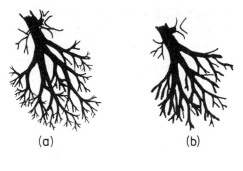

(a)   (b)

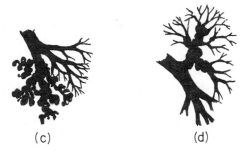

(c)   (d)

Fig. 12.1. *Bronchiectasis.* Diagram of appearances of bronchogram: (a), (b) and (c) left lower lobe; (d) left upper lobe. (a) Normal. (b) Bronchiectasis. The normal graceful tapering of bronchi is lacking; bronchi are crowded and the finer peripheral branches do not fill. (c) Gross saccular bronchiectasis. (d) Proximal bronchiectasis with normal peripheral bronchi accompanying allergic aspergillosis.

usually anxious about such things as: whether they are infectious to others, whether frequent cough damages their lungs, whether they will become disabled by breathlessness, or die prematurely—perhaps from haemoptysis. Reasonable reassurance can be expressed on all of these points in most patients. Treatment comprises:
1 Postural drainage
2 Antibiotic and chemotherapy
3 (Very rarely) Surgical excision.

1 Postural drainage

The patient should be encouraged to 'tip' for at least 10 minutes up to three times daily regularly if by doing so additional sputum is produced.

In mild cases this will apply for a week or two after colds and in severe cases it will be necessary indefinitely. Intelligent patients will discover the most productive position by trial and error. Usually a steep head-down position is most satisfactory. Exercise and 'huffing'—forced expiration continued to residual volume—may also be very helpful in encouraging sputum production.

2 Antibiotic and chemotherapy

WHEN?

Mild cases require an antibiotic after a cold and this will usually render the sputum mucoid. Moderately severe cases require an antibiotic after colds and more frequent courses of treatment may be worthwhile if this succeeds in rendering the sputum clear for some weeks. If the sputum does not become clear then antibiotics should be reserved for acute exacerbations. In severe cases antibiotics may be worthwhile on a long-term basis if this appears to reduce the volume and purulence of the sputum and prevent pneumonic episodes. The long-term use of antibiotics carries some hazards (including candidiasis and the fostering of resistant strains of bacteria) and these must be weighed against the observed benefits.

WHICH ANTIBIOTIC?

Amoxycillin, tetracycline and cotrimoxazole are all effective in standard dosage. In long-term use the development of resistant strains can theoretically be discouraged by changing the antibiotic at regular (say monthly) intervals. Almost always cotrimoxazole will be found to be most effective whatever the results of bacterial examination.

Severe illness

When a patient with bronchiectasis becomes severely ill the possibility of pneumonia or septicaemia from staphylococcus, pseudomonas or kleb-siella should be considered.

Surgical excision

This is only very rarely appropriate because medical management is quite satisfactory in most cases and because the condition tends to be diffuse.

Prognosis

This is obviously related to the severity. The vast majority of patients are able to lead normal lives and have a life expectancy which is nearly normal. The outlook is much less certain in those with extensive lung destruction or airways obstruction.

CHAPTER 13 / CYSTIC FIBROSIS

Cystic fibrosis is caused by a genetic defect and the most distinctive feature of the disease is an abnormally high concentration of sodium and chloride in the secretions of all of the exocrine glands of the body. The most striking clinical features arise from lung damage due to impaired mucociliary clearance and from malnutrition due in part to pancreatic failure.

Inheritance

The gene for cystic fibrosis is carried by about 1 in 20 of the population and is recessive. Affected individuals are homozygous for the gene. Cases of recognized cystic fibrosis arise in about 1 in 2000 live births. A quarter of the sibs of affected individuals would be expected to have the disease and about half would be expected to be carriers.

The basic defect

The flaw in the make-up of the human genome which is responsible for cystic fibrosis has not yet been identified. It seems possible that the genetic defect expresses itself by the control of chloride reabsorption at a number of critical sites in the body. Work on sweat glands has shown that the fluid produced deep in the gland is normal in composition but that there is a failure to reabsorb chloride and sodium in the more distal parts of the gland so that the sweat has an abnormally high concentration of these electrolytes. Other secretory organs in the body may have abnormal electrolyte compositions and, in the case of the lung, it seems likely that this may be sufficient to interfere with the composition of the fluid in which the cilia beat and to alter the state of hydration of the mucus gel. Impaired cilial performance and altered mechanical properties of mucus are probably early factors in the evolution of the lung lesion. The end result in the lungs, pancreas and liver may be that the secretions are thick and viscid and this has led to the use of the term 'mucoviscidosis', but it is probably misleading to regard cystic fibrosis as due to a primary defect of the mucus itself.

The pulmonary lesion

This takes the form of a more-or-less severe widespread bronchiectasis affecting peripheral airways. Lung damage results from failure of secretions to be cleared, which leads in turn to chronic infection by both saprophytic and potentially pathogenic bacteria. The sputum is purulent and produced in large amounts from hypertrophied mucus glands. Bacterial decomposition plays some part in reducing the viscosity of the sputum which tends to be viscid only briefly during severe exacerbations. Once bronchiectasis is established and the mucosa damaged mucociliary transport becomes further compromised and clearance increasingly dependent upon cough and gravity. Permanent colonization by *Pseudomonas aeruginosa* is inevitably present when lung damage is well established. This organism and *Staphylococcus aureus* appear to be important in causing lung damage and severe illness during severe exacerbations. In addition to bronchiectasis, small areas of parenchymal consolidation develop from impaired clearance and associated infection. Eventually there is increasing destruction of lung tissue and emphysema develops. Malnutrition secondary to malabsorption and sometimes dietary inadequacy lowers resistance to pulmonary infection in advanced cases.

The pancreatic lesion

The pancreas is almost always affected although about 10% of patients have no evident pancreatic deficiency. The exocrine tissue atrophies and the ducts remain as dilated cysts giving the disease its name. Pancreatic failure causes malabsorption and steatorrhoea.

Other associated disorders

The liver may be affected by intrahepatic bile duct obstruction caused by abnormal inspissated bile. Cirrhosis may result. Nasal polyposis is common in cystic fibrosis, the mechanism being poorly understood. In males there is almost always a defect of development of the Wolffian system so that epididymis and vas deferens may be rudimentary and obstructed. This defect is present from earliest childhood. The high concentration of electrolytes in sweat may lead to salt depletion in hot climates and during severe illness but this is uncommon.

Clinical features

Meconium ileus

About 10% of children affected by cystic fibrosis present in this way. The meconium is inspissated and sticky and the disorder presents the picture of intestinal obstruction evident within the first few hours of life. True meconium ileus is only seen in the first day or so after birth but a related disorder known as 'meconium ileus equivalent' may be seen at any age. Obscure abdominal colic is associated with threatened intestinal obstruction. Most episodes resolve without intervention.

Failure to thrive

About half of the total new cases presents in infancy or early childhood with the combination of retarded growth and respiratory symptoms. In some of these there is severe malnourishment and steatorrhoea. It is important to note that the other half of new cases presents with normal or near normal development and respiratory symptoms only.

Respiratory disease

1 SUPPURATIVE LUNG DISEASE

The symptoms are essentially those of bronchiectasis (p. 138). Persistent cough and a history of frequent 'chest infections' are often the first clues. The cough tends to be rattly but ventilatory function in the early stages is good and wheeze is not prominent. Differentiation from asthma and from bronchiectasis may sometimes be difficult. Once the diagnosis is suspected the crucial test is the sweat test. With progressive disease the volume of sputum increases and if produced by the patient it is seen to be green or khaki coloured. By this stage there are usually radiological changes and clubbing is likely to be present. On auscultation crackles are generally but not always audible. When they are coarse they are generally prominently early inspiratory in timing.

2 OTHER LUNG CHANGES

Pneumothorax is not uncommon and may be recurrent. Colonization of lung spaces by *Aspergillus fumigatus* and frank allergic bronchopulmonary aspergillosis may develop. Pulmonary tuberculosis develops more frequently than in the population at large, and it may be overlooked because of the abnormal radiological shadowing already present.

There is evidence that atopy is commoner amongst individuals with cystic fibrosis and some have asthma.

Pulmonary function

Although the pathological process involves an element of fibrosis, the physiological defect is one of airways obstruction. The lung becomes effectively emphysematous. There is evidence of overinflation with expiratory airways collapse, and spirometry reveals the expected obstructive pattern (p. 64). Airways obstruction becomes progressively more severe and in advanced cases chronic hypoxia and hypercapnia develop. Cor pulmonale (p. 273) may follow.

Radiographic features

The chest X-ray may be normal in the early stages. In mild disease a few flecks of irregular fine blotchy shadowing may be seen bilaterally on the lung fields particularly in the middle and upper zones. Later small areas of consolidation with shaggy outlines become widespread in the lung fields. Thickening of the bronchial walls may be evident in the form of parallel shadows representing medium sized bronchi and there may be streaky linear shadows reflecting fibrosis. Other features include over-inflation and prominence of the pulmonary artery.

Diagnosis

The association of features suggesting bronchiectasis and pancreatic failure make the diagnosis very probable. The chest radiograph can provide information which is virtually diagnostic when the disease is already well established. In the end, however, the diagnosis hinges on the result of the sweat test. In normal children the mean concentration of sodium and of chloride in the sweat is approximately 20 mmol/l. In adults this increases to about 35 mmol/l and the range of normal values increases. In cystic fibrosis sodium and chloride concentrations are in the range of 70 to 170. Values above 60 mmol/l are suggestive of the diagnosis and above 70 mmol/l the diagnosis is highly likely. Single spurious false positive results may be obtained in the presence of other serious disease or as a consequence of drying of the specimen. The test should be carried out by skilled hands and, where there is serious diagnostic doubt, it should be repeated.

Opinion is divided over whether it is necessary to investigate pancreatic dysfunction. Where there is diagnostic doubt with borderline sweat test results it may contribute useful information, but in obvious disease it is often omitted. It is now unnecessary to carry out duodenal intubation to assess pancreatic dysfunction. Two newer tests in use are the detection of urinary para-aminobenzoic acid (PABA) after ingestion of benzoyl-tyrosyl-PABA and the detection of exhaled $^{14}CO_2$ after ingestion of ^{14}C palmitate.

Management

Treatment is based firstly on measures to promote bronchial clearance and to control pulmonary infection and secondly on measures to support nutrition. Parents, older children and young adult patients in particular require a good deal of regular counselling and emotional support.

Pulmonary disease

The management centres on two elements: (i) bronchial clearance and (ii) antibiotic treatment.

BRONCHIAL CLEARANCE

At all stages of the disease the importance of effective bronchial clearance needs to be stressed. Postural drainage is the most effective adjunct. This involves lying in a steep, head-down position for periods of at least 10 minutes twice daily. Postural drainage is carried out for longer and more frequently in the day and in other positions if this proves necessary and productive. It may be accompanied by 'huffing'—slow forced expiration to residual volume with gentle coughing near full expiration—or by a vibration by a family member or physiotherapist. Huffing is quite effective on its own but gravity is the most effective single agent. It is difficult to persuade older patients with few symptoms to undertake postural drainage. Daily vigorous exercise may have more appeal.

ANTIBIOTIC TREATMENT

Regular treatment with an antibiotic is widely advised during early childhood. Flucloxacillin may offer some protection from potentially harmful infection by *Staphylococcus aureus*. Later in childhood and in adults practice varies considerably. Usually antibiotic treatment is reserved for obvious exacerbations when the volume and nature of sputum changes and there is accompanying malaise. Where there are persistent symptoms and the sputum volume is large it is usually found that long-term use of an agent such as cotrimoxazole will reduce sputum volume and increase well-being. Benefit may result even if the treatment is not apparently effective against *Pseudomonas aeruginosa* in the laboratory. During severe exacerbations intravenous antibiotic treatment is necessary and effectiveness against *Pseudomonas* appears to be important. In recent years carbenicillin combined with gentamicin has been the most frequently used combination, but this has given way to azlocillin (very expensive) combined with tobramycin and both may now be superceded by the newer cephalosporins such as ceftazidime. Once present it is not possible to eradicate *Pseudomonas aeruginosa* from the sputum. Regular sputum culture is a rather poor guide to the need for or likely effectiveness of antibiotic treatment.

OTHER MEASURES

A few patients have an important reversible element to their airways obstruction and some have asthma. Treatment with bronchodilators by inhalation may be helpful. Large doses may be required. Inhaled or systemic steroid treatment is sometimes necessary.

There is no convincing evidence that mucolytic agents are helpful in cystic fibrosis. Measures aimed at humidifying the inspired air are probably also irrelevant. Except under unusual circumstances the air in the bronchi is adequately saturated anyway and measures to supersaturate the air are poorly tolerated over a long period and of no definite benefit.

Nutrition

PANCREATIC EXTRACT

Pancreatic replacement therapy can be taken in the form of tablets or granules containing pancreatic extract derived from pig or cow. Treatment is taken before or with meals; the dose depends on the age of the patient and the clinical response, and may amount to over 20 tablets daily. Pancreatic extract is degraded by acid digestion in the stomach and some individuals have persistent steatorrhoea despite large oral doses. The effectiveness of pancreatic extract treatment can be enhanced by administration of H_2 blocking drugs (e.g. cimetidine). This is expensive.

DIET

There has been some enthusiasm in recent years for an elemental diet designed to be absorbed without predigestion. The protein is provided as beef hydrolysate, the fat as medium chain triglyceride and calories are provided in the form of a polymerized polysaccharide. To these ingredients are added vitamin and mineral supplements. The diet is not very palatable and tolerance in older children is limited. In general, patients with cystic fibrosis eat large quantities of food according to their own preferences. Vitamin supplements are sensible although overt deficiency is unusual. Where there is serious weight loss or failure to gain weight it is often due to anorexia secondary to chronic ill health associated with suppurative lung disease or breathlessness rather than to malabsorption. Attention should then be focused on intensive physiotherapy and antibiotic treatment.

Counselling and emotional support

Continuity is important. Cystic fibrosis is a chronic disabling and threatening disease of young people and considerable stress is generated in both patients and families. Reducing worry to reasonable proportions takes time.

Parents of an affected child need to know that the risk of a subsequent child having the disease is 1 in 4. At present there is no reliable antenatal diagnostic test. A test of albumin in the meconium is available and this may provide early warning in high risk babies. An expertly conducted sweat test should be conducted in such circumstances. There is at present no simple and reliable screening test which would be suitable for use in new babies generally.

Unaffected sibs have a 1 in 2 chance of being a carrier. The carrier state cannot be recognized by any laboratory test. Offspring of unaffected sibs have about a 1 in 80 chance of being affected if nothing is known about the other partner.

Adult male patients are inevitably sterile and females have reduced fertility. There have now been many recorded pregnancies in affected females and contraceptive advice may be necessary. Offspring of an affected mother have about a 1 in 40 chance of having the disease where nothing is known about the family history of the father.

Serious emotional problems may result in teenage from failure of sexual development and retarded growth. These add to the difficulties imposed by chronic ill health as patients struggle to make an independent existence for themselves. Where disability is already advanced, employment can be difficult. Circumstances at the place of work are almost always such as to discourage the patient from coughing and it is unusual for regular postural drainage to be possible at work.

Patients generally know when death is approaching and may need opportunities to talk about this and specific fears they may harbour. When terminal symptoms threaten to be intolerable regular treatment with an opiate becomes more important than vigorous resuscitative measures.

Prognosis

Until recently survival beyond the mid 'teens was rare. Most children still die before this age but survival into the mid-twenties is now common and there are well documented patients in their fourth and even fifth decades. It seems likely that improved nutritional status and antibiotic treatment have been powerful influences in bringing this about. It is not easy to see why mildly affected older patients have managed to escape the severe damage that affects others. Such patients have not necessarily had more or prompt treatment in their younger years. The disease seems to express itself with differing degrees of severity and this variation may result from chance, from environmental factors, or from some aspect of the individual's genetic make-up.

CHAPTER 14 / LUNG ABSCESS

This term is customarily reserved for localized suppurative lesions of the lung parenchyma which are not obviously due to tuberculosis or other specific infections.

Aetiology

ASPIRATION

This is the commonest cause of lung abscess. Inhalation of food, vomitus, sputum or other material is particularly likely to occur in association with:
1 States of impaired consciousness
2 Alcoholism
3 Incompetence of the larynx due to paralysis or sensory impairment (Myasthenia gravis, bulbar palsy, local anaesthesia etc.)
4 Oesophageal obstruction
5 Persistent vomiting
6 Severe bronchiectasis
7 Infection in the mouth or sinuses (particularly dental sepsis in the elderly).

BRONCHIAL OBSTRUCTION

Partial or complete bronchial obstruction leads to retention of sputum and subsequent pyogenic infection. Common examples are bronchial carcinoma and foreign body (especially peanuts and extracted teeth).

POST-PNEUMONIC

The centre of an area of destructive pneumonia may break down to form a lung abscess particularly when the pneumonia is due to *Staphylococcus aureus* or *Klebsiella pneumoniae* (see p. 114).

TUMOUR

Cavitation is quite common in bronchial carcinoma and this results in what is effectively a lung abscess lined with tumour tissue.

EMBOLIC INFECTION

This may result from secondary infection of a pulmonary infarct or from embolization of infected material from other sites of sepsis in the body or from contaminated intravenous infusion fluids and catheters. Intravenous injection of unsterilized material by drug addicts is especially likely to cause lung abscesses.

OTHER CAUSES

Trauma to the lung may rarely cause a haematoma which may become infected. An amoebic abscess may develop in the right lower lobe following trans-diaphragmatic spread from an amoebic liver abscess.

Clinical features

Fever and obvious systemic upset are present at least in the initial stages and a leucocytosis is almost invariable. Later when the abscess opens into a bronchus there may be a cough with expectoration of large amounts of foul material which is variably blood-stained at first and later brown or green. Fever and malaise may recede as the abscess becomes chronic.

Investigations

CHEST X-RAY

The diagnosis of lung abscess is almost always confirmed by the chest X-ray, which shows one or more round lesions of almost any size which with time cavitate and may contain fluid levels. Abscesses due to inhalation most commonly develop in the apical segments of the lower lobes (especially the right) and the lateral and posterior parts of the upper lobes (especially the right).

SPUTUM

Culture may yield *Staphylococcus aureus* or other common respiratory pathogens. Anaerobic bacteria may predominate in foul sputum which commonly yields no growth on standard culture. The tubercle bacillus must always be sought. Cytological examination for malignant cells is unrewarding when sputum is largely pus.

BRONCHOSCOPY

When carcinoma or a foreign body is suspected bronchoscopy may be relevant.

Diagnosis

Most lung abscesses develop during the course of serious disease and the mechanism of their causation may be evident. Thoracotomy may be necessary to exclude a cavitated carcinoma where such evidence is lacking or where the abscess increases in size. If a cavitated abscess is due to tuberculosis the sputum almost invariably contains acid-fast bacilli on direct smear.

Management

Management comprises:
1   Postural drainage
2   Antibiotic and chemotherapy
3   (Rarely) Surgical excision or drainage.

POSTURAL DRAINAGE

The most satisfactory position will be evident from the radiological localization of the abscess.

ANTIBIOTIC AND CHEMOTHERAPY

In the initial phase of acute illness therapy will be guided by bacteriological examination of the sputum and the results of blood culture. Staphylococcus, pseudomonas and klebsiella will require special measures (p. 114–5). Later penicillin in large doses orally, perhaps with the addition of probenicid to block renal excretion, will generally show gradual healing. When the patient is no longer seriously ill there is less call to treat gram-negative organisms recovered from the sputum as they are unlikely to be responsible for the persistence of the abscess. As an alternative to penicillin cotrimoxazole may be found satisfactorily empirically and should be continued for several weeks if improvement occurs. Metronidazole is also useful. Flucloxacillin should be added if *Staphyloccus aureus* is regularly recovered. The great majority of lung abscesses heal with medical treatment but this commonly takes many weeks.

SURGICAL TREATMENT

Surgical excision is only occasionally required except in the case of suspected carcinoma or where healing is delayed beyond about 4 months. Occasionally complications such as empyema or bronchopleural fistula require surgical intervention.

CHAPTER 15 / ASTHMA AND ALLERGIC DISORDERS OF THE LUNG

CLASSIFICATION OF HYPERSENSITIVITY REACTIONS

The classification introduced by Gell & Coombs (1958) is still very useful.

Type I

The antibody involved is principally of IgE class. It becomes fixed in certain tissues and particularly to the walls of mast cells. Challenge with specific antigen causes an alteration of the cell wall which permits the escape of histamine and certain other locally active substances which are collectively known as mediators. The effects of challenge by the antigen are prompt and Type I is sometimes referred to as 'immediate' hypersensitivity. This type of reaction is involved in anaphylactic responses and in extrinsic asthma.

Type II

In this form of hypersensitivity the antibody involved is fixed to the surface of circulating blood elements and the reaction takes place intravascularly (e.g. transfusion reaction). Type II reactions are not known to be of importance in respiratory disease.

Type III

The antibody involved is of IgG class and circulates in the serum and permeates the connective tissue when there is local inflammation. When antibody and specific antigen come together in a tissue they combine to form immune complexes which activate complement to set up a tissue-damaging local reaction mediated by leucocytes. This sequence of events takes some hours to evolve and Type III reactions are sometimes referred to as 'delayed' hypersensitivity. Some IgG can be demonstrated *in vitro* by formation of a precipitate with specific antigen. Antibodies of this type are known as precipitins.

Type IV

In this category the immune response is mediated by the action of lymphocytes rather than by antibody. The best example of this form of response is the tuberculin reaction. It takes 2–3 days to evolve. The behaviour of sensitized lymphocytes is the subject of intensive research. There is some evidence that cell-mediated (Type IV) hypersensitivity may play some part in asthma and allergic rhinitis but the nature and significance of this involvement is poorly understood.

Types I and III are established as being of some importance in respiratory disease.

ASTHMA

Definition

Asthma is a disease characterized by variable dyspnoea due to widespread narrowing of the peripheral airways in the lungs, varying in severity over short periods of time, either spontaneously or as a result of treatment (Ciba 1959).

Extrinsic/intrinsic asthma

Much emphasis has been laid upon the distinction between extrinsic and intrinsic asthma. In practice the distinction is rather blurred and of limited value. In extrinsic asthma the identity of the external allergen is known or strongly suspected on the evidence provided by the patient's history or response to skin-testing. In intrinsic asthma such evidence is lacking.

Atopy

IgE (tissue-fixed, immediate reacting antibody, also called reagin) is normally produced in very small amounts and only in response to substantial exposure to an external allergen. Certain individuals possess a constitutional tendency to produce important amounts of IgE following mere trivial exposure to everyday antigens. Such individuals are referred to as atopic and they tend to exhibit asthma, hay fever and other forms of allergic rhinitis, urticaria and eczema. Usually the atopic diathesis is evident from an early age.

Sometimes the term atopy is used merely to indicate that the individual has positive reactions to two or more common inhaled antigens on prick skin-testing.

Control of bronchial muscle tone

CYCLIC AMP

Cyclic adenosine monophosphate (cyclic AMP) is present within cells throughout the body and appears to be the principal factor controlling many different specialist functions. There is now a good deal of evidence to suggest that the tone of bronchial smooth muscle is mainly controlled by the intracellular level of cyclic AMP. Increased levels of cyclic AMP are associated with bronchodilatation and decreased levels with bronchoconstriction. The level of cyclic AMP is itself regulated by the effect of transmitter substances acting at specific receptor sites on the cell wall. Cyclic AMP is degraded by an enzyme, phosphodiesterase, and substances which inhibit this enzyme (e.g. theophylline) increase the level of cyclic AMP and act as bronchodilators.

The liberation of histamine and other substances from mast cells (see below) is also controlled by or modified by intracellular cyclic AMP and GMP levels. Low levels of cyclic AMP are associated with discharge of intracellular granules and high levels with relative stability of the mast cell wall.

AUTONOMIC NERVOUS SYSTEM

1 *Sympathetic nervous system*
Surprisingly there seems to be no sympathetic innervation of the airways in man. Nevertheless, bronchial smooth muscle carries receptors which are stimulated by circulating adrenaline. Stimulation of β-adrenergic receptors on bronchial smooth muscle causes an increase in cyclic AMP and bronchodilatation. Stimulation of α-adrenergic receptors results in reduction of cyclic AMP and bronchoconstriction.

2 *Parasympathetic nervous system*
Cholinergic receptors are also present in bronchial muscle and vagal parasympathetic stimulation causes bronchoconstriction, perhaps by altering intracellular levels of another nucleotide (cyclic GMP).

3   NANC nerves

There is now good evidence for the presence of non-adrenergic, non-parasympathetic (NANC) nerves supplying human bronchial muscle. It seems probable that the transmitter released by these nerves is vaso-intestinal peptide (VIP) which has already been shown to be of import-ance in the gut. It appears to exert a bronchodilator effect.

Other receptors probably exist which are specific for other substances released locally in the course of immediate or delayed hypersensitivity reactions.

MEDIATORS

Intermediary substances released or activated in the course of the asthmatic process are referred to collectively as mediators. Neurotrans-mitters (see above) are sometimes considered as mediators although it is felt unlikely that excess or shortage of these is a fundamental part of the asthmatic process.

Histamine

Histamine is a potent bronchoconstrictor and, moreover, asthmatic subjects are many times more sensitive to histamine-induced broncho-constriction than normals. Histamine provocation is used as a tool in epidemiological and pharmacological research and occasionally in diag-nosis on this account. The degree of sensitivity can vary from time to time depending on the degree of instability or quiescence of the in-dividual's asthma. Histamine sensitivity is not the fundamental abnorm-ality in asthma and antihistamine drugs have proved disappointing in its management.

Kinins

Kinins are bronchoconstrictor substances formed from circulating pre-cursors by the action of enzymes released by mast cells and some tissue secretions. The role of kinins in the asthmatic process is unknown.

Leukotrienes

For many years it was known that mast cells, in addition to releasing a relatively short-acting bronchoconstrictor (histamine) also produced a substance which produced a persistent and marked bronchoconstrictor effect. The name 'slow-reacting substance of anaphylaxis (SRS-A)' was used to describe its effect. Recent work has revealed that it is composed of several substances derived from one limb of the complex biochemical pathways which make up arachidonic acid metabolism. Leukotrienes are released by mast cells but, unlike histamine they are formed at the time of release by breakdown of arachidonic acid in the wall of the cell and not derived from preformed material in intracellular granules.

Prostaglandins

Prostaglandins are also formed by metabolism of arachidonic acid by a different pathway (the cyclo-oxygenase pathway). Prostaglandin E_2 has a bronchodilator effect and prostaglandin F_2 has a bronchoconstrictor effect which is particularly exaggerated in asthmatic individuals. Prostaglandin E_2 has sometimes bronchoconstrictor and sometimes bronchodilator effects and the action depends in part at least on the recent history of stimulation of the bronchial smooth muscle. A simple hypersensitivity to prostaglandin bronchoconstriction seems unlikely to explain much of the asthmatic process. Aspirin-like inhibitors of prostaglandin synthetase have been unpredictable and unimpressive in the treatment of asthma, and the fairly common phenomenon of aspirin sensitivity is difficult to incorporate into any hypothesis proposing a causative role for prostaglandins.

Other mediators

Neutrophil chemotactic factor (NCF) is of interest because it can be measured in the blood and circulating levels can be shown to increase during bronchial challenge with specific antibody. Its role in the asthmatic process is poorly understood. Platelet activating factor (PAF acether) is a further measurable substance of uncertain importance in the asthmatic process. It is known to cause a marked increase in capillary permeability. Little is known either about eosinophil chemotactic factor or about the role of eosinophils themselves.

Mechanism of the asthmatic response

A schematic representation of some of the factors referred to which may be important in the evolution of the asthmatic response is shown in Fig. 15.1. The mechanism of asthma is the subject of much research and this abbreviated version will require modification with time.

1   IgE is produced by lymphoid tissue in response to the extrinsic allergen. IgE becomes fixed to mast cells in the bronchial walls.

2   Exposure to further allergen results in an antigen–antibody reaction occurring on the surface of the mast cell which produces a profound effect upon the permeability of the cell wall.

3   This results in the liberation of mediator substances stored in

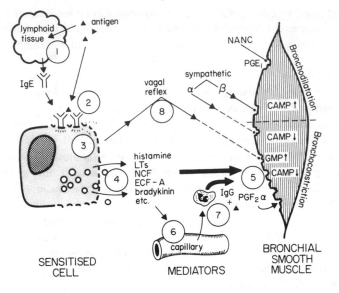

Fig. 15.1. *Some of the factors involved in the evolution of the asthmatic reaction.* The numerals are referred to in the text.

ECF–A, Eosinophil chemotactic factor.

LTs, Leukotrienes.

NANC, Non-adrenergic non-cholinergic nerves.

NCF, Neutrophil chemotactic factor.

PGE_1, Prostaglandin E_1—bronchodilator in action.

$PGF_2\alpha$, Prostaglandin $F_2\alpha$—markedly bronchoconstrictor in action in asthma.

granules within the mast cell and generation of other mediators from arachidonic acid metabolism in the wall of the mast cell.

4   Mediators include: histamine, leukotrienes which produce prolonged bronchoconstriction, eosinophil chemotactic factor (ECF-A), neurophil chemotactic factor (NCF), platelet activating factor, bradykinin and others.

5   The mediators react at specific receptor sites on smooth muscle cell membranes and this is followed by reduced intracellular levels of cyclic AMP and bronchoconstriction.

6   Mediators also cause alteration in capillary permeability.

7   This may result in the entry of IgG and leucocytes (attracted by NCF) into the bronchial connective tissue. A Type III delayed complement-fixing reaction may then occur leading to leucocyte damage, release of lysosomes, local tissue damage and release of prostaglandins and other mediators.

8   Vagal nerve endings may be irritated by mediators, local inflammation leading to a reflex parasympathetic bronchoconstrictor response.

Pathological features

In fatal cases of asthma the main changes are found in the bronchial wall:
1   Eosinophil infiltration
2   Increase in number of goblet cells
3   Plugging of the bronchi with viscid mucus containing eosinophils
4   Thickening of the epithelian basement membrane
5   Possibly bronchial muscle hypertrophy.

The lungs are overinflated but otherwise normal. Eosinophilia of the bronchial wall, sputum and sometimes of the blood is characteristic of asthma but the function of the eosinophil remains obscure.

A minor degree of the same changes are known to be present in patients with apparently well-controlled asthma who die suddenly from another cause. Quite widespread bronchial plugging may be present.

Prevalence

Asthma is common. It is estimated that perhaps 5% of the population has recognizable asthma in the course of a lifetime. Prevalence is greatest amongst children.

Mortality

Until comparatively recently asthma was regarded as a fairly minor complaint which did not cause death. Asthma is, however, responsible for about 1500 deaths annually in the UK and many of these occur in young people. For many years the mortality has remained remarkably constant. During the 1960s there was a striking increase in the death rate particularly amongst young people. The possible cause of this 'epidemic' has been the subject of protracted debate (see p. 176).

Most deaths from asthma occur outside hospital. In many the apparent period of worsening before death is very brief—minutes or a few hours—although confirmatory measurements of well being shortly before death are lacking. Characteristically deaths occur in individuals who were not thought by their family doctors to be suffering from severe asthma (actual measurements of ventilatory performance are rare in such individuals). There is strong evidence that those who die are, as a group, relatively undertreated particularly with respect to steroid treatment. Deaths occur most commonly at night or in the early hours of the morning. Mortality in the UK is significantly increased in the summer.

Age of onset

Asthma may occur for the first time *at any age*. Males predominate in childhood and females in later life. In childhood extrinsic factors and associated atopy are much more likely to be encountered than later in life. When asthma occurs for the first time in the elderly it is commonly misdiagnosed.

Clinical features

The main features are wheezing dyspnoea, a sense of chest tightness, cough and an increase in sputum volume and viscosity. Sometimes the patient describes a sensation of choking in the neck or of tightness in the chest rather than wheezing. Sometimes the cough is given more emphasis than wheezing particularly when it occurs at night.

Patterns of variability in asthma

THE ACUTE ATTACK

Distressing wheezing of more or less acute onset is the hallmark of asthma. The majority of patients have such attacks at some time and often refer to them as 'spasms'. Some patients with asthma do not have abrupt attacks and suffer more or less persistent symptoms.

The patient sits or stands bracing the shoulders on the knees or on the arms of a chair. The expression is one of preoccupation with the business of breathing breath by breath. Inspiration is snatched and expiration prolonged; both are wheezy. Examination reveals over-inflation of the chest, use of accessory muscles of respiration and marked recession of the lower part of the chest during inspiration. There is a tachycardia and usually pulsus paradoxicus; cyanosis may be present. Auscultation usually reveals universal inspiratory and expiratory rhonchi. Sometimes in very severe acute asthma wheezing is unimpressive or absent despite obvious distress and laboured chest distortion. This is a sign of dangerously severe airways obstruction.

Most attacks subside spontaneously in minutes but some are prolonged for hours despite treatment (see p. 191).

Unconsciousness is occasionally encountered in an acute attack. Sometimes this is brief and suggestive of cough syncope and sometimes actual asphyxia accompanied by impairment of venous return due to overinflation seems a more probable explanation. Attacks of unconsciousness suggest very severe asthma and inadequate treatment.

Sometimes an acute attack is completely unheralded in a completely symptom-free patient but more usually attacks occur on a background of less severe symptoms.

EXACERBATIONS OF INTERMITTENT ASTHMA

One of the commonest patterns is that of exacerbations lasting several days or a few weeks after upper respiratory infections with long periods of relative freedom from symptoms.

CHRONIC ASTHMA

Some patients have persistent symptoms which may be mild or severe. Virtually always there is a characteristic diurnal variability.

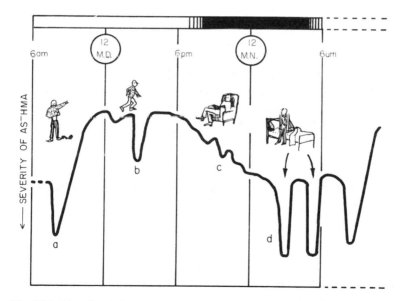

Fig. 15.2. *Diurnal variation in symptoms in asthma.* The most striking features are usually (a) chest tightness and wheezing dyspnoea on waking, improving during the morning, and (d) nocturnal attacks. In addition there may be exercise-induced asthma (b) and worsening of symptoms whilst resting in the evening (c).

Diurnal variation in symptoms is one of the most important diagnostic features of asthma and it is seen in chronic asthma as well as during exacerbations. The characteristic pattern is illustrated in Fig. 15.2. The main elements are:

Morning tightness
The patient notices tightness and wheezing usually within seconds of waking and this takes minutes or hours to subside. Coughing exacerbates symptoms.

Nocturnal attacks
Attacks at night are also characteristic of asthma. The patient generally wakes between 2 and 3 a.m. with tightness, cough and wheezing dyspnoea. He may sit up or rise to sit by an open window. Nocturnal attacks may be prolonged or repeated. Such episodes are commonly misdiagnosed as 'paroxysmal nocturnal dyspnoea due to left ventricular failure'. One of the most useful features which distinguishes this last type of nocurnal attack is the lack of morning tightness.

SEASONAL VARIATION
Marked seasonal variation is characteristic of extrinsic asthma. In the UK aggravation of asthma in the months May–July is typical of grass-pollen sensitivity. Aggravation in the winter months is common and probably due to two factors—frequent upper respiratory tract infections and house dust mite sensitivity. Patients with sensitivity to mould spores are generally worst in the autumn.

Trigger factors

A number of factors are known to aggravate asthma although they are not regarded as primary causes of the condition:
1   Exercise
2   Non-specific irritants
3   Infection
4   Drugs
5   External allergens
6   Emotional factors.

EXERCISE-INDUCED ASTHMA
Severe exercise may provoke asthma especially in young subjects.

Wheezing and tightness are experienced a minute or two after the end of exercise and are quite different from the hyperpnoea of the effort. If exercise is prolonged asthma may come on whilst it is still in progress. In some patients, especially children, exercise-induced wheezing is the only expression of asthma.

The underlying mechanisms of exercise-induced asthma are the subject of much research. It has been shown that the hyperpnoea of exercise may cause cooling of the trachea and perhaps bronchi. If respiratory heat loss is prevented by breathing warm humid air then exercise-induced asthma may be prevented. There is uncertainty over whether cooling itself or evaporation of secretions (and local osmotic change) may be the trigger. After an episode of exercise-induced bronchoconstriction there is a refractory period during which it is much harder to induce the phenomenon. The discharge of mast cells may be one part of the reaction. Exercise-induced asthma can be blocked by prior medication with a β-adrenergic stimulant drug or disodium cromoglycate.

PROVOCATION BY NON-SPECIFIC IRRITANTS

Patients with asthma demonstrate hyper-reactivity by developing bronchoconstriction in response to non-antigenic dusts, smoke, histamine and acetyl choline in concentrations which produce no detectable effect in normal individuals. Asthma may also be provoked by laughing, coughing and forced expiration.

PROVOCATION BY INFECTION

It is doubtful whether asthma is caused by specific allergy to common respiratory infective agents but it is certainly aggravated by viral and bacterial infections.

PROVOCATION BY DRUGS

A full account of drug-induced asthma is given in Chapter 25 (p. 316). Particular note should be made of the importance of **aspirin hypersensitivity**. A proportion of asthmatic individuals may develop sudden very severe asthma after consuming aspirin. The following points are relevant:

1   Aspirin sensitivity should be considered whenever sudden severe asthma develops within a few minutes on a background of very good control of symptoms (symptom-free nights and mornings).

2   Patients are commonly unaware of the relationship between aspirin and attacks of asthma.

3   The association of intrinsic asthma and nasal polyposis increases the likelihood of aspirin sensitivity.

4   Susceptible individuals should be warned never to take aspirin again and taught how to recognize preparations which contain it.

5   The hypersensitivity extends to other non-steroidal anti-inflammatory agents such as indomethacin, ibuprofen, etc.

6   Susceptible individuals also react to tartrazine which is used to give yellow colouring to foods and some drugs.

Other drugs causing aggravation of asthma include beta-blocking agents, cholinergic drugs, radiocontrast media, anaesthetic agents and muscle relaxants.

PROVOCATION BY EXTERNAL ALLERGENS

Airborne allergens in minute quantities may provoke asthma. In the UK the most common airborne allergens are grass pollen and house dust mite. Other pollens, moulds, animal danders, etc. may also provoke asthma but these are numerically relatively unimportant.

Acute exposure to the airborne antigen in a hypersensitive individual generally produces an almost immediate onset of cough, chest tightness and wheeze. This may improve over some minutes or hours if exposure is modest. Some individuals develop a delayed reaction (Fig. 15.3) reaching its height at 6–8 hours after exposure. Occasionally a biphasic response is seen in which early and late phases are both present. Early

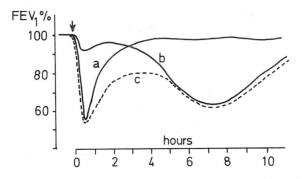

Fig. 15.3. *Immediate and delayed responses to bronchial challenge.* FEV_1 as a percentage of the resting value plotted against time after antigen inhalation (arrow). Stylized representations of three different types of response from three individuals: (a) immediate response; (b) delayed response; (c) biphasic response. Most individuals with a later response show some immediate reaction. Cromoglycate pretreatment typically blocks both immediate and delayed rections. Steroid pre-treatment blocks only the delayed response.

reactions tend to be IgE-mediated and late reactions may be accompanied by the presence of circulating precipitins against the antigen in question but this is by no means invariable. The delayed response is particularly important in the investigation of occupational asthma because the relationship between symptoms and work may be complex (p. 306). Patients with grass-pollen sensitivity, as well as experiencing seasonal asthma, commonly have hay fever and are aware that proximity to grass particularly when newly cut is likey to induce symptoms. Camping is especially likely to provoke an exacerbation.

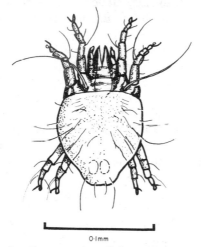

0·1mm

Fig. 15.4. *Dermatophagoides pteronyssinus:* the house dust mite.

The house dust mite (*Dermatophagoides pteronyssinus*) and its close relative the kitchen mite (*Dermatophagoides culinae*) are minute 8-legged arthropods about 0.15 mm in length (Fig. 15.4). They are almost universally distributed and are responsible for the antigenic properties of house dust. *D. pteronyssinus* is found in highest concentration in the superficial layers of mattresses where it finds ideal requirements of warmth, moisture and its principal foodstuff—desquamated human skin scales. Subjects sensitive to the house dust mite tend to suffer aggravation of their asthma:
1 at night, though not all nocturnal asthma is due to house dust
2 during bed-making and household cleaning
3 at week-ends (but excessive smoking, beer and wines may cause aggravation at this time).
4 in the early winter.

Occupational asthma, see p. 306.

Allergy to foodstuffs
This is relatively uncommon but hypersensitivity to beer, wines, shellfish, eggs, etc. is occasionally encountered.

PROVOCATION BY EMOTIONAL DISTURBANCE
The relationship between psychogenic factors and asthma is complex but the following points may be made.
1   Severe asthma is frightening and chronic severe asthma is, in addition, depressing. It commonly results in chronic loss of sleep which aggravates symptoms of anxiety. In chronic childhood asthma in particular very great strains are put upon parents and child alike. Emotional disturbance in this situation is as likely to be a consequence of the asthma as it is to be the cause.
2   Psychogenic factors may undoubtedly aggravate the severity of established asthma and may provoke actual attacks. Anger, frustration and acute anxiety are particularly potent in this context.
3   It is widely believed that asthma is 'due to nerves' and this sometimes results in patients being rather unsympathetically treated by friends and relatives.
4   Some asthmatic patients are undoubtedly able to self-induce attacks. Usually this is brought about by repeated forced expiration near residual volume and this appears to produce reflex bronchoconstriction. This may sometimes be done more or less subconsciously to attract sympathy or avoid unpleasant tasks.
5   Patients with asthma are generally very appreciative of a straightforward 'organic' approach to the management of their disease. If asthma is adequately treated and if patients understand their treatment 'psychogenic factors' almost always subside.

Asthma in children

Most of the discussion above refers equally to asthma in childhood. Treatment in children is covered on p. 190.

DIAGNOSIS
One of the most important aspects of childhood asthma is the extent to which it is underdiagnosed. There is a strong tendency for children with recurrent cough and wheeze to be labelled as suffering from 'bronchitis'. Where cough and wheeze really are recurrent the diagnosis is

virtually always that of asthma. Cough is often much more prominent as a symptom in childhood and it may be the only complaint offered by the parent. The eliciting of diurnal variation, exercise-induced attacks, coexistent features of rhinitis, eczema or of a family history may provide useful additional evidence pointing towards the correct diagnosis. Simple spirometry or peak flow measurement may provide further support by confirming airways obstruction, but a formal demonstration of exercise-induced asthma may be even more useful in suspected asthma. Peak flow rate is measured before and at intervals after a 6 minute spell of very vigorous running free out of doors. The characteristic post exercise bronchoconstriction—and its relief by bronchodilator aerosol—provides valuable objective support for a diagnosis of asthma particularly when the presentation has been atypical.

WHEEZING UNDER THE AGE OF THREE

Not all babies who have important wheezing go on to show features of asthma later. Acute rhinorrhoea, cough and obstructed breathing in the first year may be due to bronchiolitis secondary to the respiratory syncytial virus or sometimes other viruses (p. 102). There is no very clear relationship between this and the subsequent development of asthma. Where there is a persistent or recurrent tendency to wheeze with severe exacerbations very young children (under 2 years) show a resistance to the usual bronchodilator treatments which are effective later.

Course

CHILDHOOD ASTHMA

About 70% of those who develop asthma during childhood develop symptoms before the age of 5 years. The majority of children with asthma improve as puberty approaches. About three-quarters of children who suffer only occasional episodes related to simple upper respiratory infections will be free from symptoms by the age of 15. Those with the most persistent symptoms, the earliest onset and the most impressive atopic features show the least and the most postponed improvement.

ADULT ASTHMA

The outlook is similarly unpredictable. It is usually most helpful to suggest to patients that they will always have some tendency to asthma, that this may undergo spontaneous variation and that, with adequate attention to details of treatment, reasonable control of symptoms can be expected.

Tests for specific hypersensitivity

SKIN-TESTING

Skin-testing is of limited value. It is undertaken for a variety of reasons:
1 To provide confirmation of immediate hypersensitivity to external allergens with a view to their subsequent exclusion so far as this is possible, or with a view to subsequent specific desensitization.
2 To provide an indication of atopic status or to allow classification into extrinsic or intrinsic groups. This may not be of great importance to the individual patient but it may be relevant when comparing the results of treatment in different groups of patients.

There are two widely-used methods.

Intradermal method
An extract of the antigen is injected intradermally using a tuberculin syringe and a fine needle raising a wheal about 3 mm in diameter. This method may reveal immediate and delayed reactions but tends to produce a high incidence of positive results of doubtful significance. In very allergic individuals severe local reactions, asthma or even anaphylaxis may be induced.

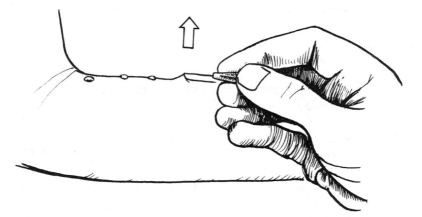

Fig. 15.5. *Modified prick skin-test.* Drops of antigen extracts and antigen-free control solution are placed on the flexor surface of the forearm. Each drop is pricked with a fine needle. The needle is held parallel to the skin surface, advanced slightly and a tiny fold of skin lifted briefly as shown. Deep stabs and bleeding should be avoided. Wheal and flare are measured after 10–20 minutes. Fine disposable needles are adequate if cleaned and dried between each prick. Vigorous preparation of the skin is undesirable.

Modified prick skin-test
A drop of each solution to be tested is placed upon the skin and a prick made by the method illustrated in Fig. 15.5. There are fewer false positive results with this method and the results correlate well with circulating levels of specific IgE. The quantity of antigen introduced is minute and the method is safe. It is much more convenient in practice than the intradermal method. Delayed responses are almost never seen.

Note
Immediate skin-test responses are suppressed by antihistamines but not by steroid treatment. Delayed reactions are suppressed by steroid treatment. Patch-testing is not relevant to the assessment of immediate hypersensitivity.

OTHER TESTS FOR SPECIFIC HYPERSENSITIVITY

RAST test
The radio-allergo-sorbent test (RAST) is a means of measuring the level of circulating IgE which is specifically directed towards a particular antigen. It is performed on serum in the laboratory. It is expensive and of very little relevance to the management of patients with asthma. Exceptionally it may be useful where it is necessary to know whether an individual is highly sensitive to a particular substance and it is at the same time considered dangerous to try even skin prick tests (e.g. in possible penicillin anaphylaxis).

Bronchial challenge
This too is of no relevance in the management of the great majority of patients with asthma. It involves the patient inhaling nebulized solution or a powder aerosol of the substance in question. Control inhalations on different days are generally required. In possible occupational asthma it may be important to support clinical suspicion with a challege test when decisions regarding employment are to be made. Bronchial challenge may be dangerous. Bronchoconstriction may be delayed and hospital admission is advisable where the level of hypersensitivity is not known.

Physiological changes in asthma

1 Airways obstruction

A REDUCTION OF FEV₁

FEV_1, vital capacity and FEV_1/VC ratio are reduced and there is reduction of peak expiratory flow rate.

B PROLONGATION OF FORCED EXPIRATORY TIME

This is generally evident even in mild cases with only slight reduction of peak expiratory flow rate or FEV_1/VC ratio.

C OVERINFLATION

This may be evident clinically and reflected by increase in total lung capacity, functional residual capacity and residual volume.

D REVERSIBILITY

Airways obstruction in asthma is often referred to as 'reversible' by bronchodilators. In fact, airways obstruction is usually only partly reversible by a bronchodilator aerosol and the degree of reversibility tends to vary from time to time and between individuals (Fig. 15.6).

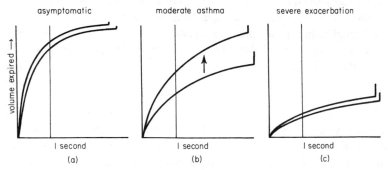

Fig. 15.6. *'Reversibility' of airways obstruction.* Forced expiratory spirograms obtained from a patient with asthma on three different occasions. The upper of the two tracings was obtained some minutes after inhalation of a bronchodilator aerosol. (a) When asymptomatic, performance is almost normal and the aerosol produces little improvement. (b) During a moderate exacerbation of asthma the aerosol produces a major improvement. (c) During a severe exacerbation there is relative resistance to sympathomimetic treatment and there is little or no response to a bronchodilator aerosol.

Very large responses to bronchodilator aerosol such as shown in (b) are only encountered in patients with asthma. Lesser responses are seen in asthma and also in patients with airways obstruction related to chronic bronchitis and are thus of limited diagnostic value.

Trivial asthma
There may be little response to a bronchodilator as there is hardly any airways obstruction to reverse.

Moderate asthma
There may be a very large response to bronchodilator therapy.

Severe asthma
Little response is usually seen during severe exacerbations.

Although a very large reversible component (50% increase in FEV_1 for example) is seen only in asthma, lesser degrees of reversibility are seen both in asthma and in chronic non-specific airways obstruction associated with chronic bronchitis and are of little diagnostic importance.

2 Ventilation

Asthma generates a very powerful drive to breathe so that in exacerbations hyperventilation is the rule and the P_{CO_2} is found to be low. Only in critically severe exacerbations does the P_{CO_2} become elevated and this is a serious sign.

3 Oxygenation

Hypoxia is an almost inevitable accompaniment of severe exacerbation of asthma owing to the presence of areas of underventilation. Cyanosis denotes severe asthma and unless it is relieved rapidly (e.g. by intravenous aminophylline) it should be taken as an indication for hospitalization.

4 Chronic respiratory failure in asthma

Chronic respiratory failure and cor pulmonale are rarely seen except in neglected, inadequately-treated cases of asthma. Hypercapnia, congestive cardiac failure and right ventricular hypertrophy can all disappear after treatment with corticosteroids.

Management of asthma

Management of asthma is based firstly on the patient having a reasonable understanding of the nature of the disorder and, secondly, on the use of a very few highly effective treatments which, if used skilfully by the patient, can result in a very good measure of control of symptoms. Most patients with asthma can expect to be able to lead normal lives.

Understanding the nature of asthma

Asthma is frustrating and frightening and the subject of myths and widespread misunderstanding. It is vital that the patient with asthma should have some reasonable concept of what asthma is. The terms in which this is presented and the detail of the description will obviously vary considerably depending on the background knowledge and character of the patient. Time spent in this discussion is very worthwhile. Some patients feel guilty about suffering from asthma when they have been told that it is a 'nervous complaint'. When asthma has only recently developed the patient may be hell-bent on finding a once-and-for-all cure which will restore him or her to the pre-existing state. Such an individual will not be sympathetic to the idea of carefully tailored treatment to suppress and relieve asthma unless the practicability of the hoped-for cure is discussed fully. Many other entrenched attitudes may be revealed if discussion is unhurried.

Control of extrinsic factors

In a small proportion of cases where there is an identifiable extrinsic cause it may be possible to treat asthma satisfactorily by merely reducing exposure to the allergen. Unfortunately, most patients with regularly troublesome asthma are unaffected by manipulation of the environment even if specific allergens are identified. Complete avoidance of grass pollen is not possible but exposure can be reduced. It is extremely difficult to avoid exposure to the house dust mite, although measures such as daily airing of the bed, frequent vacuum-cleaning of the bed and bedroom floor, discarding old mattresses, etc. may have some effect. On the whole the result of these efforts is disappointing. It is very unwise to advise patients with asthma to move to a different house or climate or to dispose of pets or to change employment on account of asthma unless the indications are particularly compelling.

DESENSITIZATION

There is only a very limited place for desensitization in the management of asthma. The treatment comprises repeated subcutaneous injections of weak extracts of specific allergen and it appears to act by inducing 'blocking antibody' of IgG type. Response to treatment is variable and difficult to assess because pollen exposure varies from year to year, and because the patient will usually be receiving a number of other treatments concurrently. Sometimes improvement follows after several seasons of repeated desensitization.

Desensitization to several allergens using a mixture of extracts is even less likely to be successful than the use of a single antigen.

Review of available treatments

The drugs used in the treatment of chronic or frequently recurrent asthma can be divided into three broad groups:

1   Treatment for **relief**. Bronchodilators by aerosol or, less effectively, orally.
2   Treatment for **'prevention'**. A steroid aerosol or cromoglycate by inhalation.
3   **Reserve** treatment. Oral prednisolone, preferably started by the patient on his/her own initiative in the event of deterioration (see below).

Most patients with chronic asthma can be managed very satisfctorily with regular inhalation of a steroid aerosol to control the asthmatic process, a bronchodilator aerosol to reverse wheezing when this occurs, and training to initiate emergency oral steroid treatment. The management of acute severe asthma will be considered separately after a review of the main groups of drugs.

Bronchodilators

Frequent or persistently troublesome asthma should *not* normally be managed exclusively with bronchodilator drugs. They are most useful when asthma is mild or already well-controlled and they lose effectiveness during exacerbations.

BRONCHODILATOR AEROSOLS

Aerosol preparations of β-adrenergic sympathetic stimulant drugs are extremely useful for the prompt relief of attacks of wheezing (Fig. 15.7). For example, their use may abbreviate a nocturnal attack to a minute or two when it might otherwise last for half an hour or more, and aerosol treatment is particularly effective in curtailing symptoms of 'morning tightness'. Bronchodilator aerosols are best employed in putting the 'finishing touches' to asthma which is already well controlled. They

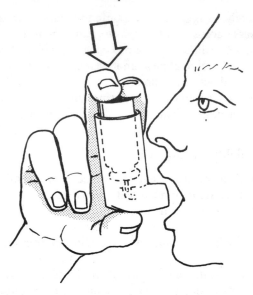

Fig. 15.7. *Pressurized aerosol in use.* The active preparation and an inert propellant gas solution are contained in a small pressurized canister which is housed in a plastic casing in an inverted position. Downward pressure on the base of the canister as shown releases a single standard 'puff' of aerosol. It is helpful if the inhaler is distanced slightly from the mouth, provided the aim is accurate. It is absolutely essential that the 'puff' is synchronized with inspiration (see text for note on technique).

should *not* be relied upon for the control of severe asthma when they are anyway ineffective. Salbutamol (Ventolin) and terbutaline (Bricanyl) are greatly preferable to isoprenaline as they are relatively selected β-2-sympathetic stimulants and cause little cardiac acceleration. They also have a longer action of up to 5 or more hours. The usual dose is 2 puffs three or four times daily or as required. If asthma is well controlled (spontaneously or because of other treatment) then bronchodilator usage will fall or cease. If more than about 8 puffs a day are required this probably indicates the need for regular prophylactic treatment with cromoglycate or a steroid preparation (see below).

Cautionary note
During the early 1960s there was an alarming increase in the incidence of sudden death from asthma which seemed to parallel the increasing use of isoprenaline aerosols. Extensive publicity led to reduction in consumption and this was accompanied by a decline in mortality. The

relationship between isoprenaline aerosols and the sudden deaths was probably complex. The great majority of the sudden deaths were un-expected and occurred in patients who had received no steroid treat-ment and may have been attributable to the following causes:

1   Excessive use of isoprenaline may have caused ventricular tachy-arrhythmias and sudden death from this cause.

2   Some individuals develop 'rebound' bronchoconstriction after the initial bronchodilator effect of isoprenaline and this may lead to escalating consumption.

3   Intensive use of isoprenaline aerosols may have disguised the sever-ity of the asthma, allowing the patients to tolerate progressive very severe asthma which might otherwise have been recognized as such earlier and treated with steroids.

4   During an exacerbation of asthma bronchodilators may cause a *fall* in arterial oxygen tension (due to relaxation of pulmonary arterioles in underventilated zones). The fall is generally only a few mmHg and is probably only of importance in the very critically-placed patient.

Experience with salbutamol and terbutaline in the high doses com-monly employed in nebulizer therapy (see below) suggests that they are very safe drugs indeed. Probably the major danger lies in their exclusive use in cases where it would be preferable for the asthmatic process to be suppressed by regular steroid or cromoglycate inhalation. Nevertheless, a proportion of the general public sees inhalers as dangerous and refusal to countenance inhaled treatment is fairly common. Inhaled treatment can be extremely important and unhurried discussion of the question of hazard is necessary so that it can be seen in proper perspective.

A note on technique—pressurized aerosols

It is important to ensure that the device is used properly and this requires a demonstration by the prescribing doctor who should also observe and comment upon the patient's first attempts.

The patient first exhales and then positions the device in front of the open mouth (Fig. 15.7). An unhurried inspiration begins and during the inhalation the aerosol is discharged—the inhalation continuing to a position of almost full inspiration where the breath is held for about 10 seconds. The standard adult dose is two 'puffs'—each puff being delivered in a separate breath. Skilled users can take the first puff early in inspiration and the next puff late in inspiration with some advantage. If vapour is visible escaping from the mouth, nose or the top of the device then coordination is faulty and the puff should be repeated.

Chapter 15

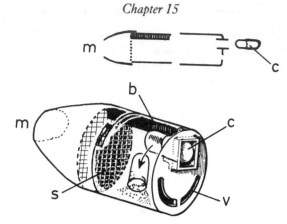

Fig. 15.8. *Breath-activated inhaler (Rotahaler: Allen and Hanburys) for the administration of dry powder aerosol.* Both bronchodilator and topical steroid treatment may be administered in this way. The powdered aerosol is prepared in a gelatin capsule (c) which is inserted into the inhaler at the opposite end to the mouthpiece (m). The two parts of the inhaler (which are shown separated in the upper part of the diagram) are then rotated relative to each other and a bar (b) knocks off the inner end of the capsule (arrow), liberating the powder into the inside of the inhaler. A vigorous inhalation causes air to be drawn into the vents (v) and the resulting turbulence draws the powder into the inspiratory airstream. The free half of the capsule is retained within the inhaler by a perforated screen (s).

Synchronization

Small children and elderly, uncoordinated or uncritical patients may be unable to synchronize discharge with inspiration. One effective answer to this problem has been the development of dry powder devices such as that shown in Fig. 15.8. Dispersal of the aerosol is brought about by the inspiration itself and synchronization is assured. Another approach has been the development of spacer devices. The Spacer Inhaler shown in Fig. 15.9(a) is an extendible compartment into which the aerosol is discharged; inspiration can take place within a second or two afterwards and perfect synchronization is no longer necessary for effective inhalation of the drug.

Particle size

At the point of release of a metered dose inhaler the drug is contained in a jet of liquid propellant travelling at high speed (estimated to be about 70 miles per hour!) As it travels this liquid jet breaks down into droplets of finer and finer size; the propellant in effect 'boiling' because of its low vapour pressure. If the spray impinges upon an object (teeth, palate,

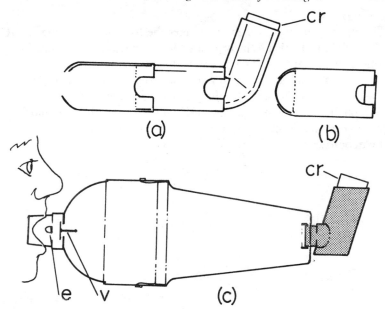

Fig. 15.9. *Spacer devices for use with metered dose inhalers.* (a) The Spacer-inhaler (Astra) is convenient and collapsible (b), and allows the patient to inhale after discharge of the aerosol; (c) the Nebuhaler (Astra) is a large-volume device designed to allow even freer dispersal of the discharged material so that a high proportion of it forms particles small enough to be inhaled. It also allows large doses of aerosol to be inhaled relatively efficiently (see text). cr, canister of pressurized aerosol; v, valve which closes on expiration; e, expiratory port.

tongue for example) within a centimetre or so of the point of discharge then a large part of the medication will be deposited as a liquid splatter. Proper angulation of the inhaler—or removal from the mouth so that it is held a few centimetres away from the tongue (Fig. 15.7)—results in more of the material being inhaled as fine respirable droplets. Even greater efficiency can be obtained with the use of a spacer device, particularly one of the large volume spacer devices such as that illustrated in Fig. 15.9(c). The shape of the device is designed to allow as much as possible of the discharged material to be distributed in an effective aerosol. This form of spacer device has proved to be a particularly efficient way of delivering larger than standard doses of aerosol and in some circumstances offers an alternative to the use of a nebulizer (see below).

NEBULIZERS

The most usual type of nebulizer takes the form shown in Fig. 15.10 where the mechanism is incorporated in a face mask and operated by a source of compressed air or oxygen. In the home the usual pressure source is a small electrically driven compressor (cost about £90; not available via UK National Health Service). The medication (which can be bronchodilator, cromoglycate, antibiotic, etc), is added in liquid form to the reservoir. Sometimes, instead of a mask, a mouthpiece is fitted to the nebulizer via a T piece.

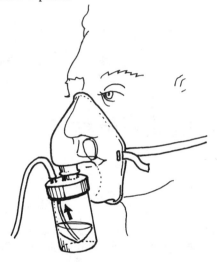

Fig. 15.10. *Mask incorporating a nebulizer.* A number of masks of similar design are available (Bard, 'Minineb' illustrated) which work on the same principle as Wright's nebulizer. Oxygen or air from a small compressor enters via the piping at the top of the transparent container and escapes from a pinhole. The vicinity of the pinhole is guarded by a tiny chamber into which fluid is drawn upwards from the reservoir (arrow) by the venturi effect. The outlet from the small chamber is a second pinhole opposite the first which directs the gas-fluid mixture at high speed onto a small plastic sphere, the impact producing a fine mist. The larger particles are flung against the wall of the container and recirculate but a proportion of the finest particles form a respirable aerosol. Used with oxygen this is effectively a 'high-concentration' mask; it may be driven with compressed air in ventilatory failure if the patient is intolerant of oxygen.

The most usual application of nebulizers is in the administration of a bronchodilator for acute asthma in the home or in hospital where the usual relieving dose of bronchodilator has failed to bring relief. Some patients with severe chronic asthma benefit from regular use. Bronchodilator treatment using a nebulizer is very effective. This is not due to special properties of the apparatus but because of the dose of broncho-dilator employed. In practice between 10 and 50 times as much bronchodilator is used in nebulizer treatment as is used in the standard 'relieving' dose of two puffs of a salbutamol pressurized aerosol (see Fig. 15.11).

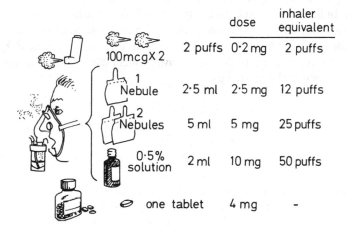

	dose		inhaler equivalent
100mcgX2	2 puffs	0·2 mg	2 puffs
1 Nebule	2·5 ml	2·5 mg	12 puffs
2 Nebules	5 ml	5 mg	25 puffs
0·5% solution	2 ml	10 mg	50 puffs
one tablet		4 mg	-

Fig. 15.11. *Nebulized salbutamol.* Diagram to illustrate the relationship between doses of salbutamol commonly administered by nebulizer and those delivered by metered dose aerosol and in tablet form. *Note:* All nebulizers retain some of the solution even when nebulization has ceased. This commonly amounts to about 0.5 ml. The amount of drug retained depends upon the dilution used. Other volumes of solution and other bronchodilators such as terbutaline are in general use (*Nebule: Allen and Hanburys*).

Nebulizers have a valuable place in the management of more severe asthma in childhood where proper coordination of pressurized aerosols is often lacking. Only a few adults really need nebulizers. This is because (i) the same effect can be obtained with an ordinary pressurized aerosol if an equivalent dose is used efficiently—for example, twelve puffs used with a large volume spacer (Fig. 15.9); (ii) patients who appear to have a requirement for large doses of bronchodilator are often found to be having insufficient (or inefficient) inhaled steroid treatment; attention to this may remove the apparent requirement for nebulizer treatment.

Dangers of nebulizers
The danger of nebulizer treatment lies in the fact that it is usually extremely effective, it is popular and it fits in with what the patient and relatives perceive as being appropriate for the management of difficult

breathing. Preoccupation with this form of treatment may, however, allow poorly suppressed gradually deteriorating asthma to be tolerated despite progressive plugging of bronchi, until a stage where further deterioration may be suddenly critical. It follows that where nebulizer therapy is in use, it is important to ensure that regular suppressive therapy is being exploited properly rather than neglected.

Nebulizer bronchodilator treatment itself seems to be safe. Important increase in pulse rate is unusual even with the high doses of bronchodilator used. There does not seem to be an important drop in PO_2 so that in ordinary use it is all right to give bronchodilators using air rather than oxygen as the driving gas.

ORAL BRONCHODILATOR DRUGS

Intelligent use of aerosol treatment (prophylactic and/or bronchodilator) is so effective that in most patients oral bronchodilator treatment is unnecessary. Introduction of an oral bronchodilator brings about no further improvement whereas, by contrast, aerosol bronchodilator treatment is usually able to bring about better control of symptoms than is achieved with an oral bronchodilator drug. Where asthma is very mild or already well controlled by other means or where the patient is disinclined to use aerosol treatment oral brochodilators may be helpful. The most useful oral bronchodilators are the long-acting theophylline preparations which are able to achieve therapeutic effect over 24 hours with twice daily dosage. Other oral agents in use include agonists such as salbutamol or terbutaline. All oral bronchodilators have a tendency to cause tremor. Theophyllines may cause nausea. Patients with severe asthma need to understand that initiation of oral bronchodilator treatment will not reverse the progress of a severe exacerbation. Oral bronchodilators are used to apply the 'finishing touches' in the treatment of asthma and are not of fundamental importance.

Steroid aerosols

Steroid aerosols form the hinge-pin of the management of chronic asthma. The substances used are highly-active steroids of inherently low glucocorticoid activity which are delivered either by pressurized aerosol (Fig. 15.7) or in powder form by breath-activated inhaler (Fig. 15.8). Three preparations are available, beclomethasone dipropionate (Becotide), betamethasone 17-valerate (Bextasol) and budesonide (Pulmicort).

Improvement in chronic asthma is generally evident within a day or two and is often dramatic. Failure of steroid aerosol treatment to influence troublesome asthma is very unusual and probably means that some detail of the practical application of the treatment has been overlooked (see practical points below).

DISTRIBUTION

Only about 20% of the administered dose actually reaches the respiratory tract, the remainder being swallowed and probably largely absorbed from the gastrointestinal tract. The high degree of topical activity however allows very small total doses to be used so that in normal use there is no evidence of the usual side-effects of steroid therapy and no evidence of pituitary-adrenal suppression.

DOSAGE

The usual total daily dosage of beclomethasone dipropionate is about 400 μg. The most widely used preparation contains 50 μg per puff. The inhalations are usually taken in the morning and in the evening since doses during the day tend to be overlooked, particularly when asthma is under good control. There is considerable variation in the daily requirements and many patients manage with 100 μm daily. Patients with particularly severe chronic asthma may require 2 mg daily. In such cases a preparation containing 250 μg per puff of beclomethasone dipropionate is useful (Becloforte).

Patients are encouraged to experiment patiently and systematically to determine their requirements. If morning symptoms are more than brief or if nocturnal waking is a feature, then reduction of the daily dose is undesirable because deterioration is an almost inevitable consequence.

SOME PRACTICAL POINTS

1   It is important to ensure that the patient can use a pressurized aerosol properly (p. 175) and some coaching is commonly required. The very young and very elderly may be unable to coordinate their inspiration with discharge of the pressurized aerosol and the breath-activated device for administering the drug in powder form has proved very useful in this situation (see Fig. 15.12 for description of use). Alternatively a spacer device may be used with the pressurized aerosol (Fig. 15.9 and p. 179).

2   It is essential that the patient should understand the prophylactic role of treatment.

3   The patient should understand that no immediate bronchodilator effect is to be expected.

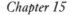

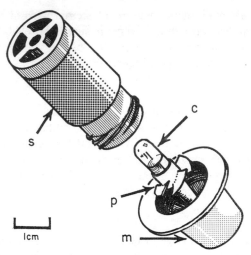

Fig. 15.12. *Inhaler (Spinhaler: Fisons Pharmaceuticals Ltd) for administration of disodium cromoglycate.* The mouthpiece (m) carries a central pin upon which a propeller (p) is free to rotate. The capsule containing disodium cromoglycate in a soluble powder base is fitted into a recess in the propeller. The two parts of the inhaler are screwed together and the capsule is pierced by two pins which are operated by a sliding sleeve (s). The patient first breathes out and then inspires vigorously through the inhaler causing the propellor to rotate. The powder is dispersed into the airstream. Two to four inhalations generally suffice to empty the capsule.

4   Treatment is required **regularly** during spells of **regular** symptoms; this may mean long-term use.

5   The dose may be reduced if symptoms are completely abolished; return of some mild morning symptoms provides useful indications that asthma would be worse on an even lower dose.

6   Steroid aerosol treatment **should not be started alone in a severe exacerbation**; it may be ineffective because of excessive secretions or imperfect distribution and the patient may become prematurely disenchanted with the treatment.

7   Severe exacerbations occurring in the course of aerosol treatment may require treatment with oral steroids; patients with severe asthma should be taught to start treatment with prednisolone themselves (see below).

8   In some cases it proved useful to use a bronchodilator aerosol a few minutes before each regular dose of steroid aerosol.

9   Patients should not run out of steroid aerosol or deterioration may be quite dramatic.

10   Particular care must be given to patients in whom long-term regular oral steroid therapy has been successfully replaced by aerosol steroids. They may be at risk both from dramatic deterioration in their asthma and from hypoadrenal symptoms during any intercurrent illness for many months after substitution.

SIDE-EFFECTS

A small proportion of patients develop patches of candidal infection on the palate or pharynx although most do not complain of this. This complication is more common when high doses are used and it responds to treatment with nystatin or amphotericin lozenges. There is no evidence that candidal infestation extends below the larynx. There is no evidence that the connective tissue of the respiratory tract suffers from atrophy of the sort observed in skin exposed to high doses of topical steroid creams.

Huskiness of the voice sometimes occurs but its mechanism seems still to be unclear.

At doses above 1.6–2 mg daily of beclomethasone, significant systemic absorption starts to occur. The only effects noted are a blunting of the adrenal response to a formal tetracosactrin stimulation test. Hypercorticoid side-effects are not seen in clinical practice.

Disodium cromoglycate (DSCG, Intal)

This substance has a prophylactic action and is usually administered by inhalation from a capsule in powder form using a special inhaler (Fig. 15.12). A pressurized aerosol preparation is also available. It is not a bronchodilator. It appears to act by stabilizing the wall of the mast cell preventing the release of intracellular mediators (p. 159) although it may have a number of less important additional effects. If it is administered before challenge with an allergen it can completely block the asthmatic response which would otherwise occur. It is extremely valuable in mild recurrent or persistent asthma and young individuals with extrinsic asthma are particularly responsive. It is effective in preventing exercise-induced asthma if taken beforehand.

SOME PRACTICAL POINTS

1   It is essential to explain the prophylactic role of DSCG to patients and to stress the importance of **regular** treatment.
2   Patients should be warned not to expect a bronchodilator effect.

3   Coexistant active bronchial infection may prevent a response to DSCG.

4   There is no point in starting DSCG during an acute exacerbation unless it is a mild one. It will probably be ineffective in a severe episode and then rejected as useless by the patient. During a severe exacerbation steroid treatment may be necessary.

The usual dose is the contents of one capsule inhaled four times daily. Trial and error may show that optimal control is obtained with between one and eight capsules daily. Some patients are irritated by the inhalation which may produce cough and reflex wheezing. In these individuals it is appropriate to use a compound preparation which contains a small quantity of isoprenaline which abolishes this effect. Patients should not be started on the compound preparation without good reason as the bronchodilator effect of the isoprenaline may make it difficult to assess response to DSCG. DSCG may also be given by pressurized aerosol and as a nebulizer solution.

Oral steroid therapy

SHORT-TERM TREATMENT

Oral steroid therapy is indicated in all alarmingly progressive exacerbations of bronchial asthma—there is no call to wait until the patient is *in extremis*. Any patient sufficiently ill to require intravenous aminophylline probably requires oral steroid therapy—at least until the exacerbation subsides over a few days or until regular prophylactic therapy with a steroid aerosol (or DSCG) can be established. Once a response to oral steroid administration is obvious the dose can be progressively reduced and often withdrawn within a week. Those who have had severe immobilizing asthma for weeks may require more protracted treatment.

Self-administration

It is important not to delay treatment of severe asthma and patients with *severe asthma* should be taught how to start treatment with a *short course* of prednisolone themselves. They need to understand the potential side-effects of long-continued treatment but also that short courses taken infrequently are safe (see below).

When? A severe asthmatic crisis may occur months after instruction of the patient and possibly away from home so that it is helpful to provide a **written** list of circumstances in which a short course of prednisolone should be started on the patient's own initiative. This might be as follows:

1   The usual bronchodilator aerosol is not working (either having little effect, or, alternatively, lasting only a very short time).

2   Asthma causes repeated or protracted waking at night (either of which tend to lead to exhaustion and depression through loss of sleep).

3   Asthma causes immobilization, even for a short period (causing the patient to have to sit motionless for some time because of distressed breathing).

4   Morning tightness persists so that it is still present at lunchtime.

5   There is progressive deterioration gradually over several days (indicating loss of control by aerosol treatment and the need to restore this by the temporary use of systemic steroid treatment).

6   Asthma sufficiently severe to require intravenous treatment with a bronchodilator drug (however impressive the short-term relief afforded by this treatment).

Some patients with severe chronic asthma find it very helpful to measure their own peak flow rate regularly and may be guided by the results in deciding when a short course of oral steroid treatment is required.

How much? If treated promptly, the majority will respond to a very short course lasting perhaps 4 days (e.g. a total of 20 mg on 1st day; 20 mg on 2nd day; 10 mg on 3rd day and 10 mg on 4th day). With experience some individuals are found to require a little more for a little longer but protracted courses are to be avoided. Over-indulgence in oral steroid treatment in a trained patient is very uncommon; it is much more usual for patients to try to defer taking a short course when one is clearly indicated. Treatment with aerosol steroid should continue during the 'short course'. The patient with severe asthma should have sufficient tablets to hand for two short courses.

LONG-TERM TREATMENT

The need for a long-term treatment with oral steroids only becomes clear when it is established that asthma cannot be satisfactorily controlled by other measures. Usually this means that short courses of prednisolone are required very frequently despite the efficient and regular use of a steroid aerosol in above-standard dosage together with supporting bronchodilator therapy. The plan should always be to maintain the dose at the lowest level compatible with reasonable (but not necessarily perfect) control of asthma and to this end it is desirable that the patient should control his own dosage. He must understand the compromise which is being attempted between disabling asthma on the one hand and the risk of side-effects on the other. There should be no hesitation in promptly increasing the dose in the event of progressive deterioration over hours or days. Prednisolone is the most widely-used preparation and there is no good reason to use other corticosteroids. In 'titrating' the lowest tolerable dose 1-mg tablets are often useful in combination with the standard 5-mg tablets.

Side-effects

The general public in the UK is very aware that steroids produce side-effects, and it is common for patients with severe asthma to put themselves at some risk through failing to restart or increase the dose of steroid because of fear of the consequences. A common fear is that use of steroid treatment will lead to 'resistance' and gradually-escalating requirements. There is no evidence that this tendency exists. Blatant over-indulgence in too high a dose is uncommon. In many patients worthwhile benefit is obtained with a regular dose of 5–7.5 mg of prednisolone daily, at which level serious side-effects are not seen. At doses up to 12.5 mg daily some cushingoid redistribution of fat and facial fullness is seen. Most patients gain weight but this is capable of control by dietary restriction. At higher doses obvious cushingoid changes are seen and predisposed individuals may develop glucose intolerance, peptic ulceration, etc. Only a very few severely in-capacitated individuals can be shown to obtain worthwhile benefit from daily doses in excess of 20 mg daily of prednisolone. Probably the most sinister complication is vertebral collapse from osteoporosis which is particularly likely to affect post-menopausal females.

REPLACEMENT OF LONG-TERM ORAL STEROID THERAPY

In more than half of patients well controlled on 7.5 mg or less of prednisolone daily, the use of an aerosol steroid preparation will enable oral treatment to be withdrawn. In most of the remainder some reduc-tion in oral treatment is possible. Withdrawal of regular oral steroid therapy which has been in progress for many years should be especially gradual as there is some risk of hypoadrenal crisis which may accompany a dramatic relapse of asthma or some other intercurrent illness. Hypo-adrenal symptoms may not be recognized as such: they may include profound lethargy, anorexia, vomiting, diarrhoea, headache and mus-cular aching.

Where these features are encountered it may be necessary to with-draw steroids over a year or more. The use of ACTH or tetracosactrin does little to help this withdrawal as the failure is not merely adrenal but involves the pituitary-adrenal axis as a whole. The patient must be encouraged to endure mild withdrawal symptoms and to reduce the dose exceedingly slowly particularly over the last 5 mg of prednisolone. A return of allergic rhinitis or eczema sometimes accompanies withdrawal of oral steroid treatment. It is sometimes safer to leave a patient on a small oral dose of prednisolone if understanding is limited.

Antibiotics

Antibiotics have a relatively minor part to play in the management of asthma. It is difficult to be certain when active bronchial infection is playing an important part but the best guide is probably the production of yellow sputum. Bacteriological examination is not very helpful. If yellow sputum is produced it is reasonable to prescribe a 5-day course of cotrimoxazole, tetracycline or amoxycillin (but beware penicillin-sensitive individuals) as well as advising an increase in suppressive therapy which is usually indicated.

Education of the patient

It is very desirable that patients with frequent or persistent asthma— and those who have demonstrated a capacity to develop acute severe asthma—should manage their own treatment as far as possible. For this to be successful (and safe) the patient must understand the use of each preparation employed and must have a plan of action prepared for unexpected changes in his condition. Just as in the management of diabetes, doctor and patient become involved jointly in an educational exercise which takes time—merely writing prescriptions is not enough. Quite a large number of items of information are required for self-management, and training requires to be fortified by written material. Experience has shown that a diagrammatic form is useful and that it helps if this is made out afresh in the presence of the patient rather than merely photocopied and handed out (see Brewis, further reading).

Asssssment of progress in chronic asthma

Because of the striking diurnal and day-to-day variation in the severity of asthma, spirometric measurements made at infrequent intervals may not be particularly helpful in assessing progress (Fig. 15.13). It is relevant to make a note of:

1   Number of nocturnal attacks (for example, in a week).
2   The length of time taken for the chest to feel clear in the mornings.

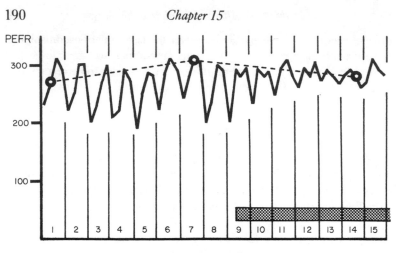

days

Fig. 15.13. *Fallibility of isolated ventilatory tests in asthma.*
Solid line: Record of peak expiratory flow rate (PEFR) measured four times daily. The shaded area represents the start of new treatment (e.g. cromoglycate or steroid aerosol). Typical diurnal variation is present over the first 9 days. Thereafter there is progressive disappearance of the early morning 'trough' although values obtained later in the day remain similar to those recorded earlier.
Interrupted line: This line connects three isolated recordings of PEFR made at three separate visits to a doctor. The doctor viewing only these results might have been tempted to conclude that at the second visit there was some improvement and that there had been deterioration between the second and third visits. The erroneous conclusions might have been that the new treatment was ineffective. In this situation adequate questioning of the patient would almost certainly lead to the clinician reaching the correct conclusion despite the PEFR recordings he had obtained.

3   Absence from work or school.
4   Consumption of bronchodilator preparations.
When assessing the effect of changes in treatment it is sometimes helpful for the patient to use a peak flow meter or gauge at home making recordings twice or three times daily. Improvement is usually accompanied by 'ironing out' of the morning and sometimes evening troughs.

Treatment of asthma in childhood

Below the age of about 18 months β-agonist bronchodilators are ineffective whether given orally or by nebulization. In the 2–5 years age group oral salbutamol may be useful. Regular asthma at this age can be suppressed by DSCG by nebulizer. More severe asthma in childhood requires regular steroid aerosol treatment, usually in adult doses. Children below school age are not usually good at using pressurized aerosols whether for bronchodilators, DSCG or topical steroid treatment and either a dry powder device or a spacer will be required. These may become difficult to use during an exacerbation. One effective method of administering a bronchodilator aerosol is to fit a pressurized inhaler into the bottom of a polystyrene coffee cup and to give multiple puffs with the wide end of the cup near to the face as the child breathes normally. The arrangement resembles the right hand half of Fig. 15.9(c).

SEVERE CHILDHOOD ASTHMA

An isolated severe exacerbation may be managed with a short course of oral prednisolone. Inhalation of salbutamol, terbutaline or equivalent by nebulizer is very effective in acute exacerbations in childhood—partly because of the relatively large dose delivered and partly because children find it particularly difficult to use inhalers when they are distressed. It is important that patient and parents do not come to rely solely on a nebulized bronchodilator when asthma could be treated more securely by suppression using steroid aerosol treatment.

Severe chronic asthma in childhood is sometimes not obvious. The usual marked fluctuations in severity and overt wheezing may be lacking and the parents and child may become accustomed to a limited level of activity. Stunting and chest deformity (Fig. 15.14) are indicative of severe asthma. As it may be difficult to judge the severity of asthma spirometry is very important. A very small number of children are not adequately controlled by regular treatment with DSCG or aerosol steroids. In this situation oral prednisolone or regular injections of ACTH or tetracosactrin may be necessary (the latter two on grounds of alleged lesser effect on growth).

Asthma in pregnancy

Asthma usually poses no particular problems in pregnancy. Occasionally exacerbations occur in the first few weeks but the last two trimesters are often marked by unusually good control. It is common for exacerbations to occur 4–6 weeks after delivery.

Acute severe asthma (status asthmaticus)

A severe, progressive, prolonged attack of immobilizing asthma which is

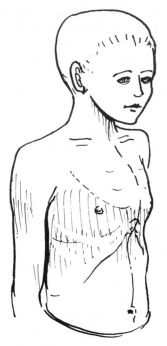

Fig. 15.14. *Chest deformity in childhood asthma.* The sternum is pushed forwards (pigeon-chest deformity) and there is a groove approximately in the position of the sixth rib (Harrison's sulcus). Deformity of the type shown is always indicative of severe asthma. It is to a considerable extent reversible if asthma is treated adequately and sufficiently early.

unresponsive to bronchodilator preparations is termed acute severe asthma. This is synonymous with status asthmaticus. Treatment may be started in the home but hospitalization is indicated. Management is based upon giving large doses of bronchodilator and corticosteroid drugs and ensuring adequate oxygenation of the patient until the attack abates.

Initial treatment

STEROID THERAPY

It is sensible to give hydrocortisone (100 or 200 mg intravenously) immediately. In fully developed acute severe asthma there is unlikely to be any appreciable effect from this treatment for many hours, and even then this may be slow. Dramatic improvement should not be expected.

Once the patient is able to take tablets, prednisolone should be given in a moderately high dose (say 20 mg 8-hourly) until improvement is obvious and sustained.

BRONCHODILATOR THERAPY

1   *By inhalation*

By definition, acute severe asthma is relatively resistant to treatment with inhaled bronchodilator drugs. Neverthless, it may be possible to obtain important improvement by use of substantially bigger doses using a nebulizer (p. 180, Fig. 15.11). Particularly where the attack has not been very prolonged and in children this form of inhaled bronchodilator treatment may be sufficient and intravenous bronchodilator treatment avoided. Usually at least 5 mg of salbutamol or its equivalent will be used 2–3 hourly initially. Practices vary quite widely and are influenced in the individual case by the severity of the asthma and the degree of response achieved with each dose.

2   *Intravenously*

Either aminophylline or a selective beta sympathetic agonist may be used. Aminophylline is still most widely employed in the UK and has stood the test of time. The initial dose chosen should be influenced by body size and whether or not the patient is thought to have been taking long-acting oral theophylline preparations. Other factors will include pulse rate, severity of the asthma and response to other measures. In general, smaller individuals not taking long acting theophyllines will be given 50 mg by slow intravenous injection and larger individual 500 mg. A continuous infusion of intravenous bronchodilator may be continued for several days where response to treatment is slow.

REASSURANCE

The patient must be made to feel firstly that his desperate symptoms are understood and secondly that he is safe.

OXYGEN THERAPY

Hypoxia is usual in severe asthma and administration of oxygen using a mask which delivers a **high** concentration is appropriate and usually safe. Almost always the drive to breathe is well preserved; very occasionally exhausted patients who have endured a prolonged exacerbation may be in chronic respiratory failure and require controlled oxygen therapy (p. 327).

There is no place for the regular use of sedative drugs in the management of status asthmaticus. The patient in status asthmaticus needs every bit of respiratory drive he can muster.

Assessment phase

Once initial treatment is established a period of extreme vigilance follows. Progress may be assessed by observation of:

PULSE RATE

Persistent tachycardia with a rate of between 120 and 140 per minute is common. As long as this persists than danger still exists.

APPEARANCE OF THE PATIENT

Important information is provided by observing the patient's position in bed, the character of his breathing, facial expression and his own assessment of progress. The auscultatory signs are of little help—reduction in rhonchi may actually indicate deterioration.

Disappearance of inspiratory lower costal indrawing (p. 49) and the return of normal outward inspiratory movement is a useful sign of significant improvement.

PEAK FLOW RATE

Regular measurement of peak flow rate is important in acute severe asthma. It allows an estimate of severity to be made and this may be useful in comparing one episode with another. More importantly, it allows progress to be assessed objectively. If the peak flow rate is improving then the patient can reasonably be assumed to be progressing satisfactorily. Inability of the patient to meet some predetermined lower limit can serve as a formal warning to summon appropriate staff. It may be claimed that the patient is 'too ill' to perform pulmonary function tests but this argument must be resisted. If the individual is genuinely unable to perform the manoeuvre at all then observation in an intensive care unit is probably needed—as is the information that the patient tried and failed.

ESTIMATION OF BLOOD GAS TENSIONS

When IPPV is being seriously considered this is of particular value. Even borderline elevation of the P_{CO_2} is a serious sign—it means that the best efforts of the patient's respiratory drive result in inadequate ventilation. Cyanosis whilst breathing oxygen-enriched air is a particularly sinister sign and is usually a compelling argument for IPPV.

Intermittent positive pressure ventilation (IPPV)

INDICATIONS

IPPV is only rarely necessary, and is used when there is:
1 Inability to secure adequate oxygenation of the patient.
2 Exhaustion—as suggested by progressive tiredness, hopelessness and apathy accompanied by a rising PCO_2, rising pulse rate and failure to produce sputum.

PURPOSE

The purpose is to ensure adequate oxygenation of the patient until the other therapeutic measures bring the attack to an end.

MEANS

1 Control of the patient's airway ensures that oxygen administration is continuous. It is possible to administer higher concentrations of oxygen by IPPV than by mask.
2 A minimum ventilation is secured. Some underventilation is acceptable.
3 The patient can be sedated and rested once the breathing is under control by IPPV.
4 Clearing of tenacious bronchial secretions can be assisted by suction—sometimes assisted by lavage with small quantities of warmed water or saline injected into the airway.

In practice IPPV is carried out by endotracheal intubation with sedation using drugs such as phenoperidine (a short acting opiate derivative) and muscle relaxants. IPPV may be necessary for as little as a few hours or for more than a week.

Convalescence

Once improvement is obvious and sustained over 24 hours, attention can be given to reduction of the dose of steroid and other drugs and to **education of the patient** in the management of his asthma. The patient can be discharged from hospital once he is mobile and he fully understands his treatment. There is no call to wait until oral steroid therapy has been withdrawn completely. It is preferable for the last 10–15 mg of prednisolone to be withdrawn after discharge from hospital.

Prevention

Almost always acute severe asthma is preventable. Severe exacerbations requiring admission to hospital are usually preceded by a period of gradual deterioration over a period of several days which should be the signal for the patient with severe asthma to start or increase oral steroid treatment. If this is done promptly a crisis is generally averted.

BRONCHOPULMONARY ASPERGILLOSIS

Principal patterns of disease

The clinical patterns of disease related to the ubiquitous mould *Aspergillus fumigatus* are illustrated in Fig. 15.15.

ALLERGIC ASPERGILLOSIS

In allergic aspergillosis both immediate and delayed responses are usually demonstrable by intradermal skin-testing and by bronchial challenge (the latter is not part of routine diagnostic procedure). The recognition of allergic aspergillosis does not usually affect management; asthma is treated on its merits as outlined above. Asthma may well be more resistant to standard forms of treatment and a high proportion of individuals are found to have a requirement for regular oral corticosteroids. Desensitization is unhelpful and antifungal treatment has not been shown to play an important part in management. Steroid treatment either by mouth or aerosol is usually fairly effective.

MUCOID IMPACTION

Episodes of lobar collapse due to 'mucoid impaction' may be treated by bronchoscopy and bronchial lavage. Usually the collapse resolves spontaneously or with the help of steroid therapy.

MYCETOMA

Mycetomas have a characteristic radiographic appearance. They lie free within the cavity and there is a thin rim of radiolucency ('halo') surrounding the rounded mass. Mycetomas enlarge very slowly; some cause massive haemoptysis. Surgical removal is indicated if haemoptysis is threatening and lung function is not severely impaired.

SYNOPSIS OF BRONCHO- PULMONARY ASPERGILLOSIS

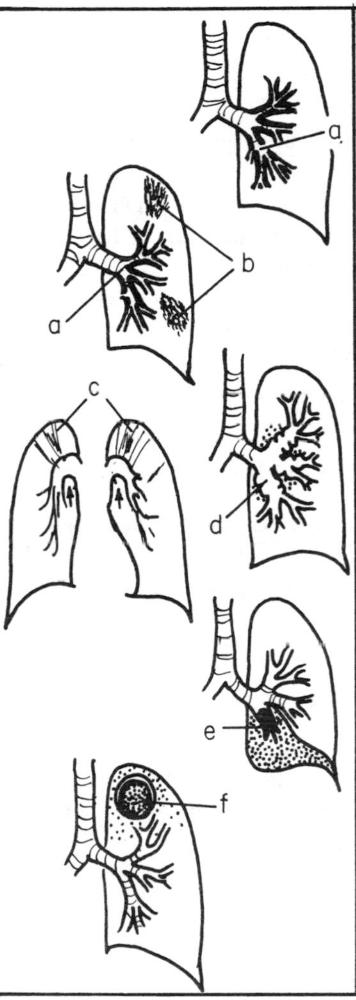

	prick test	delayed	precipitins
INCIDENTAL FINDING			
ncidental isolation from sputum	−	−	−
Isolation in atopic asthma (a)	±	−	−
ALLERGIC ASPERGILLOSIS	+	±	±
Asthma (a)			
Fleeting lung shadows (b)			
Eosinophilia			
Later:			
Upper lobe fibrosis (c)			
'Proximal' bronchiectasis (d)			
MUCOID IMPACTION	+	±	±
Recurrent segmental or lobar collapse associated with aspergillus plugs and bronchial damage (e)			
MYCETOMA (f)	±	±	++
Fungus ball in cavity — from old TB, cystic disease or ? spontaneous Haemoptysis or symptomless			

Fig. 15.15. *Synopsis of bronchopulmonary aspergillosis.*

LESS COMMON FORMS

Sometimes progressive spread of aspergillus infestation is observed over days or weeks with progressive parenchymal shadowing. The term 'invasive aspergillosis' may be used in this context. Usually this progression occurs in lungs which are already highly abnormal: for example, in cystic fibrosis or advanced fibrosing alveolitis.

Occasionally *Aspergillus fumigatus* may infect an area of necrotic lung: for example, after infarction. Generalized systemic infection by aspergillus is, however, rare and is only seen in catastrophically immunosuppressed individuals such as those undergoing radical treatment for malignant disease.

Antifungal treatment becomes an important consideration in invasive aspergillosis and in generalized systemic aspergillosis. In the latter the drug of choice appears to be intravenous amphotericin B. This may also be used in invasive pulmonary disease but ketaconazole is an alternative oral treatment which has been shown to be effective in arresting progress, even though eradication may not be achieved. Early results with inhalation ketaconazole are promising.

PULMONARY EOSINOPHILIA

This term is used to cover a variety of conditions in which radiological pulmonary shadowing is associated with a very high blood eosinophil count. The radiological shadows may be fluffy, wedge-shaped or reticulo-nodular in type.

1   Pulmonary eosinophilia with asthma

The majority of patients with fleeting isolated shadows and asthma have allergic aspergillosis and supporting evidence in the shape of skin-test reactions, the presence of serum precipitins and regular recovery of the organism is commonly forthcoming. Other antigens (e.g. house dust mite) may be capable of inducing pulmonary eosinophilia. Sometimes no obvious association with an antigen can be found.

2   Simple pulmonary eosinophilia (Löffler's syndrome)

This term refers to a transient pulmonary reaction with reticular or nodular shadowing on the chest X-ray which may be produced by drugs (e.g. sulphonamides), and various intestinal parasites. The pulmonary changes very rarely last more than 3–4 weeks.

3 Tropical eosinophilia

Pulmonary eosinophilia occurring in the tropics, with or without asthma, is usually related to sensitivity to intestinal and other parasites. Filarial infestation is probably the principal cause and most cases respond to treatment with diethyl carbamazine or organic arsenicals.

4 Polyarteritis nodosa

Pulmonary eosinophilia with or without asthma may be a feature of polyarteritis nodosa. This is rare. The diagnosis will be suggested by features such as weight loss, skin rashes, peripheral neuropathy, nephritis etc.

5 Churg–Strauss syndrome

This is uncommon. It is characterized by asthma and blood eosinophilia together with eosinophilic vasculitis and associated granuloma formation affecting several organs (for example, skin, kidney, pericardium and lung).

EXTRINSIC ALLERGIC ALVEOLITIS

This term refers to hypersensitivity reactions affecting the lung parenchyma which occur in response to inhaled organic dusts. Farmer's lung is the best-known example. Usually the exposure is heavy and occupational. The reaction is an expression of Type III hypersensitivity and precipitins can generally be demonstrated in the serum. Some examples of extrinsic alveolitis are listed in Table 15.1.

Where the condition is suspected but there is no recognizable occupational exposure to organic dust a search for a cause should include investigation of humidifiers which may be part of a central heating or air-conditioning system. A variety of obscure bacteria may inhabit recirculated water used in humidification and these in aerosol form may induce systemic symptoms (humidifier fever, p. 308).

Pathological features

The alveolar walls become thickened and infiltrated by lymphocytes, plasma cells and polymorphs. Small airways may show similar infiltrations. Advanced cases may show granuloma formation and variable degrees of diffuse lung fibrosis.

Table 15.1. *Some examples of extrinsic allergic alveolitis*

Name	Antigen responsible
Farmer's lung	Spores of thermophyllic actinomycetes in mouldy hay.
Bird fancier's lung	Avian antigens from dust from feathers, excreta etc.
Pituitary snuff taker's lung	Porcine or bovine antigens associated with extracts of posterior pituitary.
Mushroom worker's lung	Spores of thermophyllic actinomycetes in mould.
Maltworker's lung	Spores of *Aspergillus clavatus.*
Lung disease of grain-handlers	Dust derived from the grain weevil *Sitophilus granarius.*

Clinical features

The patient may notice immediate tightness in the chest with cough and sometimes wheezing on exposure to the dust concerned. This may be mild and transient. Typically exposure is followed after an interval of about 4 hours by tachypnoea, tightness and cough. Often there is associated muscular aching, malaise, headache and fever. The relationship of the illness to the dust exposure is often not appreciated, particularly when the initial reaction is trivial and the general symptoms are pronounced. Soon after exposure there may be fine rhonchi audible on auscultation but the most constant sign in all stages is the presence of persistent fine crepitations. In advanced cases there may be constant dyspnoea and exercise limitation accompanied by cyanosis and clubbing and the picture resembles that of cryptogenic fibrosing alveolitis.

Physiological changes

A pronounced restrictive defect of ventilation is the most usual finding. Variable degrees of airways obstruction may accompany this. There may be hyperventilation and arterial hypoxaemia. Transfer factor is usually significantly reduced.

Radiological features

In early cases there may be no abnormality. During regular exposure fluffy or nodular shadowing may be seen. In advanced cases there may be areas of honeycomb change and condensed masses of granuloma and fibrous tissue which may be particularly evident in the upper lobes.

Diagnosis

The diagnosis is made from the association of the total clinical picture with exposure to a suitable organic dust. Fever is an important clue. Identification of serum precipitins specific to the organic material may provide supportive evidence but results need to be interpreted with caution. In the case of farmer's lung it should be noted that about 20% of unaffected workers handling hay have serum precipitins to the thermophylic moulds responsible for the disease.

Management

Avoidance of the responsible antigen is the most important measure. This may mean a change of job or control of the exposure. It is not sufficient to advise the use of masks as these are unlikely to be used consistently by unsupervised workers. In the case of farmer's lung, improved methods of harvesting aimed at reducing the moisture content of hay are of importance. Sufferers are eligible for compensation under the Industrial Injuries Acts. Steroid therapy may be indicated on first diagnosis in a florid case, but such treatment must not be viewed as an alternative to control of exposure. Little benefit can be expected in cases with advanced fibrosis.

CHAPTER 16 / DIFFUSE LUNG FIBROSIS

CRYPTOGENIC FIBROSING
ALVEOLITIS
(also known as diffuse interstitial pulmonary
fibrosis and Hamman–Rich syndrome)

This is a rather uncommon condition in which the lung parenchyma becomes involved in a diffuse fibrotic process causing progressive impairment of gas transfer and progressive dyspnoea. The cause of the condition is not clear. It is a disease of adult life, being most common in late middle age.

Pathological features

The principal features are:
1   Thickening fibrosis and a variable degree of cellular infiltration of the interstitial tissue of the lungs which is most obvious in the lung parenchyma.
2   'Desquamation' of large numbers of cells into the alveoli. These include macrophages and other mononuclear cells, some of which may be altered Type II pneumocytes.

These changes may be irregularly dispersed within the lung and some individuals may show predominantly one form of change. As fibrosis progresses alveolar tissue becomes absorbed within condensing cellular fibrous tissue and in large parts of the lungs no alveoli may be visible at all. Because the process tends to be widespread complete collapse of large parts of lung is not generally seen; instead the lung remains aerated but the air-spaces are mainly made up of dilated bronchioles and the appearance is termed 'honeycomb lung' (Fig. 16.1).

Symptoms

In the earlier stages the patient presents with an easy panting dyspnoea and symptoms of exhaustion on effort. Sometimes an irritating unproductive cough is a prominent symptom. With progress of the disease dyspnoea can become frightening even on trivial exertion. Additional

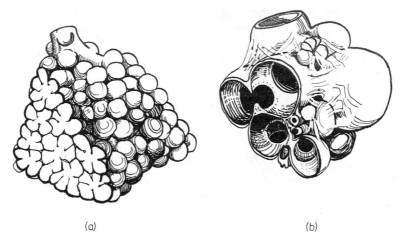

(a)   (b)

Fig. 16.1. *Honeycomb lung.* A three-dimensional impression of the structure of the normal lobule (a) and of the air spaces in advanced lung fibrosis (honeycomb lung) (b). There is dense fibrosis with disappearance of normal lung architecture. The air spaces are thick walled and much larger than alveoli. Most of them probably represent dilated terminal and respiratory bronchioles.

symptoms may develop due to hypoxia, cardiac failure, and broncho-pulmonary infection and, terminally, features of respiratory failure and pulmonary embolism may be added to the clinical picture.

Signs (see Fig. 16.2)

The patient is easily dyspnoeic, usually tachypnoeic, and may be cyanosed. Clubbing of some degree is seen in about two-thirds of cases. The chest appears normal and the costal margin moves upwards and outwards in the normal way (Fig. 16.4) but in severe cases there is an inward movement of the lower sternum on inspiration. The most consistent finding is the presence of fine crepitations on auscultation of the chest. These tend to occur throughout inspiration, being especially marked towards the end of inspiration.

Physiological changes

SPIROMETRY
A restrictive ventilatory defect is almost always evident by the time troublesome symptoms are reported.

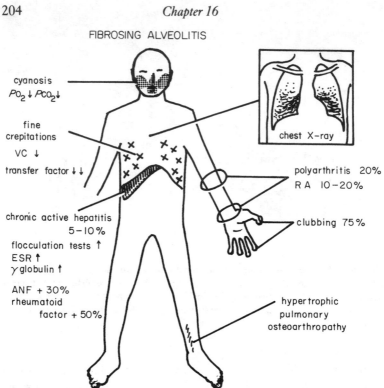

FIBROSING ALVEOLITIS

cyanosis
$Po_2 \downarrow Pco_2 \downarrow$

fine
crepitations
VC ↓
transfer factor ↓↓

chronic active hepatitis
5–10%
flocculation tests ↑
ESR ↑
γ globulin ↑

ANF + 30%
rheumatoid
factor + 50%

chest X–ray

polyarthritis 20%
R A 10–20%

clubbing 75%

hypertrophic
pulmonary
osteoarthropathy

Fig. 16.2. *Summary of features of fibrosing alveolitis.*

LUNG VOLUMES

All lung volumes are reduced but tend to maintain their relative proportions.

LUNG COMPLIANCE

This is reduced. Measurement is not essential to the diagnosis.

BLOOD GASES

At rest blood gases tend to be normal until the disease is well advanced, when arterial hypoxemia and hypocapnia (low PCO_2 due to hyperventilation) are generally found. Exercise is limited by arterial hypoxaemia and exercise tolerance may be extended by breathing oxygen-enriched air.

GAS TRANSFER

There is characteristically a pronounced impairment of transfer factor (p. 84). This is an early feature and it would be difficult to sustain a diagnosis in the presence of normal values. Normal values for transfer factor show variation between different laboratories and are dependent upon age and stature. An average normal value might be in excess of 5.5 mmol min^{-1} kPa^{-1} (16.5), moderately severe symptoms would be expected below 3.0 mmol min^{-1} kPa^{-1} (9.0) and severe disability accompanies levels below 1.5 mmol min^{-1} kPa^{-1} (4.0) (values in brackets are traditional units: ml/min/mmHg). KCO is always reduced. Traditionally the defective gas transfer has been regarded as a 'diffusion defect' due to thickening of the alveolar membrane. This explanation is undoubtedly an oversimplification and it seems likely that other mechanisms are more important and these include:

1   A much extended range of ventilation:perfusion ratios throughout the lung due to irregularly-distributed stiffness (p. 25).

2   Replacement of alveoli by fibrous tissue resulting in overall reduction in alveolar surface and capillary blood volume.

Radiological changes

The appearances vary somewhat depending upon the stage of the disease and its rapidity of onset. The most usual features are (i) a 'ground-glass' haziness especially at the bases. To this may be added (ii) streaky wisps of shadow with elevation of the diaphragms suggesting basal collapse and (iii) a generalized micronodular (miliary) mottling. The end-stage of the disease is characterized by (iv) the appearances of 'honeycomb lung' in which multiple circular areas of translucency 2–5 mm in diameter become evident within areas of opacification. Terminally there may be changes due to infection and pulmonary infarction.

Associated disorders

The ESR is usually elevated. Associated polyarthritis is common. About 10% of cases may have rheumatoid arthritis and a positive rheumatoid factor is found in the serum in about 50% of cases. Elevation of γ-globulins is fairly frequently found. A number of cases with coexisting chronic active hepatitis have been described and cirrhosis occurs more frequently than expected. Antinuclear factor may be present and other non-organ specific antibodies are found in about 30% of cases. A higher than expected incidence of thyroid disease has been reported. The relationship between cryptogenic fibrosing alveolitis and other collagen or autoimmune disorders remains conjectural.

Diagnosis

The diagnosis can usually be made on clinical grounds with the support of radiological appearances and simple tests of pulmonary function including measurement of transfer factor.

In a typical patient the diagnosis may be straightforward: a middle-aged individual with progressive panting dyspnoea and cyanosis but with no evidence of cardiac disease or airways obstruction is found to have clubbing and diffuse crepitations and a reticulo-nodular pattern of shadowing on the chest X-ray which is more pronounced at the bases; spirometry reveals a much restricted vital capacity but good early-expiratory flow rate and transfer factor is found to be markedly impaired.

DIFFERENTIAL DIAGNOSIS

In less typical cases the differential diagnosis is potentially lengthy. Miliary mottling is discussed on p. 95). Some of the more important alternatives are:

1 *Extrinsic allergic alveolitis* (p. 199). It is very important to differentiate this preventable form of alveolitis. Clinical, radiological and physiological features may be identical; points of difference are: (a) history of exposure to appropriate organic dust and presence of serum precipitins; (b) more prominent involvement of upper lobes in extrinsic alveolitis; (c) rheumatoid factor, ANF and elevation of γ-globulin are commonly found in cryptogenic fibrosing alveolitis.

2 *Bronchiectasis.* Basal crepitations, clubbing and irregular basal shadowing on the chest X-ray may cause confusion. Points of difference are: (a) cough is longstanding and productive of large amounts of purulent sputum; (b) dyspnoea if present is usually a consequence of airways obstruction; (c) cyanosis is uncommon and generally associated with chronic ventilatory failure; (d) transfer factor is not usually reduced.

3 *Chronic left heart failure.* May rarely produce reticulo-nodular shadowing and dyspnoea; clinical, radiological and ECG changes of left heart disease will generally be present.

4 *Sarcoidosis.* Differentiation may be difficult without a positive Kveim test or other features of sarcoidosis particularly in the skin and eye (p. 219). In diffuse sarcoidosis of the lungs the defect in transfer factor is often more modest than would be expected from the radiographic changes.

5 *Lymphangitis carcinomatosa.* This may produce progressive dyspnoea with striking impairment of transfer factor. There will usually be past or present evidence of carcinoma—usually an adenocarcinoma.

6 *Pulmonary embolism.* This should rarely cause confusion but repeated embolism should always be borne in mind in any patient with progressive obscure breathlessness and basal shadowing on the chest X-ray.

7 *Industrial lung disease.* Most especially diffuse pulmonary fibrosis due to asbestos (see p. 313).

LUNG BIOPSY

Biopsy confirmation of the diagnosis is not essential when the diagnosis or a particular line of action is clear. Sometimes however a therapeutic decision is impossible without a histological diagnosis.

Open-lung biopsy

This allows removal of a relatively large specimen which can be selected from a moderately affected part of the lung. The disadvantages are the hazards of anaesthetic, thoracotomy and subsequent convalescence.

Closed-lung biopsy

A number of needle techniques have been developed for obtaining specimens of aerated lung. The Jack needle shears off a tiny fragment of lung snagged by small hooks on the stylet. Steel's lung trephine is operated by a high-speed air drill and cuts a small core of lung tissue. In most instances the disturbance is slight; only about a third of patients develop a pneumothorax and of these less than half require pleural intubation. Transbronchial biopsy (Fig. 19.5) performed by fine biopsy forceps passed through a fibre-optic bronchoscope and wedged in a peripheral bronchiole offers an alternative relatively safe means of obtaining multiple samples of lung parenchyma in the diagnosis of diffuse lung disease. The main drawbacks of closed biopsy are the small size of the specimen and occasional failure to obtain a specimen. Bronchoalveolar lavage may be used to assess activity; see p. 212).

Course of the disease

The course is very variable. A small number of patients have a rapidly progressive course over only a few months and the illness may be accompanied by severe malaise and pneumonic features. A slower downhill course is more usual over a period of years. In some elderly individuals the condition is discovered by chance and appears to be completely stationary.

Treatment

CORTICOSTEROID TREATMENT

Patients with disturbing dyspnoea or clear evidence of progression should be treated with corticosteroids. It is usual to use a large dose (40–60 mg of prednisolone daily) for a period of up to 2 months if the disease threatens to disable. If any improvement is to be achieved it will generally be evident by this time. The dose is then progressively reduced to the lowest level capable of maintaining the improvement.

RESULT

Improvement of some degree is seen in about two-thirds of cases receiving corticosteroid treatment. The more acute the mode of onset and the younger the patient, the more likely it is that there will be a worthwhile improvement. However, a worthwhile response may be seen even in advanced disease with honeycomb change.

IMMUNOSUPPRESSIVE THERAPY

Azathioprine may have some effect on the disease and may be useful where there are especially compelling reasons for avoiding large doses of prednisolone. More recently cyclophosphamide has been used where the response to steroid treatment has been disappointing.

OXYGEN

This may be useful in advanced disease when even gentle exercise is poorly tolerated. A stationary cylinder in the house and long lengths of plastic piping may enable the patient to negotiate the stairs or take a bath which might otherwise be impossible. A rechargeable portable cylinder may extend the range of activities out of doors.

SUPPORTIVE MEASURES

Measures to control infection, heart failure and exhausting cough are required as the disease progresses. Opiates may be necessary to control terrifying terminal dyspnoea.

DIFFUSE FIBROSIS DUE TO
DRUGS AND POISONS

Drugs

Drugs capable of producing lung fibrosis include: busulphan, bleomycin, nitrofurantoin, cyclophosphamide and methysergide (see p. 320).

Paraquat

Poisoning with the weedkiller Paraquat induces a vicious accelerated form of diffuse lung fibrosis in which the whole range of fibrosing alveolitis, from the earliest changes to widespread honeycombing, may be condensed into a period of less than 3 weeks, by which time death from hypoxia has usually supervened. Very occasionally individuals may escape with lung changes arrested at an intermediate stage. Fatal poisoning follows accidental consumption of only a mouthful of agricultural concentrate (Gramoxone). Accidental poisoning with diluted material or the more generally available Paraquat/diquat mixture in granular form is almost unheard of. Intentional self-poisoning with various preparations accounts for about half of the fatalities.

Radiation

Therapeutic irradiation which involves the lung fields may lead to an acute pneumonitis which generally resolves within a few weeks. A variable degree of fibrosis may follow over subsequent months in the distribution of the irradiated areas.

Occupational causes (see p. 309).

RHEUMATOID ARTHRITIS

The pulmonary accompaniments of rheumatoid arthritis are summarised in Fig. 16.3.

Pleurisy and pleural effusion

These are common in rheumatoid arthritis and may tend to be recurrent. Effusions are rarely large.

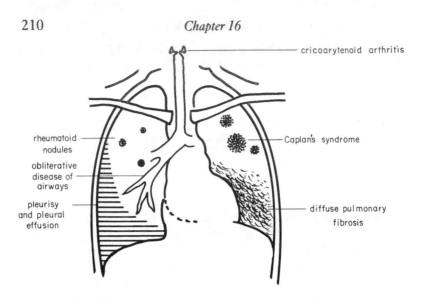

Fig. 16.3. *Summary of pulmonary complications of rheumatoid arthritis.*

Pulmonary fibrosis

This is much less common, probably occurring in no more than 2% of cases. There is a definite but ill-understood relationship between rheumatoid arthritis and fibrosing alveolitis. The fibrosis accompanying rheumatoid arthritis may appear to be stationary for many years. If pulmonary fibrosis is disabling or progressive, treatment with cortico-steroids may be indicated.

Pulmonary nodules

These are not common. The appearance is of several soft spherical nodules up to 1 cm in diameter and this may lead to the erroneous diagnosis of metastatic malignant disease. The nodules have the same histology as rheumatoid nodules elsewhere; they sometimes cavitate and may disappear spontaneously.

Caplan's syndrome

Rheumatoid arthritis occurring in association with coalworkers' pneumoconiosis may be marked by the occurrence of very large pul-monary nodules 2–3 cm in diameter. These may also break down and cavitate, sometimes leading to the suspicion of tuberculosis though tubercle bacilli are not found. Sometimes the rheumatoid arthritis is not clinically evident until years later. Other pneumoconioses may be associated with massive nodules in patients with rheumatoid arthritis.

Obliterative disease of airways

It has been recognized recently that a small proportion of patients with rheumatoid arthritis may develop rapidly progressive airways obstruction associated with obliteration of small bronchi.

Cricoarytenoid arthritis

This may lead to hoarseness or occasionally inspiratory stridor.

SYSTEMIC SCLEROSIS

This uncommon condition produces a number of pulmonary complications most of which only become evident when the disease is relatively advanced.

Diffuse pulmonary fibrosis

The clinical, radiological and physiological features of this are like those of fibrosing alveolitis, although there is some evidence that the alteration of fibrous tissue may be of a fundamentally different nature in systemic sclerosis.

Restriction of chest wall movement

This late complication may arise as a consequence of severe thickening and contraction of the skin of the trunk.

Inhalation pneumonia

Pneumonia and lung abscess may result from overspill from a dilated oesophagus secondary to stricture formation. Pneumonia is a common terminal event.

The diagnosis is made by recogniton of the characteristic changes in the skin and other organs. Where pulmonary fibrosis appears to be causing disability, corticosteroid treatment is generally tried—almost always with disappointing results.

SYSTEMIC LUPUS
ERYTHEMATOSUS (SLE)

The pulmonary complications of this uncommon multi-system disorder are as follows:

Pleurisy

Pleurisy, sometimes with a small effusion, is common and may be the presenting feature. Pleurisy occurring in young female patients who are more ill than might be expected and who have a high ESR should lead to suspicion of SLE.

Pneumonia

Patchy recurrent pneumonia is a common feature of SLE in relapse. Usually the patient is ill and there may be a characteristic rash, arthritis and other features of the disease. The diagnosis will be supported by the finding of antinuclear factor, LE cells and DNA antibody in the serum.

'Small lung syndrome'

It is uncertain whether true diffuse pulmonary fibrosis occurs in association with SLE but patients may complain of dyspnoea associated with a sensation of restriction within the chest. There may be no definite physical signs of radiological features but spirometry may reveal a restrictive ventilatory defect and transfer factor may be moderately impaired. The syndrome tends to resolve fairly promptly with steroid treatment. One factor in its causation may be impaired action of respiratory musculature.

BRONCHOALVEOLAR LAVAGE (BAL)

This is a fairly new technique with limited clinical applications which has given interesting new information about cellular activity in diffuse inflammatory lung disease. A fibre-optic bronchoscope (Fig. 19.3) is introduced under local anaesthesia and the tip is wedged in a segmental bronchus of suitable size. Several 20 ml aliquots of warm saline are then introduced and aspirated. The aspirated material is filtered, centrifuged and resuspended and then subjected to cytological examination.

Normal cell content

In non-smoking normals more than 90% of cells are alveolar macrophages; about 7% are lymphocytes (of which three-quarters are T cells, only a small proportion of which are activated) and polymorph leucocytes are about 1% of the total. In smokers about 3% of cells are polymorphs, mostly neutrophils.

Fibrosing alveolitis

In this condition and others associated with collagen-vascular diseases there is a striking increase in the proportion of neutrophils. Eosinophils and lymphocytes may also be present in increased numbers. These changes may reflect intensity of inflammatory activity but they are not diagnostically helpful.

Sarcoidosis

In sarcoidosis there is characteristically an increase in the lymphocyte percentage. There may also be an increase in neutrophils and eosinophils too. Apical fibrosis disease is associated with an increase in neutrophils rather than lymphocytes. The clinical usefulness of the lavage fluid changes is still being assessed.

Other diseases

BAL can be diagnostic in alveolar proteinosis (special staining of the secretions) and in *Pneumocystis carinii* pneumonia (microscopic identification of the organism). It can also produce evidence of unsuspected intrapulmonary haemorrhage (haemosiderin-laden macrophages). Lavage of localized lesions suspected of being due to tuberculosis sometimes results in the culture of mycobacteria when sputum culture has failed.

CHAPTER 17 / SARCOIDOSIS

The definition of sarcoidosis is based upon the presence of granulomatous tissue with a characteristic histological picture found in characteristic areas of the body. The diagnosis rests upon identification of
clinical features and in practice histological confirmation is not always
necessary.

The histological picture

The characteristic cell is a largish epithelioid cell with a pale staining
nucleus arranged in clumps or whorls of varying size and bounded by a
sparse zone of lymphocytic infiltration. The clumps of typical cells all
look strikingly the same in the various affected tissues. Caseation is not
seen even in the centre of quite large masses; but hyaline degeneration
may merge with areas of fibrosis. Occasional giant cells are present and
some may be seen to contain concentric inclusion bodies (Schaumann
bodies).

Although the histological appearances may contribute to a diagnosis
of sarcoidosis the granuloma is not sufficiently characteristic for a
confident diagnosis to be made exclusively on histological grounds.

Aetiology

The aetiology is not known. It is no longer regarded as a neoplastic type
of reticulo-endothelial proliferation akin to Hodgkin's disease and discussion centres on the possibility that it represents an atypical response
to the tubercle bacillus (and possibly other agents which are capable of
producing granulomata) or that it may be due to an unidentified trans-
missible agent. Exposure to beryllium has in the past produced granulomata indistinguishable from those of sarcoidosis (exposure is now very
strictly controlled).

A striking feature of cases of sarcoidosis is evidence of defective
cellularly mediated (Type IV) hypersensitivity. It may be difficult or
impossible to induce a response to tuberculin or other agents normally
capable of evoking this response. Despite this evidence of impaired
lymphocyte function, the lungs appear to be the site of intense activity
and contain very large numbers of T lymphocytes in active sarcoidosis.

Clinical manifestations

It is useful to consider the clinical manifestations under two headings:
1 Acute manifestations in the young which are generally benign and characterized by bilateral hilar node enlargement (BHL) and erythema nodosum.
2 Chronic or recurrent manifestations, which tend to occur in an older age-group, involve many tissues of the body and include infiltration and fibrosis of the lungs.

1. ACUTE MANIFESTATIONS—BHL AND ERYTHEMA NODOSUM
This is by far the commonest manifestation of sarcoidosis. Sarcoidosis is the commonest cause of erythema nodosum in young adults. Sometimes general malaise, mild fever and arthralgia precede the erythema nodosum for a week or two. Other accompaniments of this acute form of sarcoidosis are acute arthritis of ankles, knees or wrists with marked oedema and reddening, parotid enlargement and acute anterior uveitis. There are no signs on examination of the chest and there is no disturbance of pulmonary function.

Diagnosis
BHL accompanied by erythema nodosum is always due to sarcoidosis and no further investigations are really necessary. Where BHL is found without any helpful clues there is still rarely real difficulty in diagnosis. If BHL is slight there may be difficulty in distinguishing the appearances from those of unusually prominent pulmonary arteries. Lymphoma is sometimes suspected but this almost never shows the striking symmetry of the BHL of sarcoidosis and it is exceedingly rare for hilar adenopathy to be the sole manifestation of lymphoma. In cases of serious doubt tuberculin and Kveim tests may be helpful (but not infallible) and lymph node biopsy or mediastinoscopy may be necessary. Patients with BHL and radiologically clear lung fields probably all have microscopic granulomata in the lung parenchyma. Granuloma can be retrieved in about 80% of cases by transbronchial biopsy and this finding can be useful when there is serious diagnostic doubt.

Course
The prognosis is excellent. Erythema nodosum and arthralgia subside within a month and uveitis rarely persists much longer. Radiological signs of BHL may persist for 2–3 years but generally resolve over about 18 months. Occasionally some flecks of pulmonary infiltrate are seen to

Chapter 17

come and go during this time but only a very small percentage of cases go on to develop the more indolent forms of sarcoidosis.

Treatment
As a rule no treatment is necessary. Particularly severe arthralgia or erythema nodosum may be helped by aspirin or even prednisolone in modest dosage for 2–3 weeks. There is usually no call for hospitalization or intensive follow up, both of which foster concern and neurosis which may be potentially more disabling than the condition itself.

2. CHRONIC OR RECURRENT MANIFESTATIONS

PULMONARY INFILTRATIONS IN SARCOIDOSIS
Limited infiltrations may appear in the course of evolution of BHL with erythema nodosum but major involvement of the lungs in sarcoidosis tends to be encountered when there is already evidence of indolent sarcoidosis in various tissues of the body (see Fig. 17.1). Not all chronic indolent sarcoidosis passes through an acute phase with BHL and erythema nodosum—indeed this evolution may be rare.

There may be an alveolitis accompanying granulomatous involvement of the lung and this has been the subject of great interest in recent years since the development of bronchoalveolar lavage which permits the

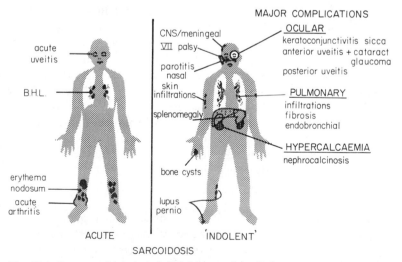

Fig. 17.1. *Summary of the principal clinical features of sarcoidosis.*

sampling of cells from alveoli (p. 212). Increased numbers of lympho-cytes are found in sarcoidosis.

Radiological appearances
These are of mottling often affecting the mid-zones principally and the mottling may be formed in radially-arranged leashes. In some instances there is generalized finer stippling.

Physiological changes
A modest restrictive defect and some reduction in transfer factor is usual if changes are widespread but the defect often seems slight when compared with the X-ray appearances (*cf.* Fibrosing alveolitis, p. 205).

PULMONARY FIBROSIS
This is quite rare and represents an end stage following granulomatous infiltration and alveolitis. It usually involves the mid-zones most severely. The X-ray appearances are of contraction of lung volume and fine spider's web-like linear shadows, with areas of condensed shadow-ing which may contain honeycomb spaces or larger cysts. Physiological tests reflect the changes; lung volumes are small, there is usually a restrictive ventilatory defect and serious impairment of transfer factor although sometimes an obstructive defect is present. Exercise is limited and there may be cyanosis. Clubbing is a rarity.

ENDOBRONCHIAL SARCOIDOSIS
Plaques of granuloma may occur either scattered throughout the bron-chial tree or as a localized deposit. Localized or occasionally diffuse airways obstruction may be produced. With the increased use of fibre-optic bronchoscopy in suspected sarcoidosis, for purposes of lung biopsy or bronchoalveolar lavage, endobronchial sarcoidosis has come to be recognized as quite a common accompaniment of chronic disease.

COURSE OF PARENCHYMAL CHANGES
Infiltrations often remain stationary for years. Perhaps a quarter of patients with extensive infiltration develop some fibrosis which may also remain constant for long periods and may not be associated with severe symptoms. Probably less than 10% with such infiltrations become disabled and a smaller proportion actually die from pulmonary involve-ment.

Indices of activity of pulmonary sarcoidosis
There is no easy way to determine whether active and progressively damaging pulmonary inflammation or granulomatous infiltration is occurring in sarcoidosis. By the time that symptoms or even obvious impairment of pulmonary function is present, progression may be inevitable. In recent years the following have been examined as possible pointers: increase in percentage of T lymphocytes in bronchoalveolar lavage fluid (p. 212) to above 28% of the total cells (normally less than 10%); increase in diffuse uptake of isotope in a gallium-67 lung scan; increase in serum angiotensin converting enzyme (ACE) and increase in serum beta microglobulin concentration. Results of lavage and gallium scanning are sometimes combined to determine whether an individual has 'high intensity' or 'low intensity' alveolitis. The usefulness of this distinction is still being assessed.

EXTRAPULMONARY SARCOIDOSIS
Some of the commoner sites are indicated diagrammatically in Fig. 17.1 and a few deserve special mention.

Ocular sarcoidosis
Anterior uveitis (iridocyclitis) is the commonest manifestation. It may be obvious because of pain, misting vision and the presence of ciliary injection but sometimes it is only revealed by slit-lamp inspection. Posterior uveitis (perivenous sheathing and chorioretinitis) is much less common. Uveitis occurs in about a quarter of all patients with sarcoidosis and sarcoidosis accounts for about 5% of uveitis presenting to ophthalmologists. Keratoconjunctivitis sicca and lacrimal gland enlargement may complicate chronic sarcoidosis.

Uveoparotid fever
This is the name given to a syndrome of uveitis, parotid gland enlargement and sometimes facial nerve palsy (usually temporary).

Central nervous system involvement
Facial palsy may also be due to meningeal involvement which may produce a variety of obscure neurological syndromes and epilepsy.

Skin involvement
Lupus pernio is a chilblain-like lesion occurring in violaceous patches on the face and limbs and it is generally accompanied by pulmonary involvement. Nodules of sarcoid granuloma may occur in the skin particularly in old scars.

Bone involvement

Bone cysts are the hallmark of established indolent sarcoidosis. Digits are commonly involved. Abnormal nail growth may occur when the terminal digit is involved. If affected, the digit is swollen; there is no point in routinely X-raying the hands in suspected sarcoidosis.

Calcium metabolism

In most cases there is abnormally increased absorption of calcium and hypercalcuria (increased calcium flux). In chronic sarcoidosis renal stones are more frequent than in normals and nephrocalcinosis is occasionally encountered. Hypercalcaemia is rare by comparison and renal failure is usually present when it arises.

Cardiac involvement

Involvement of the heart is uncommon and may be silent. It may present with heart failure or disturbances of rhythm including complete heart block.

Diagnosis

Where a number of features occur together the diagnosis may be straightforward and it is by no means obligatory to obtain histological support. Where diagnosis is uncertain biopsy of lymph nodes, liver or lung may be justified. Peripheral transbronchial lung biopsy (see Fig. 19.5) is frequently helpful even when the evidence of parenchymal lung involvement is minimal.

The limitations of histological examination must be born in mind (p. 214) and it should also be remembered that occasionally mediastinal lymph nodes may show a sarcoid form of granulomatous reaction to early invasion by carcinoma.

TUBERCULIN TESTS (p. 128)
There are negative results in over three-quarters of all patients with sarcoidosis.

KVEIM TEST
An intradermal injection of suspension of an extract of human sarcoid spleen is made into the skin and the site marked (e.g. by tattooing). After 6 weeks the site is inspected and biopsied. A positive result is indicated by the presence of sarcoid granuloma. Individual extracts have differing records of reliability but generally over three-quarters of patients give

positive results. 'False positive' results may be found in Crohn's disease and a number of disorders associated with enlargement of lymph nodes.

Treatment

The great majority of patients with sarcoidosis require no treatment at all. The generally accepted indications for treatment with oral steroids are:

SEVERE UVEITIS

Where uveitis cannot be adequately controlled by topical steroid treatment oral prednisolone may be necessary and this is the commonest indication for such treatment.

PROGRESSIVE PULMONARY CHANGES

Where there is clinical, radiological and physiological evidence of deterioration it is usual to start treatment with oral steroids. X-ray signs of infiltration often resolve promptly with little change in physiological function but sometimes with improvement in dyspnoea and cough. There is no convincing evidence that protracted control of radiological infiltrations with steroid treatment averts development of fibrosis.

HYPERCALCAEMIA

Carries the threat of progressive renal failure and it is usually controlled by a modest dose of oral steroid.

IMPORTANT NEUROLOGICAL INVOLVEMENT

Epilepsy or meningeal involvement are usually regarded as indications for steroid treatment.

Skin manifestations of sarcoidosis may be amenable to local treatment by steroid creams or local steroid infiltration which is worthwhile in cosmetically strategic areas.

CHAPTER 18 / CHRONIC BRONCHITIS, AIRWAYS OBSTRUCTION AND EMPHYSEMA

Definitions

CHRONIC BRONCHITIS. Chronic cough with production of sputum on most days for at least 3 months in the year for at least 2 years

The term refers simply to the symptoms of cough and sputum (generally excluding that due to some localized lesion in the lungs). It is an indicator of mucus hypersecretion. Simple chronic bronchitis is not accompanied by shortness of breath.

AIRWAYS OBSTRUCTION. Diffuse airways narrowing causing increased resistance to airflow

The expression denotes a disturbance of physiology, and airways obstruction is generally confirmed by physiological tests. Airways obstruction commonly accompanies chronic bronchitis and is generally responsible for the dyspnoea. Airways obstruction in chronic bronchitis is *not* necessarily due to emphysema. Some individuals (almost always smokers) develop airways obstruction without ever having the symptom of chronic bronchitis or other evidence of mucus hypersecretion.

EMPHYSEMA. Dilatation of the terminal air-spaces of the lungs distal to the terminal bronchiole with destruction of their walls

The term denotes a pathological lesion, not a clinical syndrome. Dyspnoea which occurs in association with chronic bronchitis is *not* necessarily due to emphysema. It is generally not possible to diagnose the presence of emphysema reliably in life on clinical grounds alone. Generalized emphysema is always accompanied by evidence of airways obstruction.

221

ASTHMA. A disease characterized by variable dyspnoea due to widespread narrowing of the peripheral airways in the lungs, varying in severity over short periods of time, either spontaneously or as result of treatment

As some patients with asthma present with chronic cough productive of sputum and as airways obstruction is a principal feature, it is to be expected that some patients with asthma may unintentionally be included in the group of diseases discussed here (see p. 232).

CHRONIC OBSTRUCTIVE PULMONARY DISEASE (COPD)

This term, and others rather like it, have grown into common use as a means of indicating the common clinical situation in which all of the above phenomena may be inextricably mixed. The term is convenient but lacks precision and fosters the misconception that there is a single uniform disease entity in which all elements are necessarily present. Where it appears in this chapter it should be taken to mean emphysema, with or without the symptom of chronic bronchitis and which is not believed to be due to asthma.

Prevalence

1   In the UK chronic bronchitis as defined occurs in about 15% of men and 5% of women. The ratio of males to females increases with age.
2   A huge amount of loss of work is attributable to chronic bronchitis and COPD (about 30 million working days each year).
3   The prevalence is higher in the UK than in other countries.

Mortality

1   In the UK about 30 000 persons die from COPD each year.
2   Mortality rises steeply with age but more than 8500 of the deaths occur before retirement age.
3   The mortality from COPD is higher than in other countries.

Aetiology

It is not possible to identify a single cause of chronic bronchitis and COPD but a number of factors are known to be involved.

Cigarette smoking is overwhelmingly the most important factor in the genesis of chronic bronchitis and COPD.

Symptoms
Symptoms of simple bronchitis in the general population are:
1 common in smokers
2 related to the number of cigarettes smoked per day
3 exceptional in non-smokers.

Simple ventilatory tests
Smokers, as a group, have lower performance than non-smokers of comparable age; the severity of the impairment being proportional to the number of cigarettes smoked per day. Affected smokers show a more rapid decline in FEV_1, with age than normals. Some smokers remain unaffected.

Morbidity
Work-loss and hospital admissions are much more frequent in smokers and related to the number of cigarettes smoked per day.

Mortality
The mortality from COPD is much higher amongst smokers. The risk of death from COPD in a man smoking 15 cigarettes daily is 12 times that of a non-smoker. In a man smoking 30 cigarettes daily the risk is 20 times that of a non-smoker.

ATMOSPHERIC POLLUTION

Long term
1 When the effect of cigarette smoking has been allowed for, the prevalence of symptoms, morbidity and mortality from COPD are found to be related to the degree of urbanization. They are also related to mean levels of atmospheric pollution which seems likely to be the most important element within urbanization in this context.
2 In non-smokers the effect of urbanization and atmospheric pollution is very small.
3 In smokers the adverse effects of atmospheric pollution become increasingly marked in proportion to smoking exposure, which suggests an interaction between these factors.

Short term

Exceptional episodes of heavy pollution have been associated with greatly increased numbers of admissions to hospitals and deaths because of COPD.

SOCIO-ECONOMIC FACTORS

Mortality from COPD as judged from death certification is inversely related to socio-economic status. Mortality in the Registrar General's Class V is six times greater than in Class II.

INFECTION

Virus infections are known to be associated with some exacerbations of COPD and bacterial infection of the sputum is a feature of established exacerbations. These infections may play an important role in the progress of the disease but there is no good evidence to support a causative role.

REGIONAL FACTORS

Chronic bronchitis and its accompaniments is very much more common in the UK than in most other countries. The reasons for this are probably complex and include the effect of differing diagnostic conventions.

Within the UK the prevalence and mortality from COPD tends to be higher in the North and West compared with the South and East even when allowance is made for the effects of urbanization.

CONSTITUTIONAL FACTORS

Familial tendencies to COPD are sometimes encountered but the effects of shared smoking habits, atmospheric pollution and social class obscure the relationship. Unrecognized asthma may sometimes underlie the familial tendency.

A very rare form of emphysema is due to an inherited deficiency of α_1-antitrypsin, a component of normal plasma globulin (see below).

PROTEASE – ANTIPROTEASE INTERACTION AND THE DEVELOPMENT OF EMPHYSEMA

It is now thought likely that emphysema develops as a consequence of destruction of parenchymal lung tissue (particularly elastin) by proteolytic digestion. The demonstration that intratracheal instillation of the proteolytic enzyme papain in rats resulted in the development of emphysema, and the recognition that in humans genetic deficiency of the principal anti protease (α_1-antitrypsin) is associated with severe youthful emphysema form the twin foundations for this theory.

The source of proteolytic enzyme in the genesis of human emphysema is thought to be the neutrophil. Very small numbers of neutrophils are normally present within alveoli and in relation to small airways but much greater numbers are present in smokers. Macrophages may play a part in bringing this about as macrophages from smokers are more actively chemotactic to neutrophils. The turnover of neutrophils may become such that the released enzyme exceeds the local capacity to neutralize it and, over very long periods of time, emphysema may result. The mechanisms involved are likely to be more complicated than this outline suggests. For example, it is known that protease inhibitors other than α_1-antitrypsin exist in the lung. Furthermore, it seems quite probable that the performance of the inhibitors may be chemically impaired by local oxidant reactions. Macrophages are capable of such reactions as part of their antimicrobial activity and they are, moreover, capable of releasing elastase.

Clinical features and progress of the disease

SIMPLE CHRONIC BRONCHITIS

The progress of simple bronchitis is generally insidious. Cough which may be present initially only during the first part of the day in winter months may, over several years, come to last all day throughout the year. Occasional patients relate the onset of symptoms to a single severe respiratory tract infection.

ACUTE EXACERBATIONS

Particularly in relation to colds, patients with chronic bronchitis develop increased cough productive of yellow purulent sputum with mild symptoms of general malaise. The illness may last a few days or several weeks.

DEVELOPMENT OF AIRWAYS OBSTRUCTION

Symptoms

Not all patients with simple chronic bronchitis develop airways obstruction. The cardinal symptom is dyspnoea which may be accompanied by wheezing and is generally related to effort. Dyspnoea is commonly noted for the first time after an acute exacerbation. Clinical and spirometric evidence of airways obstruction is common in patients who are quiet unaware of any symptoms apart from cough. Airways obstruction is often already severe when medical attention is sought for the first time.

Bronchial hyper-reactivity produces symptoms associated with airways obstruction and may help to distinguish dyspnoea due to this cause. The patient complains of sensations of tightness, choking or paroxysms of coughing when confronted by smoke, cold air, fog, car exhaust and other fumes. Symptoms are often related to particular weather conditions.

Signs
Clinical signs associated with the presence of airways obstruction are described on p. 58. It is important to remember that these may be unreliable. In particular the presence or absence of wheeze is not an indicator of the presence or absence of airways obstruction. It is very easy to overlook the presence of airways obstruction even when it is severe.

Measurement
Proper assessment of any patient with cough and breathlessness requires the use of a spirometer or at least measurement of peak expiratory flow (see pp. 60–71) preferably as part of the examination. Although there is in general a relationship between severity of airways obstructions as judged by the FEV_1 or peak expiratory flow rate on the one hand, and the severity of symptoms and disability on the other, there is wide individual variation. In adult males of normal stature, symptoms of exercise dyspnoea are not usually remarked upon when the FEV_1 is above 2 litres; disability is not usually critically severe above 1 litre. Some individuals are uncomplaining with an FEV_1 of under 1 litre. Most patients with an FEV_1 of 0.5 litre are very severely disabled indeed.

PROGRESS OF DISABILITY

There is generally a very gradual progression of disability extending over 10 – 40 years. It may become apparent through increasing absence from work, gradual limitation of exercise tolerance and a reduced range of activities (p. 42). The prognosis is related to severity of exercise limitation; 40% of patients who are required to walk at a reduced pace on flat ground die within 5 years.

With time, acute exacerbations become more alarming and are accompanied by breathlessness at rest, and difficulty in expectoration; admission to hospital may be required during these episodes.

CLINICAL PATTERNS IN SEVERE CHRONIC OBSTRUCTIVE LUNG DISEASE

Two patterns of disturbance may be discerned during the progress of advanced COPD which differ mainly in the extent to which ventilatory drive is preserved in the face of increasing airways obstruction. The main features are summarized in Figs 18.1 and 18.2. Most patients do not fit either pattern completely but have some features of both.

Type A ('pink puffer')

In this group ventilatory drive is well preserved even in the presence of very severe airways obstruction. Dyspnoea may be intense. Blood gases are maintained in the normal range at rest until terminally.

Type B ('blue bloater')

Individuals meeting this description have poor respiratory drive and easily drift into respiratory failure with elevation of P_{CO_2}, hypoxia and heart failure particularly during infective exacerbations (see cor pulmonale p. 273).

In simple terms, the 'pink puffer' can be regarded as 'doing his best' to breathe enough to keep the P_{CO_2} down often in the face of great difficulties, whilst the 'blue bloater' 'gives up' at a relatively early stage and settles for poor blood gases when he could breathe more 'if he tried harder'.

The reasons for the early ventilatory failure of Type B patients are not clear. The prognosis for the group is poor: about 70% die within 5 years. Patients with severe day time hypoxaemia are subject to even more severe nocturnal dips in oxygen saturation during REM sleep. Many deaths occur at night. Long-term near-continuous oxygen therapy may prolong life (see p. 330).

Emphysema

1 The term emphysema (defined p. 221) refers to a form of parenchymal lung damage and not to a clinical syndrome.
2 It is difficult to diagnose reliably.
3 Whether or not a patient has emphysema is not clinically very important—the management of the patient will only exceptionally be affected by the diagnosis.
4 Emphysema is widely over-diagnosed on inadequate evidence.
5 As emphysema is untreatable the diagnosis tends to foster an air of hopelessness in the management.

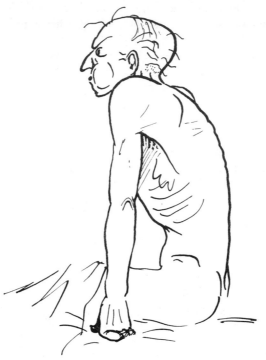

Fig. 18.1. *Type A or 'Pink puffer'—the picture of good respiratory drive.*
Individuals in this category tend to have the following features:
 Intense dyspnoea often with purse-lip breathing
 Thin and often elderly
 Small sputum volume
 Rarely develop oedema or overt heart failure
Investigations may show:
 Near-normal blood gas values (until terminally)
 Very severe airways obstruction
 Increased total lung capacity
 Radiological evidence of emphysema
 Impairment of transfer factor.

Pathological features

Two principal patterns are seen (Fig. 18.3).

1 CENTRILOBULAR OR CENTRIACINAR EMPHYSEMA

Distension and damage affect the respiratory bronchioles; the more distal alveolar ducts and alveoli tend to be well preserved.

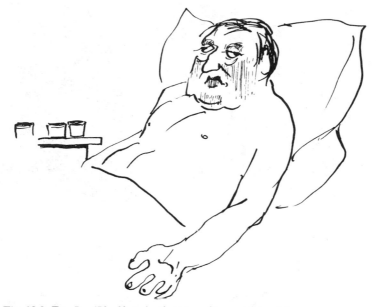

Fig. 18.2. *Type B or 'Blue bloater'—the picture of poor respiratory drive.*
Individuals in this category tend to have the following features:
   Relatively mild dyspnoea
   Often obese
   Large sputum volume and frequent infective exacerbations
   Often oedematous and easily lapse into congestive heart failure.
Investigation may show:
   Abnormal blood gases—hypercapnia, hypoxaemia with elevated plasma bicarbonate
      and polycythaemia, severe nocturnal hypoxaemia during REM sleep
   Sometimes only moderately severe airways obstruction
   Fairly normal total lung capacity
   No radiological evidence of emphysema
   Little or no reduction in transfer factor.

2 PANACINAR EMPHYSEMA

Distension and destruction appear to involve the whole of the acinus.

IRREGULAR EMPHYSEMA

This term is used to describe the very common appearance of scarring
and damage which affect the parenchyma patchily without particular
regard for acinar structure.

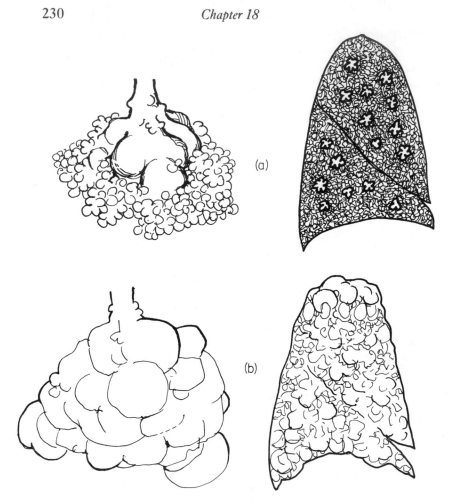

Fig. 18.3. *Emphysema.* Diagrammatic view of lobule and whole lung section in (a) centrilobular and (b) panacinar emphysema.

CLINICO-PATHOLOGICAL RELATIONSHIPS

Centrilobular emphysema of modest extent is very common and not necessarily associated with disability. More severe degrees are associated with prominent bronchitic symptoms, disturbance of ventilation—perfusion relationships and hypoxia. This may be due to the relatively well-preserved blood supply to the badly-ventilated alveoli beyond the damaged zone.

Severe panacinar emphysema is less common. The elastic network of the normal lung is badly disorganised, the lung becomes floppy leading to a severe degree of airways obstruction particularly during expiration. Changes in the blood gases tend to be less drastic, perhaps because the blood supply in damaged areas is reduced in proportion to the reduced ventilation to these areas. Ventilatory drive is generally better preserved than in cases with severe centrilobular emphysema. It is tempting to associate the 'pink puffer' with panacinar emphysema and the 'blue bloater' with centrilobular emphysema; available evidence suggests that this is an oversimplification but that some sort of loose relationship may exist.

Which patients have emphysema?

CENTRILOBULAR EMPHYSEMA

There are no helpful clinical or radiological features which allow the diagnosis of centrilobular emphysema although there are clinical situations in which its presence may be suspected.

PANACINAR EMPHYSEMA

Clinical

Most of the hallowed signs of emphysema are merely those of over-inflation which may accompany airways obstruction of any sort. Emphysema may be suspected when the features of Type A are encountered (Fig. 18.1).

Radiological

The following features are strongly suggestive of severe panacinar emphysema:

1 Bullae evident on chest X-ray.
2 Deficiency of blood vessel markings in the peripheral half of the lung fields in most areas seen on PA chest X-ray compared with relatively easily seen more proximal vessels.

These features will often be accompanied by evidence of severe overinflation—low flattened diaphragms on the PA field and a large retrosternal air-space on the lateral film.

Note

1 When interpreting a reported radiological diagnosis of emphysema it is important to know the criteria used by the radiologist. Many radiologists equate the signs of mere overinflation with the presence of

emphysema and such signs can be completely reversible if the patient has asthma.

2   Radiological diagnosis of panacinar emphysema is only possible when the disease is advanced.

3   Widespread emphysema of any type may be present despite a normal chest X-ray.

Management of chronic obstructive lung disease

Smoking

Patients should always be urged to stop smoking even when they insist that it helps them to produce sputum. Symptoms of simple chronic bronchitis may disappear but there is often no change in the symptoms in the case of more advanced disease. Smokers with impaired ventilatory performance show more rapid deterioration in performance with age than normals. On stopping smoking the rate of deterioration with age tends to return to approximately the rate experienced by normals. Important improvement in performance is unusual, however, and patients should not be led to expect it or ensuing disappointment may be followed by resumption of smoking.

Detection of unsuspected asthma

A proportion of patients diagnosed as having chronic bronchitis and airways obstruction may show dramatic improvement in respiratory symptoms when treated with corticosteroids—suggesting an unrecognized 'asthmatic' component. It is extremely important that such individuals should not be overlooked.

Trial of steroids
Prednisolone 20 mg daily for a fortnight is sufficient to determine whether or not there is responsive disease. Prednisolone in this dose for such a short duration is virtually devoid of harmful effects and minimal fuss should accompany the prescribing of the drugs; if there is no response then it may be stopped abruptly. A trial of steroid therapy should be carried out at a time when the patient is in a stable state rather than during recovery from an infective exacerbation.

Assessment
Sometimes the response to steroid treatment is dramatic and obvious and there is improvement in symptoms and simple ventilatory tests (FEV$_1$

and PEFR). Sometimes the tests show no change but enquiry reveals that exercise tolerance, nocturnal attacks and morning symptoms are improved. It is useful to give the patient a peak flow meter to record twice daily morning and evening PEFR values before, during and after the trial period. Acute bronchial infection with purulent sputum may inhibit response to steroids Where there is doubt it may be worth repeating the trial after an interval of a few weeks.

Who requires trial of steroids?
It could be argued that all patients who have chronic airways obstruction severe enough to interfere with their daily activities merit a therapeutic trial. It may be more practical to limit such a trial to those most likely to respond. Some obvious features which may suggest asthma are: onset in childhood, substantial periods of normality, a family or personal history of allergies (urticaria, eczema, asthma, nasal obstruction or operations for nasal polyposis), a family history of anything suggestive of airways obstruction. Some less obvious attributes of those who may respond are:
1   *Relatively short duration of dyspnoea.* Individuals dsypnoeic for 5 years are more likely to respond than those dyspnoeic for 25 years (except those with very early onset).
2   *Severe morning symptoms.* The more severe symptoms of tightness and breathlessness in the morning relative to the remainder of the day, the more likely is a response to steroids. Equally significant is the tendency for these symptoms to persist for a perceptible period (usually stereotyped, well recognized by the patient and sometimes up to several hours)—longer than just 'the time it takes to get the phlegm up'.
3   *Presence of eosinophilia in blood or sputum.*
4   *Nocturnal cough and breathlessness.*
5   *Tendency to be worse in summer.* But a tendency to be worse in winter is of little help in forecasting responsiveness.

Pulmonary function tests
These are of little help in forecasting responsiveness to steroids in this group; huge responses to bronchodilator inhalation are only seen in asthma, but lesser degrees of 'reversibility' do not discriminate (p. 172).

Antibiotic and chemotherapy

WHEN?
1   All patients with chronic bronchitis should receive treatment with a broad spectrum antibiotic during infective exacerbations: that is, when

the sputum is persistently purulent (yellowish or green) and increased in quantity above the usual. Antibiotic treatment shortens exacerbations and may prevent lung damage.

2   Treatment should be started promptly. It may be helpful for some patients to have a small stock of antibiotic at home so that there need be no delay in starting treatment.

3   There is no need to culture the sputum in an infective exacerbation unless the patient is gravely ill or the response to treatment is unsatis-factory. If the sputum becomes purulent it is generally safe to assume that the responsible organisms are the pneumococcus and *Haemophilus influenzae.*

4   If the sputum is mucoid in appearance there is usually no need to prescribe an antibiotic whatever the bacteriological results.

WHICH ANTIBIOTIC?
There is little to choose between the following:
1   Amoxycillin or talampicillin 250 mg three times daily *or*
2   Cotrimoxazole, two compound tablets twice daily *or*
3   Tetracycline 250 mg four times daily.
Amoxycillin and talampicillin are related to ampicillin and have the same antibacterial spectrum. They are absorbed about twice as readily as ampicillin and are gradually replacing it where treatment is by the oral route (they are actually absorbed as ampicillin). In high dosage amoxy-cillin and talampicillin (ampicillin) are potentially bactericidal against *Haemophilus influenzae.* Amoxycillin may be marginally more effective and may penetrate sputum and pus more effectively. In severe exacerba-tions or where exacerbations occur frequently in a disabled subject a dose of 500 mg may be given 6-hourly for the first 2 days. This may eradicate *Haemophilus influenzae* from the sputum for some weeks.

DURATION OF TREATMENT
Antibiotic treatment should be continued until the sputum is again mucoid and for not less than 5 days. There is little evidence that long-term treatment with antibiotics is helpful.

Bronchodilator treatment

Oral bronchodilator preparations (e.g. theophyllines) may bring about modest improvement in symptoms and are worthy of careful trial. Even slight amelioration of airways obstruction may be helpful in a disabled patient. There is no need for patients to take regular oral broncho-dilators unless they can demonstrate benefit to their own satisfaction.

The use of aerosol bronchodilators usually produces more effective bronchodilatation. A salbutamol aerosol used in a dose of 2 puffs 4 times daily or as necessary up to 3 hourly may provide valuable relief. The response is much less marked than that obtained in asthma but improvement in FEV_1 of 20% or so can commonly be obtained if higher than standard doses are used (for example, 600 μg or 6 puffs of salbutamol).

Mucolytics

These agents play a minor role in the management of chronic bronchitis. It is rare for patients to notice important symptomatic benefit. Brom-hexine in a dose of 16 mg four times daily may render sputum less tenacious and is worthy of trial in disabled patients who complain of excessive difficulty in producing viscid sputum.

Management of more severely disabled patients

In this group, in addition to measures already mentioned, the treatment of heart failure (p. 275) and the encouragement of radical weight loss in the obese become important. Patients should be encouraged to be active and to undertake regularly such exercise as they are capable of. They may need to be reassured that 'overdoing it' is more of a theoretical than a real risk and that it is not necessary to remain indoors 'to avoid catching a cold' during winter months. Practical measures such as provision of ground floor single level accommodation (or a chair lift), central heating, regular visits by a home help and (in the very limited individual), a mobility allowance to allow regular use of a taxi, may all make a difference to the quality of life.

Immunization of disabled patients against expected epidemic strains of Influenza A virus is usually recommended.

Domiciliary oxygen therapy (see p. 329) may become relevant. Patients who have chronic hypoxia and severe airways obstruction and who have been proved to have stopped smoking may be candidates for long-term near-continuous oxygen therapy which is most conveniently administered using an oxygen concentrator. This may improve well-being and survival.

Management of severely-ill patients requiring admission to hospital

Management comprises:

1   Antibiotic therapy
2   Bronchodilator therapy
3   Encouragement to expectorate
4   Supervision of respiratory failure.

Parenteral antibiotic therapy may be necessary in desperately-ill patients.

Intravenous bronchodilator therapy will be necessary in most instances. Aminophylline is effective and has stood the test of time. It may be given by continuous infusion or by slow intravenous injection over a few minutes. It causes respiratory stimulation, cardiac acceleration and frequently coughing and vomiting. It is desirable to follow intravenous aminophylline with vigorous encouragement to cough. Terbutaline or salbutamol may be given subcutaneously or intravenously as an alternative to aminophylline.

The majority of patients admitted to hospital with a severe exacerbation of chronic bronchitis accompanied by airways obstruction will recover in response to the above measures.

It may be difficult to decide whether or not the patient suffers from chronic asthma (p. 232). Where there is doubt in a severely-ill individual it is reasonable to start intravenous or oral steroid therapy. The relevance of steroid therapy can be critically reviewed during the convalescent phase.

BASIC INVESTIGATIONS

1   *Chest X-ray*
Obvious pneumonia will affect antibiotic policy. There may be evidence of pneumothorax, pleural effusion, malignant disease, etc., all of which may affect management from a quite early stage.

2   *Measurement of P_{CO_2}*
It is important to measure P_{CO_2} using arterial blood or rebreathing method at least once (p. 71).

3   *Measurement of P_{O_2}*
Very desirable if the patient is cyanosed.

4 *Blood urea and serum electrolytes*
Elevation of blood urea will suggest dehydration (common) or renal failure related to severe cardiac failure. Elevation of plasma bicarbonate level will suggest well-established chronic ventilatory failure.

5 *Sputum culture*
This is particularly relevant when the patient is collapsed or pyrexial or has already failed to respond to adequate antibiotic therapy.

6 *Detailed documentation of disability*
Particular care should be taken to obtain details of the extent and duration of the patient's respiratory disability (and his tolerance of it) by interrogating close relatives at the time of admission. The extent to which the patient has been exposed to various forms of treatment should also be noted. If the patient deteriorates a decision on whether or not artificial ventilation should be undertaken cannot be made without this information.

Management of respiratory failure

Respiratory failure is generally regarded as being present when the arterial oxygen tension is low (in round figures below 9 kPa or below 70 mmHg) and the arterial carbon dioxide tension is high (above 6.3 kPa or 47 mmHg). In exacerbations of chronic airways obstruction acompanying chronic bronchitis some degree of respiratory failure is common. Arterial P_{CO_2} is elevated because of reduced alveolar ventilation and arterial P_{CO_2} is reduced partly as a direct consequence of the reduced alveolar ventilation and partly because of regional underventilation (ventilation-perfusion imbalance, see Fig. 2.7(c) and consider Fig. 2.10). Hypoxia is potentially lethal; hypercapnia is intoxicating but not immediately lethal.

THE PROBLEM OF OXYGEN THERAPY
Oxygen should not be given to patients in presumed respiratory failure without a good deal of careful thought; most patients do not need it.

Patients with established respiratory failure who have had a raised P_{CO_2} for some days become unresponsive to the CO_2 stimulus to ventilation and rely increasingly on hypoxia to maintain the drive to breathe. If they are given oxygen to breathe, they breathe less; if they are given high concentrations of oxygen, they breathe very much less. This underbreathing results in increasing hypercapnia which intoxicates and ultimately acts as a respiratory depressant. Oxygen should therefore logically be reserved for those patients with *severe hypoxia*. Unfortunately, patients with severe hypoxia are generally those with a high PCO_2 and CO_2 insensitivity so that:

Patients who really need oxygen often cannot tolerate it
and conversely
Patients who tolerate oxygen often do not really need it.

Who has severe hypoxia?
This may be difficult to decide. The severity of hypoxia depends largely upon:

Arterial oxygen content
Cardiac output
Distribution of the cardiac output (Fig. 26.1, p. 322).

The following points are worth making:
1   Patients in respiratory failure with cor pulmonale generally tolerate arterial hypoxaemia quite well since the cardiac output is usually normal.
2   Cyanosis is **not** an indication for oxygen therapy.
3   Severe hypoxia can be assumed to be present if the PO_2 is less than 4.7 kPa (35 mmHg).
4   There is some evidence that profuse sweating, moaning and grunting may denote severe hypoxia.

Controlled oxygen therapy
If oxygen is required it is required *continuously*. Intermittent oxygen is illogical and more dangerous than either continuous oxygen or no oxygen at all (see Chapter 24).

In established respiratory failure severe hypoxia should be treated initially with 24% oxygen delivered by a venturi-type mask (Fig. 26.3); this may be enough to raise the arterial PO_2 to acceptable levels. However, in severe cases the relief of hypoxia is followed by some fall in ventilation and the PO_2 falls to a level approaching that present before oxygen administration began. The aim is to increase the PO_2 *slightly* accepting that this may mean a *slight* rise in PCO_2. If high concentrations of oxygen are used then underventilation will be extreme before the hypoxic drive reappears.

The likely response to oxygen therapy can be judged from:
1 *Level of PCO_2*. Above 9 kPa (or about 70 mmHg) underventilation will be a problem.

2 *The appearance of the patient.* If he looks as if he has a strong drive to breathe he probably has (Fig. 18.1).

Underbreathing on oxygen may become evident within minutes but it may develop over hours or days with the patient becoming almost imperceptibly more somnolent and less inclined to clear his airways of accumulating sputum. Underbreathing on oxygen can be combated by measures to stimulate ventilation.

Respiratory stimulants
The most effective stimulant is regular encouragement to cough and take deep breaths which can be given by nurses, physiotherapsts, relatives, etc. The patient will generally breathe more effectively sitting up in bed or in a chair rather than curled up.

Doxapram is a useful short-acting respiratory stimulant which is given by continuous intravenous infusion in a dose of 1–2 mg per minute. It may be effective in combating the respiratory depressant effect of oxygen administration discussed above.

Treatment of heart failure
It is usual to digitalize patients with overt signs of cardiac failure, although these signs usually subside without specific treatment once there is improvement in the respiratory failure. Frusemide appears to have a beneficial effect in established respiratory failure with or without oedema.

Avoidance of sedatives
Patients in severe respiratory failure with hypercapnia are frequently confused and very noisy. The temptation to use sedative drugs must be resisted. There is no sedative which does not aggravate hypoventilation.

Arrested improvement
Occasionally patients relapse after an initial period of improvement and they are found to have reached a state of equilibrium with a $P\text{CO}_2$ of about 10.5 kPa (80 mmHg or so). They are seen to be asleep much of the day perhaps having intermittent oxygen and apparently remaining too ill to be got out of bed. In addition to reintroducing treatment with aminophylline and nikethamide or doxapram the following measures may prove helpful.
1 Administration of frusemide 80 or 120 mg twice daily.
2 Complete withdrawal of oxygen.
3 Venesection if the PCV is in excess of 53%.

4   Sitting the patient out of bed.
5   Administration of the carbonic anhydrase inhibitor dichlor-
phenamide 50 mg three times daily.
A proportion of patients will remain in chronic respiratory failure after
recovery with a persistent elevation of P_{CO_2}. The patient will usually be
able to say when he is back to his usual state or better and this end-point
should be heeded.

ARTIFICIAL VENTILATION

The use of intermittent positive pressure ventilation (IPPV) should be
considered when measures described so far fail to prevent deterioration
and:
1   It proves impossible to secure adequate oxygenation;
2   The patient is unable to cough up secretions through stupor or
exhaustion.
    Before embarking upon IPPV it is usual to review the patient's
previous condition. If he has been totally immobilized and in misery
despite adequate trial of available treatments it may not be kind to
restore him temporarily to this existence. Once the decision has been
taken to embark on IPPV, oxygen can be given continuously and endotracheal intubation carried out without undue delay by the most-skilled
person available. During IPPV the patient is sedated and rested and
maintained on oxygen sufficient to keep the arterial P_{O_2} at about 60
mmHg. Secretions are removed by endobronchial suction. Vigorous
mechanical ventilation is avoided because rapid lowering of the P_{CO_2}
may lead to circulatory collapse. Large volumes of intravenous fluid and
dextran are sometimes required at this stage to maintain adequate
circulatory filling as judged by central venous pressure measurement.
Usually at least 24 hours of IPPV is necessary. Attempts to withdraw
ventilatory assistance are made on each following morning. Occasionally
tracheostomy is necessary where recovery is slow and intermittent
ventilatory assistance and tracheal suction continue to be required.

DOMICILIARY OXYGEN THERAPY

Patients who have undergone a severe life-threatening exacerbation of
chronic ventilatory failure may be suitable for long-term near-continuous oxygen therapy (p. 329).

OTHER CAUSES OF CHRONIC VENTILATORY FAILURE

Chronic bronchitis with airways obstruction is overwhelmingly the commonest cause of chronic ventilatory failure.

Pulmonary disease

A few patients with chronic severe asthma (generally incompletely tested) may develop chronic hypoventilation. Occasional patients with severe lung changes associated with bronchiectasis and those in the later stages of cystic fibrosis may develop chronic ventilatory failure, as may those who have had extensive surgical lung resection in earlier life.

Progressive ventilatory failure may sometimes result from a localized obstruction of the airway, e.g. tracheal stenosis. Obstruction of the upper airway by enormously enlarged tonsils and adenoids in small children may lead to unrecognized chronic underventilation.

Restriction of chest-wall movement

Factors other than *obesity* which may restrict chest-wall movement include:
   Severe kyphoscoliosis
   Ankylosing spondylitis
   Pleural thickening and fibrosis due to tuberculosis, tumour or drugs
   Skin changes including systemic sclerosis
   Progressive muscular weakness
   Chest-wall surgery—in particular previous thoracoplasty (a now-outdated treatment for tuberculosis where collapse of the upper part of a diseased lung was achieved by removal of most of the upper 2–4 ribs).

All of the above may occasionally produce chronic ventilatory failure. Where this arises there is commonly evidence of associated airways obstruction. The normal response to the development of airways obstruction is always a degree of compensatory overinflation so that breathing occurs at a higher lung volume. This offsets the obvious effects of early airways obstruction to a remarkable extent. Patients with the above disorders limiting chest size or movement are very seriously penalized if they also develop airways obstruction of even mild degree as they are unable to compensate. It is of more than usual importance that affected individuals should not smoke.

Primary alveolar hypoventilation

This label is used to describe patients with good mechanical ventilatory function who nevertheless underbreathe and consequently show elevation of arterial P_{CO_2} and a degree of arterial hypoxia. Where obesity is a feature the term 'Pickwickian' has been applied. There appear to be three factors which may interact to produce the disorder:

OBESITY

Extreme obesity produces subtle changes in the mechanical efficiency of breathing and in particular a reduction in functional residual capacity (the lung volume at which quiet breathing takes place). This may lead to parts of the lung being closed off for much of the breathing cycle if the closing volume is within the tidal range (see p. 69); local underventilation and arterial hypoxia result.

MINIMAL AIRWAYS DISEASE

A proportion of patients who appear at first sight to have primary alveolar hypoventilation are found to have undetected mild airways obstructon or bronchiectasis on careful investigation.

FAILURE OF CENTRAL DRIVE TO BREATHE

A pure defect of central drive to breathe without obesity or minimal airways disease is rare.

The condition may present with oedema, headache, somnolence and cyanosis. The arterial P_{CO_2} is always elevated, especially during sleep and ventilatory tests yield normal or near-normal results. Patients with this condition show almost no ventilatory response to inhaled CO_2 despite good ventilatory function. They are able to exercise surprisingly well.

Sleep apnoea syndromes

TRANSIENT HYPOXAEMIA IN CHRONIC OBSTRUCTIVE LUNG DISEASE

Nocturnal dips in oxygen saturation are seen in patients with chronic obstructive lung disease (p. 228). Underventilation is one component of these episodes, but the fall in oxygen saturation is greater than would be expected from this alone and presumably some deterioration in ventilation perfusion matching takes place too. This phenomenon is not generally classified as sleep apnoea.

TRUE SLEEP APNOEA

Definition

For convenience this is defined as episodes of complete cessation of airflow for at least 10 seconds and with at least 40 such episodes in a night of 7 hours sleep.

Central sleep apnoea

Airflow and respiratory movements both cease; there is an interruption of central drive to breathe. Sometimes this is associated with degenerative brain disease, brain stem ischaemia, Parkinsons disease or acromegaly. Almost complete failure to breathe when asleep may occur in muscle disease or motor neurone disease. The cause of central sleep apnoea may be obscure.

Treatment is unsatisfactory. Oxygen external ventilatory support or IPPV at night may be necessary.

Obstructive sleep apnoea

Airflow at the mouth and nose ceases but respiratory movement continues. This form is usually associated with obesity and sometimes aggravated by alcohol and accompanying chronic lung disease. The obstruction may be partly due to the tongue falling backwards and partly to failure of pharyngeal musculature to brace the floppy redundant lateral pharyngeal walls during inspiration. Snoring and agitation as the period of obstruction is intermittently overcome can cause disturbance to other members of the household who may complain more than the patient. Drowsiness, headache, polycythaemia, heart failure and evidence of pulmonary hypertension make up the fully developed clinical picture. The diagnosis is readily overlooked, particularly as daytime blood gases may be unexceptional. Treatment is usually based on drastic weight reduction and avoidance of alcohol and sedatives. Some patients require tracheostomy. Recently treatment with continuous nasal positive pressure (by blowing air through a mould applied to the nostrils) has been shown to be effective, although not all patients can tolerate it.

Mixed types

Some patients show clear obstruction as well as phases of absent breathing movement.

CHAPTER 19 / CARCINOMA OF THE BRONCHUS

Incidence

About 35 000 people die from carcinoma of the bronchus in the UK each year. Half of these deaths occur before the age of 65. The incidence has risen progressively since the beginning of the century—partly because it was frequently misdiagnosed as tuberculosis in earlier years but probably largely because of the increase in smoking. It is about five times more common in men than women. The rate of increase in mortality rate for men is slowing down and the mortality rate for men under 65 is beginning to fall, but that for women continues to rise; women are catching up.

Aetiology

SMOKING

There is now an overwhelming body of evidence which indicates that cigarette smoking is the major cause of bronchial carcinoma.

1   The rise in deaths from carcinoma of the bronchus has reflected increasing exposure to cigarette smoking over the past 50 years, particularly when the two sexes are studied separately.

2   The risk of death from bronchial carcinoma increases by a factor roughly equal to the number of cigarettes smoked per day. That is to say that an individual smoking 25 cigarettes daily has about 25 times greater chance of dying from the disease than a non-smoker of the same age and sex. For some subgroups the relative risk is even higher; for example, in men smoking unfiltered cigarettes the risk of smoking between 30 and 40 cigarettes daily is about 80 times that of a non-smoker.

3   The risk of bronchial carcinoma is greatest in those who inhale cigarette smoke.

4   The risk of dying from bronchial carcinoma falls off dramatically if cigarette smoking stops. (The excess risk is approximately halved every 5 years after stopping smoking.) Pipe and cigar smokers have a slightly increased risk of bronchial carcinoma which is very much smaller than that of cigarette smokers.

The strength of the association between cigarette smoking and bronchial carcinoma tends to swamp other factors.

Urbanization

The incidence of bronchial carcinoma is greater in urban than in rural areas, even when cigarette smoking is allowed for. Atmospheric pollution is regarded as the most likely explanation of this difference but the relationship is poorly defined.

Occupational factors

Occupational factors appear to play a relatively small part in the causation of the disease but there is nevertheless good evidence that industrial exposure to chromates, haematite, nickel, carbonyl, arsenic, coal gas and radioactive gases is associated with an increased risk of bronchial carcinoma. Carcinoma of the bronchus may complicate established asbestosis (p. 312).

Pathology

CELL TYPES

Four main types of carcinoma may be distinguished (Fig. 19.1). Sometimes histological classification proves difficult. The cell type has some

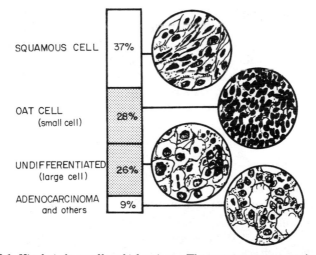

SQUAMOUS CELL	37%
OAT CELL (small cell)	28%
UNDIFFERENTIATED (large cell)	26%
ADENOCARCINOMA and others	9%

Fig. 19.1. *Histological types of bronchial carcinoma.* The percentages are approximate. Oat cell and undifferentiated large cell carcinoma are sometimes grouped together in a single 'undifferentiated' or 'anaplastic' category. Typing is often difficult owing to variation in histological appearances between different parts of the same tumour.

relationship to the pattern of growth and response to treatment. Probably the most important histological distinction is into two groups: small cell carcinoma and non-small cell carcinoma.

Small cell carcinoma. This develops from the Kulchitsky cells of the bronchial wall. These have endocrinological potential which is sometimes manifest clinically. The tumours develop rapidly and become generalized very early in their course so that surgery is almost never curative. Untreated, small cell carcinomas have a very short median survival of 2–3 months but they have been shown to be importantly susceptible to chemotherapy. The treatment of choice in virtually all small cell carcinomas is thus combination chemotherapy, whereas in other forms of bronchial carcinoma chemotherapy plays a rather minor role.

Non-small cell carcinoma. This group comprises all other types including principally squamous cell carcinoma and adenocarcinoma. The treatment of choice in this group is surgical removal whenever practicable. A proportion of squamous cell carcinomas tend to grow more slowly and metastasize later than the other varieties. Adenocarcinomas appear not to be related to smoking exposure.

SITE OF ORIGIN AND SPREAD

The majority of carcinomas originate in the larger bronchi and about two-thirds are visible on bronchoscopy (p. 251). The tumours spread by direct invasion of the lung, chest wall and mediastinal structures and particularly by metastasis to the hilar and the mediastinal lymph nodes.

Blood-borne distant metastasis is common; liver, adrenal gland and brain being particularly favoured organs. At death metastases are present in the great majority of cases.

Diagnosis

CLINICAL FEATURES

Bronchial carcinoma presents in a wide variety of ways. Commonly there are symptoms and clinical features relating to the chest but the disease may present with metastatic complications or non-metastatic neuro-endocrine syndromes or because of non-specific symptoms such as malaise and weight loss.

Chest symptoms

Cough. Chronic bronchitis is usually present anyway but a persistent aggravation of cough may be the first feature of carcinoma.

Dyspnoea. Usually this is a late symptom due to collapse of an obstructed lobe or lung, pleural effusion or extensive lymphatic infiltration of the lung.

Haemoptysis is common at any stage of the disease and occasionally massive.

Chest pain. Very common. Sometimes diffuse and poorly localized but tending to be constant. Sometimes well localized and related to chest-wall involvement. Central chest pain may be related to mediastinal gland enlargement.

Hoarseness when it is persistent may be due to involvement of the left recurrent laryngeal nerve by hilar extension of the tumour. (Sometimes unilateral laryngeal paralysis is asymptomatic.)

Chest signs

Commonly there may be no physical signs on examination of the chest.

Lymph node enlargement may be apparent, particularly nodes behind the medial ends of the clavicles.

Signs of collapse (p. 56).
Signs of consolidation (p. 56)
Signs of pleural effusion (p. 56).

A particularly characteristic and sinister sign is *stridor* (p. 47) which usually reflects extensive involvement of a main bronchus or the trachea. Where the tumour arises in the trachea or a main bronchus the resulting dyspnoea may occasionally be confused with that due to diffuse airways narrowing—particularly if the chest X-ray is not obviously abnormal (see pp. 69 and 70).

Clinical situations

Carcinoma is strongly suspected in cases of unresolved pneumonia or recurrent pneumonia and pleural effusion (especially if large, recurrent or bloodstained). There is an increased incidence of bronchial carcinoma in conditions causing diffuse pulmonary fibrosis (p. 202).

Metastatic complications

The range of syndromes encountered is large and includes cerebral tumour, paraplegia, painful hepatomegaly, obstructive jaundice, pathological fractures and bone pain, skin nodules, etc. Some syndromes deserve particular mention.

Superior vena caval obstruction (Superior mediastinal syndrome)
This causes venous engorgement of the upper part of the body with
facial congestion, oedema and headache particularly in the morning.
Examination reveals a suffused facies and static, filled jugular veins with
distension of the veins of the chest and upper limbs. Fine veins around
the chest just above the costal margin are prominent and major collateral
veins may be seen running down the axillae. SVC obstruction is particularly likely to complicate carcinoma near the right hilum. These
cases are inoperable but symptoms of venous compression may be
resolved by radiotherapy (p. 259) or, in the case of small cell carcinomas,
by chemotherapy (p. 259).

Pancoast's tumour
This term refers to carcinoma which extends upwards from the apex of
the lung to invade the structures of the axilla. The lower part of the
brachial plexus is particularly likely to be involved and this produces
distressing pain down the inner surface of the arm.

Horner's syndrome
Involvement of the sympathetic ganglia or the thoracic sympathetic
fibres may result in the production of Horner's syndrome.

NON-METASTATIC EXTRA-PULMONARY MANIFESTATIONS
With the exception of clubbing, these manifestations are uncommon.

Endocrine disturbances
These are most frequently associated with small cell carcinomas. they
include the following:
   Hypercalcaemia. Of obscure causation; causes polyuria.
   Inappropriate ADH secretion. This usually presents with stupor, acute
confusion or psychosis, sometimes accompanied by epilepsy. The
feature may fluctuate. Some patients are misdiagnosed as suffering from
intracranial metastases. A cardinal feature is the very low serum sodium
level.
   Cushing's disease. Bronchial carcinomas may be the site of inappropriate ACTH secretion.
   Melanosis.
   Gynaecomastia.

Neurological disturbances
  Diffuse encephalopathy
  Cerebellar degeneration
  Myelitis
  Peripheral neuritis
  Myasthenic syndrome
  Polymyositis producing proximal weakness and wasting particularly of the trunk muscles
  Dermatomyositis comprising polymyositis with a violaceous telangectatic skin eruption.

These neurological features sometimes appear before there is any evidence of the bronchial carcinoma. They may regress after removal of the tumour.

Thrombophlebitis migrans
Bronchial carcinoma may present like other malignancies with repeated multiple peripheral venous thrombosis. Thrombosis in an upper limb is always suspicious.

Hypertrophic pulmonary osteoarthropathy
This is a rare complication. It presents with dull aching and sometimes swelling of the wrists or ankles. X-rays of the ends of the radius or tibia reveal subperiosteal new bone formation in the form of linear opacities parallel to the outer surface of the bone. Usually it is associated with advanced clubbing. Other disorders which cause clubbing may rarely cause hypertrophic pulmonary osteoarthropathy.

Investigation

In most cases investigation is indicated to confirm the diagnosis as a prelude to considering treatment, and as a means of excluding other treatable alternative diagnoses. In older patients who have little or nothing in the way of symptoms, however, investigation may often be irrelevant to management. If it is clear that because of age or frailty only palliative treatment would be given (and if there are no symptoms this will not be needed) confirmation of the diagnosis may with benefit be deferred until such time as the gravity of the position is starting to become obvious. This may allow the patient some months of normal life unencumbered by premature hopelessness and forboding. Sometimes, however, worry and uncertainty about the diagnosis are themselves the most disabling consequences of the disease and here investigation and

frank discussion of the position may be helpful even if therapeutic
potential is limited.

The chest X-ray usually provides the most compelling early evidence of
bronchial carcinoma. A wide range of appearances is encountered.

Rounded shadow
This is the most common X-ray finding at the time of presentation.
Occasionally the carcinoma is a tiny nodule when first seen. Usually it is
already in excess of 2 cm in diameter and may have a fluffy or spiked
appearance at its border, or there may be radially-arranged shadows
indicating infiltration or patchy collapse peripheral to the mass. Where
there is evidence that a carcinoma is slow-growing or where there is
cavitation a squamous cell carcinoma becomes more probable. Slower-
growing squamous carcinoma may have a relatively smooth contour.
Cavitation within the rounded shadow is common.

Collapse of a lobe or lung
In smoking adults this finding is most usually due to carcinoma of the
bronchus although there are of course many other possible causes.

Hilar or mediastinal enlargement
These changes are usually the result of lymph node metastases. Where
there is evidence of prominent and very rapid growth of lymph node
metastases a small cell carcinoma becomes more probable.

Pleural effusion
Particulary if it is large or accompanied by other features outlined above,
a pleural effusion always raises the possibility of bronchial carcinoma.

Lymphangitis carcinomatosa
This term refers to diffuse spread of carcinoma through the lymphatic
channels of the lungs. Carcinomas of various types, particularly adeno-
carcinomata of stomach and breast, may present this picture especially
after mediastinal involvement. There is usually fairly severe dyspnoea.
The X-ray appearances are of streaky micronodular mottling which is
generally radially arranged and which may be very widespread. The
diagnosis may be made by peripheral transbronchial biopsy (Fig. 19.5).
When bronchial carcinoma is the cause the shadow is usually asym-
metrical and there may be a solid lesion. Localized streaky shadowing

suggestive of lymphatic obstruction or infiltration is common in the immediate neighbourhood of bronchial carcinomata.

No abnormality

The chest X-ray is found to be normal in only a small proportion of patients. In these the lesion is sometimes very tiny (in cases presenting perhaps with remote metastatic syndromes) or situated proximally in main bronchus or trachea. A tumour may lie posteriorly and medially and be obscured by the heart or hilar shadows.

Tomography

Sometimes better visualization of a lesion is possible with this technique. Narrowing of the trachea or main bronchus may be revealed. Tomography is expensive, rarely furthers the diagnosis appreciably and it should not be regarded as obligatory when a localized abnormality is detected on plain films.

Bronchography

This may occasionally be useful particularly in localizing tumours prior to surgery.

HISTOLOGICAL-CYTOLOGICAL CONFIRMATION

The diagnosis may be near-certain from clinical and radiological features alone but an attempt should normally be made to obtain histological or cytological confirmation.

Sputum cytology

The diagnostic yield from cytological examination depends upon the experience and interest of the pathology service and upon the provision of adequate fresh specimens of true sputum. In about half of patients with advanced bronchial carcinoma diagnostic apparances are evident if at least three good specimens are examined. The yield in small peripheral lesions is very low.

Bronchoscopy

Bronchoscopy is usually indicated in suspected bronchial carcinoma. The aim is (a) to obtain histological confirmation of the diagnosis and (b) to assess operability. About two-thirds of tumours can be seen at bronchoscopy and biopsied. The introduction of the fibre-optic bronchoscope has increased this figure, especially in the case of upper-lobe tumours which are particularly difficult to inspect and biopsy with the standard rigid instrument. Bronchoscopy may be omitted in superior vena cava obstruction and in terminal cases where there is no possibility of surgical treatment and the diagnosis has already been obtained by cytological or other measures. Rigid bronchoscopy is generally carried out under general anaesthesia with intravenous agents and muscle relaxants (Fig. 19.2). Ventilation is maintained by venturi entrainment of air with a nozzle injecting high-pressure oxygen at intervals into the bronchoscope.

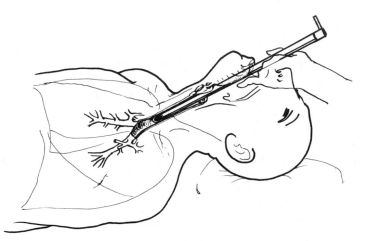

Fig. 19.2. *Bronchoscopy using a rigid bronchoscope.* Depending upon its size, the instrument can be passed most of the way down the main bronchi. Views of the orifices or the segmental bronchi are obtained (with the aid of angled telescopes in the case of the upper lobes). Rather less of the bronchial tree than is shown in the diagram is available for inspection.

The fibre-optic bronchoscope (Fig. 19.3) is now widely used in diagnosis, sometimes passed through a rigid instrument but more usually introduced transnasally in the conscious seated patient using topical anaesthesia. It is convenient, causes minimal upset to the patient and permits improved visualization particularly of the upper lobes.

The following findings all suggest that the lesion may be inoperable:
1   Involvement of the proximal part of a main bronchus particularly the left.
2   Widening of the carina (Fig. 19.4) or tracheal compression from mediastinal lymph nodes and left vocal cord paralysis due to left recurrent laryngeal nerve involvement.

Peripheral transbronchial biopsy

This technique is used for obtaining specimens of lung parenchyma by means of very small biopsy forceps which are passed to the lung periphery through a flexible bronchoscope (Fig. 19.5). It may be useful in the diagnosis of diffuse lung involvement by bronchial carcinoma, alveolar cell carcinoma and by lymphangitis carcinomatosa. Histological material may sometimes be obtained in more localized parenchymal involvement. The technique is useful in the diagnosis of non-malignant diffuse infiltrations and infections of the lung.

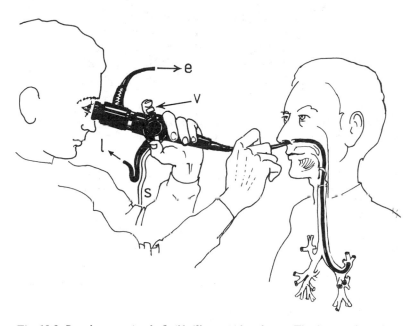

Fig. 19.3. *Bronchoscopy using the flexible (fibre-optic) bronchoscope.* The diagram shows the arrangement for transnasal examination in the conscious subject. The distal tip of the instrument is controlled by a lever which is moved with the left thumb. It can be moved through an arc of about 180 degrees in one plane. The range of movement is extended by rotating the instrument as a whole. The section nearest to the operator's eye is a beam-splitting attachment (Lecturescope, Olympus Optical) which allows a second observer to view the bronchial tree via an additional eye piece (e). The bronchial tree is illuminated by light conducted to the instrument from a mercury vapour light source (l) by fibre bundles which continue to the tip. All but the smallest calibre instruments have a hollow channel. This connects to a suction line (s) by a valve (v) which operates the suction when the finger is applied. Small biopsy forceps and brushes for cytological sampling may also be passed through the channel (see also Fig. 19.5).

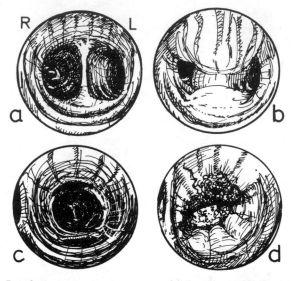

Fig. 19.4. *Bronchoscopic appearance in carcinoma of the bronchus.* (a) Sketch of normal
appearances at the lower end of the trachea showing sharp carina with a view down the
right main bronchus and of the origin of the left main bronchus. (b) The appearances of
mediastinal involvement by tumour in the subcarinal and related lymph nodes with
widening of the carina, bulging posteriorly and anteriorly and narrowing of both main
bronchi. (c) Sketch of normal right intermediate bronchus. (d) Typical appearances of
narrowing caused by tumour encircling the bronchus; there is also tumour occluding the
narrowed lumen and invasion of the mucosa posteriorly. R, right; L, left.

Needle biopsy

Percutaneous aspiration needle biopsy may produce diagnostically useful cytological material from peripheral solid tumours. If such lesions
are large a Tru-cut needle can be used which removes a small core of
tissue. A trephine biopsy may be used in diffuse lung involvement.

In the case of smaller peripheral shadows there may be no need to
persist with attempts to obtain histology because an early thoracotomy is
almost always indicated if pulmonary function permits. Carcinoma is the
commonest cause of small rounded shadows and this group has the best
chance of successful surgical treatment.

Pleural aspiration

When there is an effusion valuable evidence may be obtained from the
cytological content of the fluid. Cytogenetic study of pleural fluid is also
very useful. If stereotyped chromosomal abnormalities are identified in

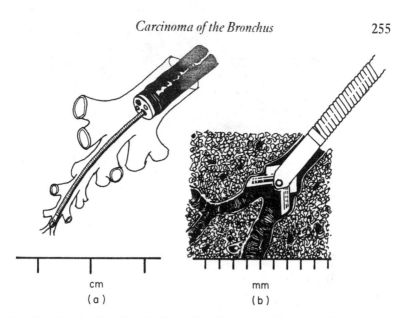

Fig. 19.5. *Peripheral transbronchial biopsy.* A small specimen of lung parenchyma is obtained by passing a long biopsy forceps through a flexible bronchoscope and beyond visual range into the lung periphery until it wedges (a). It is then withdrawn slightly and opened (b). The sample comprises the small tongue of lung tissue between two limbs of a branching small bronchus or bronchiole and it is obtained by closing the forceps as the patient breathes out.

cells obtained from the fluid then malignancy is virtually certain (see p. 294). It is desirable for the patient to roll about and tip head down immediately prior to aspiration, otherwise cells tend to sediment to the bottom and only clear fluid may be aspirated. Pleural biopsy should always be carried out.

Pleural biopsy

The usual technique employs the Abrams punch (Fig. 19.6). This is introduced into the pleural space under local anaesthetic. Where the pleura is greatly thickened good specimens may be obtained with the air-driven trephine.

Mediastinoscopy and scalene-node biopsy

Mediastinoscopy comprises inspection of mediastinal structures, particularly lymph nodes by blunt dissection downwards from the suprasternal notch sometimes using a modified laryngoscope. Biopsy of mediastinal nodes may provide confirmation of the diagnosis (and of

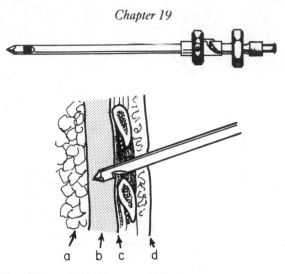

Fig. 19.6. *Pleural biopsy using the Abrams punch.* The instrument is in two parts. The outer pointed sheath has a notch near the tip and carries a spiral groove at the proximal end. The inner cylinder has a sharp cutting edge at its distal end and a lateral peg at its proximal end which fits into the spiral groove. When the two parts of the instrument are rotated relative to each other the spiral groove causes the inner cutting cylinder to close the notch, cutting off any tissue engaged in its mouth.

Below the instrument is shown in position for obtaining a pleural biopsy. After aspirating fluid the instrument is withdrawn until the notch snags on the pleural surface. The cutting edge is then rotated into the closed position and the instrument withdrawn. (a) lung; (b) pleural fluid; (c) parietal pleura; (d) skin surface.

inoperability) prior to radiotherapeutic or chemotherapeutic treatment, particularly when bronchoscopy is negative despite obvious mediastinal or hilar enlargement. Scalene-node biopsy may be performed with the same aim. These techniques are useful when Hodgkin's disease, lymphosarcoma or occasionally sarcoidosis are likely alternative diagnoses.

Liver biopsy
Where there is liver enlargement or jaundice liver biopsy may provide histological confirmation. The yield from this investigation can be improved by carrying out a liver scan and directing the biopsy needle to any accessible 'cold area' which is revealed.

Thoracotomy
In some cases the diagnosis may not be confirmed until thoracotomy is performed. Where all the evidence points to an operable bronchial

carcinoma and there are no major contraindications, thoracotomy should not be unnecessarily delayed as the danger of metastasis increases with every day which passes.

Treatment

The options comprise:
1   Radical surgery
2   Palliative surgery
3   Radical radiotherapy
4   Palliative radiotherapy
5   Chemotherapy
6   Palliative medical and nursing measures
7   No treatment.

Each case will require careful individual consideration and the choice of treatment will be affected by such considerations as extent and type of the tumour, the age of the patient and presence of other (especially cardio-pulmonary) diseases, the nature of the symptoms and also upon the patient's wishes.

1 RADICAL SURGERY

This offers the best chance of long-term survival in non-small cell carcinoma where the tumour is apparently well localized to a lobe or lung and the patient can tolerate the excision. Unfortunately, half of the patients with bronchial carcinoma are unsuitable for resection because of obvious spread to the mediastinum or beyond, or because of co-existent cardiopulmonary disability. Of those who are operated upon half are found to have unresectable disease. Of those in whom the tumour is apparently resected at operation about 25% are still alive at 5 years (Fig. 19.7). The operative mortality is generally 15–20% depending upon how aggressive the selection policy is.

Preoperative functional assessment

Chronic bronchitis and associated airways obstruction frequently accompany bronchial carcinoma and the latter may make resection impossible. No single test permits prediction of feasibility of pneumonectomy and the decision depends on the balance of clinical and laboratory evidence taken in conjuncton with the likelihood of successful removal of tumour. Greater risks are justified in the case of a small squamous cell carcinoma.

The following features are associated with a high mortality and

BRONCHIAL CARCINOMA

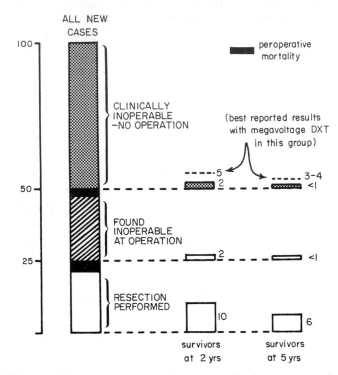

Fig. 19.7. *Operability and survival in bronchial carcinoma.* The figures are approximate and no account is taken of histological type.

intolerable disability after pneumonectomy. An FEV_1 of less than half the predicted value, single-breath transfer factor of less than half the predicted value and evidence of chronic respiratory failure (elevated Pco_2). Exercise dyspnoea of Grade II or worse.

2 PALLIATIVE SURGERY

This is rarely carried out but it may be useful in Pancoast's tumour where severe pain results from involvement of the brachial plexus or in the management of broncho-pleural fistula, severe haemoptysis, etc. Laser treatment is finding a limited place in the palliative treatment of tumorous narrowing of the main bronchi or trachea. Various neuro-surgical procedures such as tractotomy and thalamectomy may be occasionally indicated for terrible pain from other areas.

3 RADICAL RADIOTHERAPY

The advent of megavoltage techniques has allowed larger doses to be given in shorter time and with relatively less unwanted tissue damage. Various techniques exist; most aim at a total dose of 4000–6000 rads over the course of 3–4 weeks. Radical radiotherapy has found its principal application in patients who are in good general condition, but who have inoperable disease which is nevertheless relatively well localized within the thorax. Mean 3-year survival in this group is about 15% in squamous carcinoma and adenocarcinoma and 4% in the case of anaplastic tumours.

4 PALLIATIVE RADIOTHERAPY

This is undertaken for the relief of symptoms. A particular indication for palliative treatment is the presence of superior vena caval obstruction especially when due to non-small cell carcinoma. The obstruction generally subsides dramatically after a few days and usually it does not recur as the disease progresses. Pain due to chest-wall invasion, lymph node enlargement or bone metastases may be susceptible to radiotherapy.

Non-radical radiotherapy does not extend survival. There is thus no reason to subject patients to radiotherapy merely because of the presence of a carcinoma. When the diagnosis is known, however, some patients and their doctors find inaction unbearable and speculative 'palliative' radiotherapy is sometimes prescribed as a result.

5 CHEMOTHERAPY

Chemotherapy is the treatment of choice in small cell carcinoma and is offered to all except the elderly and debilitated. It is fairly demanding and requires full understanding and cooperation on the part of the patient. Three or four drugs are always used together. Those most freuently included are: cyclophosphamide, vincristine, doxorubicin, VP-16 (etoposide) and methotrexate. Treatment is given in pulses at intervals of about 3 weeks and is usually continued for at least 6 months. A variety of schedules has been evolved; all seem to have rather similar rates for the induction of remission. A process of refinement through controlled clinical trial is in progress. Some schedules incorporate radiotherapy to the primary and some include cerebral radiotherapy because of the high incidence of cerebral secondaries in patients who survive the initial phase of chemotherapy. The treatment produces nausea, malaise, alopecia and weight loss together with variable marrow depression.

About 80% of patients show clear evidence of tumour response which, initially at least, is often associated with gratifying improvement in tumour symptoms. Where the tumour is limited to one hemithorax and associated cervical glands (limited disease) about 40% of patients will achieve apparent disease-free remission. Where the tumour has spread beyond these bounds (extensive disease) half as many achieve apparent complete remission. Remission lasts as long as 2 years in about 10% of patients with limited disease and 5% in extensive disease. About 7% and 2% respectively may become 'long-term' survivors of 5 years or more.

6 PALLIATIVE MEDICAL AND NURSING MEASURES

Pleural effusion
Rapidly recurring pleural effusion can be satisfactorily treated in about three-quarters of patients by one treatment with a pleural sclerosing agent. Three methods are in general use involving instillation of either tetracycline, bleomycin or *Corynebacterium parvum.* The purpose in each case is to generate an inflammatory pleurisy. Results are similar in all three methods and are improved if particular efforts are made to aspirate the chest to dryness. A variable degree of temporary pain and malaise may be produced.

General
The patient's principal need from his medical and nursing attendants is their time. Many patients want to talk about what is happening to them and to know more about the way ahead but it may be an impossible topic for discussion unless unhurried opportunities are created.

There is great scope for alert symptomatic treatment in progressive bronchial carcinoma, particularly in connection with cough (which usually responds to methadone linctus if necessary in large doses) and pain (which may require strong analgesics). Where wasting and anorexia are themselves the focus of distress it is worth prescribing a modest dose of oral steroids. In terminal stages if anxiety, pain and dyspnoea are prominent, *regular* injections of diamorphine are usually the most reliable means of producing calm and equanimity without undue sedation.

7 NO TREATMENT
In very old or disabled individuals with few symptoms the discovery of inoperable carcinoma does not usually demand any treatment.

Alveolar cell carcinoma

This rather uncommon tumour arises from alveolar or bronchiolar epithelium and spreads along the alveolar and bronchiolar surfaces. The affected areas tend to become filled with whorls of tumour cells but the essential architecture of the lung parenchyma is preserved in the early stages at least. The tumour shows some resemblance to adeno-carcinomas and may be difficult to differentiate from metastatic adeno-carcinoma from stomach, pancreas, etc. The tumour presents with cough, haemoptysis or non-specific symptoms. Occasional tumours produce a large amount of mucin and, at an advanced stage, the patient may report increasing production of large volumes of glary sputum. The chest X-ray may show irregular rounded or shaggy shadows which are unevenly distributed in one lobe or lung. The tumour sometimes appears to be disseminated or perhaps multi-focal in origin. Mis-diagnosis is common (most usually as tuberculosis) and the correct diagnosis may only become apparent by means of peripheral trans-bronchial lung biopsy or after thoracotomy. Cytological examination of the sputum is sometimes helpful. The tumour is somtimes slow growing and in localized tumours the results of surgery are appreciably better than for bronchial carcinoma. Occasional patients may survive for over 5 years with relatively localized disease. Diffuse tumours do not respond to radiotherapy and are always fatal.

Bronchial adenoma

These uncommon tumours normally present with haemoptysis, cough and sputum and sometimes there is bronchial obstruction with distal collapse. Half may be biopsied at bronchoscopy. The great majority are bronchial carcinoids which are slow growing, locally invasive and which only rarely metastasize. Clinical evidence of secretory activity—the carcinoid syndrome—is rare and suggests the presence of metastases. The majority of the remaining tumours are cylindromata. These tumours are also slow growing and locally invasive but at least 10% show malignant features. The overall mortality amongst patients with bronchial adenoma is of the order of 10%. If there are no metastases evident at the time of the operation and histological examination reveals no atypical features, long-term survival is the rule.

Mesothelioma (see p. 314)

CHAPTER 20 / PULMONARY EMBOLISM AND PULMONARY HYPERTENSION

PULMONARY EMBOLISM

Pulmonary embolism is **important** in that it is potentially fatal, often preventable and sometimes treatable. The mode of presentation depends to a large extent on the size of embolus (Fig. 20.1).

Source

Thrombosis—the systemic veins and occasionally the right side of the heart are the usual source of emboli.

VENOUS THROMBOSIS

A number of factors predispose to venous thrombosis.

1 *Damage to vein wall.* Due to local trauma or inflammation.

2 *Slowing of the circulation.* Immobility, local pressure, venous obstruction, varicose veins, congestive cardiac failure, shock, dehydration, hypovolaemia, etc.

3 *Hypercoagulability of the blood.* Associated with recent trauma, childbirth or operations, thrombocythaemia, oral contraceptives, malignant disease, etc.

Clinical evidence of venous thrombosis
Thrombosis in deep veins of the legs, pelvis or abdomen may be completely silent and be unsuspected until pulmonary embolism ensues (phlebothrombosis). The relative lack of local inflammatory reaction in the vessel wall may result in the clot being only loosely attached. Where there is more local inflammation of the vein (thrombophlebitis) the characteristic features of local *warmth*, tenderness, oedema and superficial venous dilation are more evident and the clot may be more securely adherent. *The severity of the local signs is a relatively poor indication of the risk of pulmonary embolism.*

Confirmatory tests of venous thrombosis
    Ultrasonic probe. Occlusion of major leg veins may be revealed by this means. An ultrasonic probe is placed over a major vein (popliteal or

262

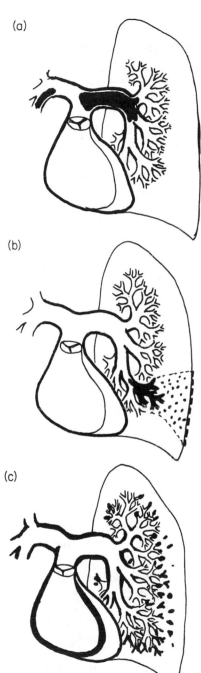

(a) MASSIVE PULMONARY EMBOLISM
Sudden circulatory collapse:
    hypotension, unconsciousness, cold mottled
    periphery. Cyanosis.
Central chest pain.
Hyperventilation.
Engorged neck veins.
ECG Sometimes S_1, Q_3, T_3 pattern.
CXR. Usually unhelpful.
Angio. Shows obstruction.
Scan. Not done.

(b) MEDIUM-SIZED EMBOLI
With infarction
    Pleural pain haemoptysis, effusion, fever,
      hyperventilation.
    CXR. Segmental collapse/consolidation.
Without infarction
    May be 'silent'.
    ? dyspnoea, hyperventilation.
    ? fever.
    CXR may be normal.
ECG. Unhelpful.
Angio. Usually shows obstruction if early.
Scan. Usually reflects obstruction.

(c) REPEATED SMALL EMBOLI
Progressive breathlessness, hyperventilation
? effort syncope.
Clinical features of pulmonary hypertension.
ECG. Right ventricular hypertrophy and axis
    deviation.
CXR. Prominent pulmonary artery.
Angio. May be normal or show slow circulation or
    peripheral 'pruning'.
Scan expected to show some patchy irregularity of
    perfusion.

Fig. 20.1. *Synopsis of pulmonary embolism.*

iliofemoral) and the calf or thigh distal to the probe is compressed. The probe will produce a signal if blood accelerates through the vein beneath and absence of the signal (generally an audible one) suggests venous occlusion. The test is crude but rapid and atraumatic.

Venography. Radiopaque contrast material is injected into a vein on the foot and films taken as it traverses the veins higher in the leg. This technique gives good evidence of major venous occlusion but is time-consuming, expensive and moderately uncomfortable.

I^{125} *fibrinogen.* The isotope is injected intravenously and the uptake in the legs compared with the uptake in other regions of the body. Preferential uptake suggests the incorporation of the fibrinogen into fresh thrombus. The test is very sensitive. Most postoperative patients show some uptake. Large proximal thromboses may be missed.

Clinical features, diagnosis and management

The consequences of pulmonary embolism depend very much upon the **size** of the emboli. Massive pulmonary embolism presents with circulatory collapse. Medium-sized pulmonary emboli tend to cause pulmonary infarction and a 'pneumonic' picture; multiple very small emboli cause gradual obstruction of the circulation and pulmonary hypertension leading to gradually progressive dyspnoea and right heart failure.

These broad categories will be discussed separately.

Massive pulmonary embolism

CLINICAL FEATURES
Massive pulmonary embolism causes its effects by suddenly plugging up the pulmonary circulation producing catastrophic drop in cardiac output. It present with sudden collapse—the patient becomes shocked, pale and sweaty and usually strikingly tachypnoeic. Consciousness may be lost, usually transiently, and there may be fitting. The pulse is feeble and rapid and the blood pressure low, a third or fourth heart sound may be audible. The periphery becomes pale and cold and there may be mottled cyanosis especially in dependent areas. The cyanosis is generally central and may be unresponsive to oxygen administration. Where consciousness is preserved severe crushing chest pain may be present. The neck veins are usually strikingly engorged.

When the circulation is more or less completely arrested death ensues rapidly, and the picture is that of a 'cardiac arrest' and ventricular fibrillation may in fact be present. In this desperate situation there is a notably poor response to external cardiac massage even when promptly applied.

DIAGNOSIS

This is commonly obvious from the circumstances (e.g. associated with postoperative venous thrombosis). The other conditions which often have to be considered are:

1 *Myocardial infarction.* Distinction may be difficult in the early stages especially (when typical ECG changes of infarction might not have developed). Acute right bundle branch block and T-wave depression in V_1-V_4 suggest embolism but *the ECG is often normal.* Excessive dyspnoea without signs of pulmonary oedema may suggest embolism.

2 *Acute internal blood loss.* The most helpful distinguishing feature is the state of the neck veins which will be barely filled, even in the recumbent patient, if blood loss is the explanation for profound collapse and well filled in acute massive embolism.

2 *Acute bacteraemic shock or pancreatitis.* Onset is generally less rapid, there may be evidence of the primary cause and central venous pressure will be low.

4 *Cardiac tamponade.* Tamponade due to pericardial effusion will generally appear more gradually, there may be paradoxical variation of venous (up in inspiration) and arterial (down in inspiration) pressures. Haemopericardium may be due to ruptured myocardial infarction, cardiac surgery, trauma, pericarditis (especially on anticoagulants), and involvement of the pericardium by bronchial carcinoma. Diagnosis of sudden tamponade may be difficult. The size of the heart shadow on a chest X-ray may be helpful. Echocardiography can provide firm evidence of the presence of pericardial fluid.

5 *Dissecting aortic aneurysm* may mimic pulmonary embolism. Sometimes the chest X-ray shows widening of the aorta.

6 *Pneumothorax and massive collapse of a lung.* May produce sudden shock but will normally be identifiable by careful examination of the chest and by chest X-ray.

Where sudden death is averted there is usually some improvement in the patient's condition over minutes or hours attributable to movement of the clot further into one or both lungs.

CONFIRMATORY TESTS

The most satisfactory investigation is pulmonary arteriography which will usually demonstrate the obstructed zone. Lung scanning may be indicated if the patient's condition is good and there is serious doubt about the diagnosis. It is not normally carried out in this situation. A normal lung scan excludes significant embolism. In massive acute pulmonary embolism, hypoxia is almost invariable and hypocapnia usual; normal blood gases make significant acute massive embolism very unlikely.

TREATMENT

1 *Emergency treatment* comprises the administration of oxygen; there is very little else that can be done.

2 *Fibrinolytic therapy.* Where the patient's condition continues to give cause for concern but he is considered likely to survive at least 24 hours fibrinolytic therapy is indicated. Streptokinase or urokinase is administered intravenously and an infusion continued for up to 72 hours. This treatment provokes the thrombolytic mechanisms and greatly accelerates clearing of clot.

3 *Embolectomy* is now rarely carried out but may be necessary where the peripheral circulation fails to be restored after a few hours and hypotension persists. Angiography may be of some assistance in highlighting those individuals who require surgical treatment. Thrombolytic therapy has made embolectomy a rather rare measure.

4 *Anticoagulant treatment.* This is instituted after fibrinolytic therapy is complete.

PROGNOSIS

The short-term prognosis is very variable but about 30% of truly massive emboli prove fatal. The outlook is usually clear within a few hours of the onset and is obviously related to the rapidity of recovery. Commonly an acute massive embolus occurs on a background of several preceding emboli which may have blocked off much of the remaining pulmonary circulation. Anticoagulation reduces the risk of further embolism to about half.

Long-term anticoagulation is not necessary after complete recovery from acute massive infarction. Recurrence of this form of embolism is rare. Long-term outlook is good.

Medium-sized pulmonary emboli

Usually embolization presents with pleural pain perhaps accompanied by breathlessness, fever and cough productive of blood-streaked sputum. There may be signs of pleural effusion and a pleural rub or evidence of localized consolidation. Repeated medium-sized emboliz-ation may occur relatively silently in recumbent ill patients particularly in the elderly. The only clinical feature may be tachypnoea.

The diagnosis depends upon thinking of pulmonary emboli whenever 'pneumonia' is the preliminary diagnosis. Aspiration of the pleural effusion usually yields a modest amount of blood-tinged fluid but sometimes the fluid is clear.

INVESTIGATIONS

The chest X-ray commonly shows elevation of the diaphragm with linear areas of atelectasis in the basal zones but may show no ab-normality. The appearances of bilateral basal shadowing in a breathless patient should always suggest pulmonary embolism if no other cause is evident.

Pulmonary function tests

Nearly always the patient is found to be hyperventilating and the P_{CO_2} is low. Other tests of pulmonary function are not very helpful—there may be increased deadspace ventilation but this is tedious to measure, the normal range is very wide and it is found to be increased in many forms of pulmonary disorder.

The lung scan (V/Q scan)

In essence, the lung scan involves the use of a gamma camera which builds up a plot of the distribution of radioactivity within the lung, firstly whilst the patient breathes a radiolabelled gas which emits gamma rays and, secondly, after injection of radiolabelled albumin which displays the distribution of pulmonary perfusion.

1 *Ventilation images.* Radiolabelled xenon is added to the breathing circuit of a closed-circuit spirometer. As the patient breathes from this apparatus the gamma emission from well ventilated zones of the lungs builds up rapidly. Any less well ventilated zones show a more gradual increase in radioactivity (slow 'wash-in'). At equilibrium the camera image shows the distribution of aerated lung. When the patient breathes in from the room once more there is a wash-out phase which can also reflect the speed of regional ventilation. Very elegant studies can be undertaken using radioactive krypton, which has a very short half-life enabling rapid appreciation of regional ventilation; it is also possible to obtain images in many different projections. In practice it adds little to information obtained with xenon.

2 *Perfusion images.* Macroaggregated particles or microspheres of human albumin are labelled with a gamma-emitting radioisotope (generally Technetium 99^m) and a dose is injected intravenously with the patient lying down so as to minimize the effect of gravity. The particles of the preparation are of such a size that they impact in pulmonary capillaries. (Only about 1 in 1000 capillaries are obstructed and no detectable harm results. The albumin particles are broken down after a few hours.) The patient is seated in front of the gamma camera and an image is built up which reflects the distribution of pulmonary perfusion. Anterior, posterior and oblique images are usually obtained. In the normal the lateral images will show a preponderance of perfusion inferiorly and posteriorly as a consequence of the influence of gravity on the normal pulmonary blood flow in the supine position.

Uses. 'Cold areas' are evident on the scan wherever there is a large area of defective blood flow and this is obviously useful in supporting a diagnosis of pulmonary embolism. Patchy cold areas are common in severe airways obstruction—especially in asthma where they may change hour by hour without any accompanying clinical or radiological changes. Other localized conditions of the lung such as pneumonia or carcinoma are associated with localized defects of perfusion. The lung scan does not differentiate between embolism and other causes of defective perfusion associated with obvious radiological abnormality. It is, however, very useful:

1   If it shows clear areas of defective perfusion which are not the site of obvious collapse or consolidation on the chest X-ray (Fig. 20.2) or of reduced ventilation as judged from the ventilation images.

2   If it shows completely normal distribution of pulmonary perfusion— this is strong evidence against the presence of pulmonary embolism.

Theoretically is might be expected that a ventilation scan would always show striking diminution of perfusion relative to ventilation in the case of embolism and impairment of both ventilation and perfusion in other lung disease. In practice the disinction remains difficult; pulmonary embolism may be accompanied by local reduction of both ventilation and perfusion.

In summary, the evidence which lung scans produce concerning distribution of perfusion must be interpreted in the light of the chest X-ray appearances and the clinical circumstances.

Pulmonary arteriography

If performed within a few days pulmonary arteriography will usually demonstrate embolized zones if they are large enough. The extent to

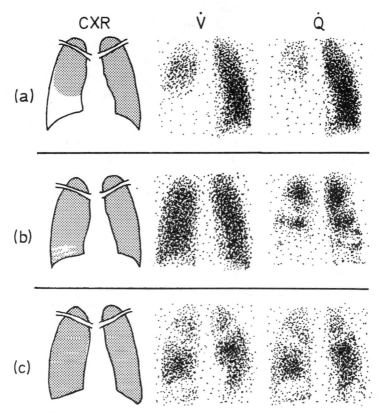

Fig. 20.2. *Diagrammatic representation of the chest X-ray (CXR) appearances together with ventilation ($\dot{V}$) and perfusion ($\dot{Q}$) images obtained with a gamma camera in three patients. Only anterior projections are shown.* In practice posterior, lateral and oblique projections would be obtained for perfusion images (and, less commonly, ventilation images). In the diagram, ventilation images are shown at a stage before complete equilibrium is established.
(a) *Large right pleural effusion.* Ventilation is reduced on the right as expected. Perfusion is also reduced as expected. Even though perfusion seems proportionately more reduced than ventilation, the diversion of blood flow is in keeping with that commonly seen in pleural effusion and the overall distribution of perfusion resembles that of ventilation— there is a 'matching defect'.
(b) *Pulmonary embolism.* In this particular case the chest X-ray shows only trivial changes at the right base. Ventilation is uniformly distributed but there are several major defects in the distribution of perfusion. These are 'non-matching defects'. Such defects are typical of pulmonary embolism and the appearances shown are diagnostic of multiple pulmonary embolism. Radiological shadowing in the lung fields, of whatever cause, is almost inevitably accompanied by abnormality of ventilation and/or perfusion at that site. The interest, as in case (b), then centres on the other radiologically normal areas of lung.
(c) *Severe airways obstruction.* It is common for quite marked regional defects of ventilation and perfusion to accompany severe airways obstruction. The chest X-ray may show only overinflation. Usually the distribution of perfusion and that of ventilation are broadly similar (matching defects) as in (c).

which these investigations are employed in providing confirmation of the diagnosis depends upon the extent to which the diagnosis is in doubt and also upon the condition of the patient. For example, arteriography and lung scanning can hardly be regarded as essential to confirm clinically obvious embolism in the post-operative period or in association with manifest leg vein thrombosis. On the other hand, in a patient being treated for bleeding peptic ulcer it would be important to have the advantage of all the evidence available from special investigations to be absolutely certain that embolism *was* occurring before embarking upon anticoagulant therapy which would carry substantial hazard in these circumstances.

TREATMENT

Immediate
Measures to relieve pain are required in the early stage when pleurisy may be extremely distressing. Opiate drugs are most useful. Anticoagulation is usually obligatory. If the patient is breathless and there are signs of extensive embolism, fibrinolytic therapy may be employed before anticoagulation.

Long-term—how long should anticoagulants be continued?
Where embolism occurs in the postoperative period or in association with an acute thrombophlebitis an arbitrary period of 2–3 months is usually sufficient. Where there is repeated embolism with either long-established venous disorder or with no obvious primary site for thrombosis it may be necessary to continue anticoagulant indefinitely.

PROGNOSIS
Anticoagulant therapy is generally effective in preventing new thrombus formation but further embolism from existing clot is always possible for several days after starting treatment. Usually healing of the lung is near-complete, the affected areas re-expand or contract to linear scars. Sometimes pleural adhesions produce lingering painful tethering of the chest and the vital capacity may be slightly reduced. Haemoptysis sometimes continues for a week or more.

If numerous repeated medium-sized emboli occur, significant obstruction to the pulmonary circulation and pulmonary hypertension may develop (see below).

Repeated small emboli

CLINICAL FEATURES

Very small emboli (microemboli) will go unnoticed until a large part of the pulmonary circulation has become impacted. If repeated embolization continues over weeks or months pulmonary hypertension develops. The outstanding symptom is dyspnoea on exercise which is generally an easy, panting dyspnoea resembling that seen in cardiac disease. Severe pulmonary hypertension is eventually accompanied by clinical ECG and radiological evidence of right ventricular hypertrophy (Fig. 20.3). Tiredness, syncope on effort and angina reflect a critically limited cardiac output. Usually there is no obvious peripheral source of emboli, although many of the patients with this disorder are found to have extensive varicose veins. A proportion of the remainder may follow pregnancy or use of oral contraceptive agents. Rarely tumour emboli (e.g. trophoblastic tumours or carcinoma of the breast) may lead to the appearance of pulmonary hypertension.

INVESTIGATIONS

Electrocardiogram
This will generally show clear evidence of right ventricular hypertrophy (Fig. 20.3 and p. 274).

Chest X-ray
This will generally reveal prominence of the pulmonary arterial conus and proximal pulmonary arteries; there may be a suggestion of undervascularization of the peripheral lung fields.

Pulmonary arteriography
This is generally unhelpful and merely shows dilated proximal pulmonary arteries and a rather slow pulmonary circulation.

Lung scanning
This is similarly unhelpful. There may be relatively poor perfusion of the bases but by the time severe symptoms are present the whole of the pulmonary circulation is involved and regional underperfusion is not seen.

Cardiac catheterization

This is important: (i) the presence of pulmonary hypertension is confirmed; (ii) by measuring wedge pressure, left heart disease (particularly unsuspected mitral stenosis) is excluded; (iii) by measuring the oxygen content of blood in the right heart, a left to right shunt may be excluded.

TREATMENT

Long-term anticoagulant treatment is the only really important treatment apart from anti-failure measures where they are necessary.

PROGNOSIS

The outlook depends upon severity and duration but is generally poor. Once established, pulmonary hypertension is usually progressive. Patients who lack an obvious source for pulmonary emboli fall into the group labelled idiopathic primary pulmonary hypertension.

FOOTNOTE

Postmortem studies have shown that failure to diagnose pulmonary embolism is common. A substantial proportion of patients who die from potentially treatable pulmonary embolism which has not been diagnosed in life have been thought at some stage of the illness to have a psychogenic cause for their breathlessness. The lack of a clear cause for breathlessness in terms of obvious cardiac or pulmonary disorder together with normal simple pulmonary function tests should lead to the suspicion of pulmonary embolism until this is excluded, for example by lung scan.

IDIOPATHIC PRIMARY PULMONARY HYPERTENSION

This rare disorder presents in precisely the same manner as microthromboembolic pulmonary hypertension and usually the cause is unknown. In 1957–59 a large number of cases appeared in central Europe which seemed to be related to consumption of aminorex fumarate—an anorectic agent used to assist weight loss.

The course is almost always progressive and the disease is fatal within a few months or years. Exceptional individuals survive 10 years. Death either occurs suddenly, probably from syncope, or gradually with intractable heart failure. Anticoagulants are generally used because it is virtually impossible to exclude microthromboembolism. Vasodilators such as tolazoline may provide some relief and dipyrimadole may help, perhaps by exerting an effect upon platelet function.

COR PULMONALE

Some confusion arises from the differing ways in which this term is employed. Essentially it means heart disease secondary to primary disease of the lungs. Some (particularly American) clinicians use the term to indicate any cardiac change—especially ECG evidence of right ventricular hypertrophy. Others reserve the term to describe episodes of overt heart failure especially those which accompany chronic airways obstruction with respiratory failure. Pulmonary embolism is not usually included in the group labelled cor pulmonale.

In practice, persons who develop right-sided heart disease have chronic hypoxia in common. In persons with airways obstruction cor pulmonale (however defined) is almost confined to individuals who are chronically hypoventilating and have elevated levels of arterial PCO_2 as well as hypoxia. In diffuse parenchymal disorders such as fibrosing alveolitis cor pulmonale develops at a late stage when there is chronic hypoxia. In this instance the patient is usually not underventilating and the PCO_2 is normal or low until terminally.

Hypoxia is of course a potent cause of pulmonary arteriolar constriction.

Evidence of right ventricular hypertrophy

CLINICAL

1   In the absence of airways obstruction the signs comprise a prominent parasternal heave, a loud pulmonary second sound (the last component of a split-second sound on inspiration) and sometimes a right atrial protodiastolic gallop. In very severe pulmonary hypertension pulmonary valve incompetence and tricuspid incompetence may supervene.

2   Where pulmonary hypertension is secondary to obstructive airways disease, right ventricular hypertrophy is difficult to diagnose clinically because overinflation of the chest almost invariably obscures the physical signs.

ECG

The best evidence is provided by the chest leads—other features merely provide helpful support. Letters in brackets refer to Fig. 20.3.

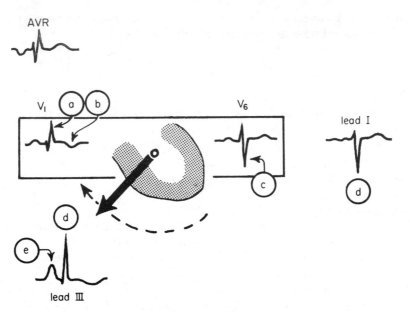

Fig. 20.3. *ECG changes in right ventricular hypertrophy.* The solid arrow represents the mean QRS vector in the frontal plane; it is deflected to the right as indicated by the interrupted arrow. See text for description.

Leads V_1–V_2

The appearance of a QR complex or an RSR' complex in which the upward (R or R') deflection is dominant constitutes strong evidence of right ventricular hypertrophy (a). Widening of the QRS complex is also suggestive; the T wave is commonly inverted (b).

Lateral chest leads (V_5–V_6)

Deep S waves suggest right ventricular hypertrophy (c). Usually this is accompanied by 'clockwise rotation' with the QRS complex becoming mainly positive only in V_5 or V_6 (V_3 or V_4 in the normal).

Other supporting evidence

This may take the form of *right axis deviation* (a mean QRS vector in the frontal plane of greater than 100°—crudely detected by observing the dominant QRS to be directed downwards in lead I and upwards in lead III (d) 'pointing towards each other'). ST depression and T-wave inversion may be present in the inferior leads (II, III, VF). Right atrial hypertrophy may be reflected by *P. pulmonale*—tall peaked P waves with a vertical axis best seen in inferior leads (e).

Treatment

HEART FAILURE

Treatment of overt heart failure is the same as for any form of congestive heart failure and is based upon the use of diuretics. Digoxin is commonly used—particularly for the control of atrial fibrillation.

VENTILATORY FAILURE

Where the cor pulmonale is a consequence of chronic ventilatory failure associated with airways obstruction there may be limited scope for improvement in some cases. More vigorous treatment of airways obstruction by the use of higher doses of inhaled bronchodilators, by the encouragement of radical weight loss and progressive exercise in the obese, together with cessation of smoking and appropriate prompt treatment of infective exacerbations may all help. In the few cases in which cor pulmonale is the consequence of unrecognized asthma, appropriate treatment may be followed over many months by gradual resolution of all of the clinical and electrocardiographic features. Where failure of ventilation is primarily due to muscular weakness or to deformity of the thorax (for example in severe kyphoscoliosis or following thoracoplasty) long-term ventilatory support, particularly at night, may be employed using external negative pressure ventilation (ENPV) by means of a cuirasse which envelops the chest and which is evacuated at intervals by a pump.

HYPOXIA

Reversal of hypoxia is important in the management of overt heart failure; where this arises in the setting of chronic ventilatory failure it is usually necessary to use low inspired concentrations of oxygen together with infusion of a respiratory stimulant (p. 239). Patients with respiratory failure who have suffered an episode of oedema and particularly those who have recurrent or resistant heart failure should be considered for treatment with long-term (near-continuous) domiciliary oxygen treatment (p. 332).

SOME UNCOMMON CONDITIONS AFFECTING PULMONARY VASCULATURE

Pulmonary arteriovenous aneurysm (arteriovenous fistula)

The lesion takes the form of a lobulated swelling connecting pulmonary artery and pulmonary vein. Small or medium-sized fistulae produce no symptoms and tend to be found on routine chest X-ray. Large fistulae may cause arterial desaturation and be associated with telangectasia elsewhere (e.g. nose, causing epistaxis). There is a risk of embolism and cerebral abscess. Surgical treatment is indicated if the lesion is large.

Polyarteritis nodosa

This condition is characterized by arteritic lesions in many organs due to deposition of antigen–antibody complexes in the walls of small vessels. The pulmonary circulation may be involved leading to the devlopment of multiple nodular infarcts which may be evident on the chest X-ray. Polyarteritis is sometimes associated with asthma. The diagnosis becomes evident by virtue of associated arteritic lesions in the skin, kidney or nervous tissue. The ESR is always high and there may be blood eosinophilia. Treatment with corticosteroids is indicated.

Wegener's granuloma

This rare condition is generally regarded as a variant of polyarteritis nodosa. The principal features are: (i) nasal or aural granulomata causing ulceration, crusting, pain and bone erosion; (ii) pulmonary nodules 0.5–1.5 cm in diameter; (iii) renal involvement. The diagnosis may be made from the features described and supported by biopsy. The condition was formerly invariably fatal but prolonged survival is regularly achieved with corticosteroid and immunosuppressive drugs.

Goodpasture's syndrome

The combination of glomerulonephritis and intra-alveolar haemorrhage is called Goodpasture's syndrome. Haemoptysis may be striking or slight and mottling is generally evident on the chest X-ray. Transfer factor may be increased because of the increase in intrapulmonary haemoglobin. The pulmonary lesion may precede the onset of nephritis. Differentiation from polyarteritis nodosa depends on whether there is evidence of arteritis in other areas apart from the kidneys. The distinction may be artificial. The associated glomerulonephritis is generally very severe.

Idiopathic pulmonary haemosiderosis

This rare condition is characterized by treated intra-alveolar capillary haemorrhage of obscure cause. It presents in childhood or young adult life with either anaemia or haemoptysis. The chest X-ray generally shows a miliary mottling pattern. The diagnosis may be confirmed by lung biopsy or by bronchoalveolar lavage, both of which may reveal the presence of large numbers of iron-laden alveolar macrophages. Treatment with corticosteroids is generally tried but may have little effect. Death may follow a massive haemoptysis.

CHAPTER 21 / PULMONARY OEDEMA

In its simplest terms, pulmonary oedema may be regarded as an increase in the fluid content of the extravascular tissues of the lung. Pulmonary oedema may occasionally follow interference with the normal functioning of the pulmonary capillaries and alveolar lining cells by a variety of insults (see p. 285) but much the commonest cause of pulmonary oedema is increased capillary pressure due to impaired performance of the left heart.

PULMONARY OEDEMA WITH RAISED CAPILLARY PRESSURE

PRIMITIVE VIEW OF PULMONARY OEDEMA

Until fairly recently the prevailing view of pulmonary oedema was that increased capillary filtration led immediately to fluid entering the alveoli and that this fluid then caused bubbling sounds (crepitations). This simple model ignores the important effects of the interstitial space and the function of lymphatic channels.

INTERSTITIAL OEDEMA

Electron microscopy has shown that a very thin continuous space exists between the alveolar cells and capillary endothelium and that this space is continuous with the interstitial connective tissue surrounding airways and larger blood vessels in the lungs. The osmotic pressure exerted by plasma proteins drains any fluid from the space so that the space is of negligible size. In the normal situation hydrostatic osmotic and tissue time pressures are nicely balanced (Fig. 21.1a). Increase in capillary

Fig. 21.1. *Pulmonary oedema*. Diagram of an alveolus and pulmonary capillary. (a) *Normal situation:* approximate values for hydrostatic and colloid pressures in mmHg. These forces are in equilibrium or slightly in favour of fluid reabsorption so that the interstitial space is negligible at alveolar level. (b) *Pulmonary oedema*. Increase in pulmonary pressure leads to increased transudation of fluid. Increase in lymphatic fluid transport. At this stage interstitial oedema involves mainly the bronchovascular connective tissue (Fig. 21.2). (c) *Severe pulmonary oedema*. There is now separation of the fluid film from the alveolar surface and intra-alveolar oedema.

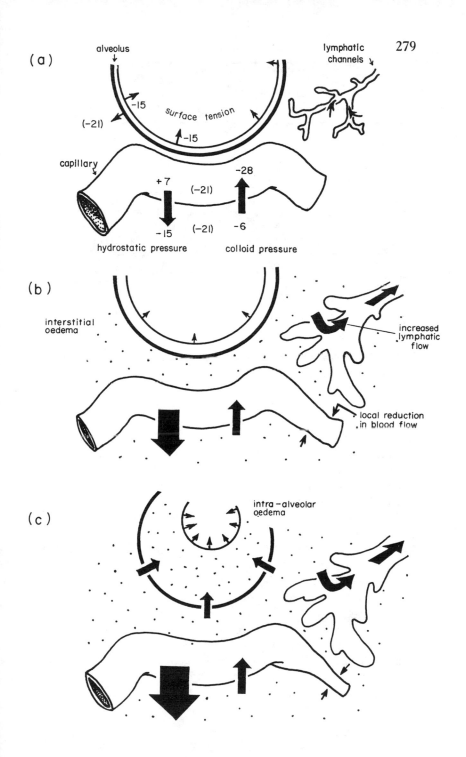

(a)

alveolus

lymphatic channels

−15

surface tension

(−21)

−15

capillary

+7

(−21)

−28

−15

(−21)

−6

hydrostatic pressure

colloid pressure

(b)

interstitial oedema

increased lymphatic flow

local reduction in blood flow

(c)

intra-alveolar oedema

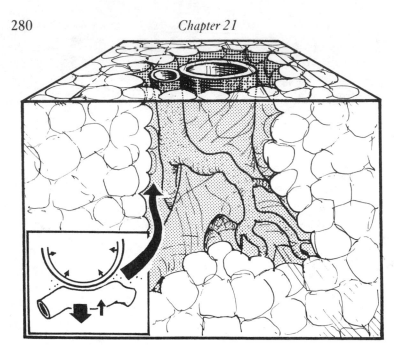

Fig. 21.2. *Diagrammatic representation of the formation of interstitial oedema extending in the form of a 'cuff' around the bronchovascular bundle.*

pressure may cause increased filtration and interstitial oedema which may initially be limited to lymphatic drainage. Further increase in filtration may lead to substantial oedema of the interstitial space. The interstitial oedema extends in the form of a cuff around small airways and blood vessels (Fig. 21.2). This produces important local changes in ventilation and perfusion.

1   Small airways become narrowed by interstitial oedema.

2   The lung tissue becomes firm and non-compliant—less air enters the zone on inspiration; during expiration closure of the airways occurs early leading to the production of rhonchi.

3   On inspiration when the airways eventually open they do so with a click—producing crepitations (p. 54).

4   Reduced ventilation of the firm non-compliant zone leads to local hypoxic and reflex arteriolar constriction and in addition the accumulated interstitial oedema may compress vessels resulting in reduced perfusion to the zone (blood is directed to less affected areas—an appropriate compensation).

5   Defective perfusion may lead to defective local production of surfactant.

6   Distortion of the cuffed bronchiolar/vascular bundles in the lung may cause irritation of vagal sensory endings ('J' receptors) leading to reflex stimulation of ventilation.

Because of the effect of gravity, capillary filtration is always greatest in the lower zones and interstitial oedema, cuffing, crepitations, etc. are all more marked at the base of the lungs. Ventilation and perfusion become directed increasingly to the upper zones.

ALVEOLAR OEDEMA

Further increase in interstitial oedema which overloads the capacity of the lymphatics to preserve a state of balance may lead to alveolar oedema. The surface tension of the lung layer draws fluid into the alveoli (Fig. 21.1c). In doing so the diameter of the alveolar bubble becomes reduced and surface tension increases. The effect of surface tension is to some extent counteracted by the surfactant layer but this may become defective with reduced blood flow. When imbalance becomes severe, fluid may pour into the alveoli and accumulate in the airways. In florid pulmonary oedema pink fluid and foam are coughed up in large quantities.

Symptoms of pulmonary oedema

Shortness of breath is the principal symptom. This may be accompanied by:
   Exercise dyspnoea
   Tachypnoea
   Cough
   Orthopnoea and paroxysmal nocturnal dyspnoea
   Cheyne-Stokes respiration
   Finally, extreme dyspnoea, cyanosis, coughing up of foaming sputum, haemoptysis.
   Mild pulmonary oedema may cause no symptoms at rest but exercise dyspnoea is inevitable. More severe oedema causes breathlessness at rest and often an irritating cough.

ORTHOPNOEA

Typically orthopnoea is present (but also occurs in other forms of dyspnoea).

PAROXYSMAL NOCTURNAL DYSPNOEA (PND)

PND may occur—the patient characteristically wakes in the early hours with wheezy cough and severe dyspnoea. This episode may sometimes be indistinguishable from nocturnal attacks of bronchial asthma. One of the most helpful distinguishing features is the complaint of *morning* tightness, cough and dyspnoea by the asthmatic patient which is generally lacking in the patient with PND due to pulmonary oedema. The precise mechanism of production of orthopnoea and PND is debatable and probably complex but one important factor may be the effect of gravity causing spread of basal pulmonary oedema to relatively oedema-free areas of the lung when the patient reclines, without important improvement in the bases.

CHEYNE–STOKES RESPIRATION

This is waxing and waning ventilation generally with periods of apnoea. Cyclical breathing is commonly present in pulmonary oedema but is rarely sufficiently striking to be remarked upon. It is an expression of unstable ventilatory control due to a slowed circulation time, increased ventilatory drive and hypoxia. Fulminant pulmonary oedema is characterized by extreme respiratory distress with wheezing and commonly a rattling sound on breathing.

CYANOSIS AND THE COUGHING UP OF FOAMY PINK SPUTUM

In this situation ventilation may be impeded and the P_{CO_2} may rise.

Signs

The character of the breathing may be laboured and wheezing or rapid and panting and sometimes with a fine rattling sound audible. In mild pulmonary oedema the only sign may be fine crepitations at the bases. Generally these are mainly mid- or end-inspiratory in timing (p. 54). In some cases widespread fine rhonchi are audible.

There may be obvious signs of the cause of the oedema—particularly mitral or aortic valvular heart disease or cardiac enlargement with the characteristic sustained impulse of left ventricular enlargement. A third or fourth heart sound (or gallop) is a particularly valuable sign when the cause of the dyspnoea is in doubt.

X-ray changes

The heart may be enlarged and pulmonary vessels may appear to be prominent, particularly those to the upper lobes. Mild pulmonary oedema may cause no radiological features. Kerley 'B' lines are very useful evidence of established pulmonary oedema (Fig. 21.3). These comprise short horizontal linear opacities which are found next to the pleural surfaces in the costo-phrenic angles. They are probably caused by dilated lymphatic channels in interlobular septa. Blotchy lung shadowing is common in severe pulmonary oedema. Very striking perihilar oedema may be somewhat fancifully referred to as a 'bat's wing' pattern; it is not of any special signficance. A fine mottling is occasionally seen in persistent pulmonary oedema.

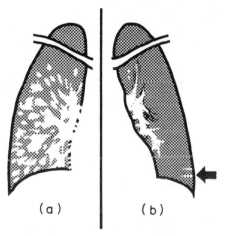

Fig. 21.3. *Radiographic appearances in pulmonary oedema.* (a) Severe pulmonary oedema. (b) Early pulmonary oedema. The arrow indicates the appearance of Kerley 'B' lines. The vascular shadows passing up to the upper zones are more prominant than in the normal resting erect individual.

Functional disturbance

Spirometry usually reveals a restrictive pattern of ventilatory impairment but prolonged respiratory time and reduced FEV_1/VC fraction are common. Hyperventilation is usual and the P_{CO_2} is low in all but the most severe cases.

Arterial P_{CO_2} is almost always reduced—sometimes to critically low levels—but the reduction is often modest when the radiological extent of the pulmonary oedema is considered (a testimony to the efficiency of the redistribution of the pulmonary circulation away from oedematous underventilated areas).

Treatment

PRIMARY DISTURBANCE

Where pulmonary oedema results from valvular heart disease, renal failure, hypertension or other obvious primary disturbance, special measures will be required.

OXYGEN

Oxygen should be given in as high a concentration as practicable (see p. 325).

DIURETIC

Intravenous frusemide (40–80 mg) is generally very effective within a few hours. Sometimes improvement is dramatic and evident within 15 minutes before any notable increase in urine formation by the kidneys— an effect attributable to a peripheral effect of frusemide causing increased venous capacitance.

DIGITALIZATION

This may be helpful when failing left ventricular function is important, particularly when atrial fibrillation is present with a fast ventricular rate.

OPIATES

Morphia is particularly useful and opiates perhaps act by reducing fear and ventilatory drive and possibly also by inducing relaxation of sympathetically-mediated peripheral vasoconstriction.

EXCEPTIONAL MEASURES

Inotropic agents such as salbutamol or dopamine may be relevant in overwhelming heart failure.

Venous cuffs applied to the arms and legs may improve the situation for a short time in the critically ill patient.

α-adrenergic blocking agents have recently found a place in the management of serious pulmonary oedema, particularly if it persists despite other measures. Phenoxybenzamine and phentolamine are preparations commonly employed. Administration of these agents and of others such as nitroprusside is by carefully regulated continuous infusion. Peripheral vasodilation is induced which improves the effectiveness of left ventricular emptying at the expense of some fall in blood pressure. Use of these agents requires continuous pulmonary arterial or at least central venous pressure measurement and considerable expertise.

IPPV. In patients overwhelmed by fulminating pulmonary oedema intermittent positive pressure ventilation (IPPV) is occasionally life-saving. The principal benefits which follow are: (i) improved clearing of foam and secretions by bronchial suction; (ii) the ability to administer really high concentrations of oxygen continuously if necessary; (iii) the relief of exhaustion and terror by the use of powerful sedation. Some authorities support the use of high inflation pressures throughout the breathing cycle with the aim of 'pushing' fluid back into the pulmonary capillaries. Such measures can, however, cause embarrassment of the circulation as the increased airway pressure is transmitted directly to the pulmonary capillaries (and especially to those in the less oedematous areas).

Less common forms of pulmonary oedema

Pulmonary oedema which is not due to left-sided heart disease is uncommon. It is sometimes helpful to demonstrate that the oedema is not due to raised pulmonary capillary pressure by measuring the pressure recorded by a catheter in the pulmonary artery advanced into the lung until it wedges. It is not always necessary to make this measurement because the nature of the pulmonary oedema may be evident from the preceding circumstances or from features of associated illness.

Lowered plasma oncotic pressure

Pulmonary oedema may develop when the oncotic pressure of plasma is severely reduced due to hypoproteinaemia (e.g. in nephrotic syndrome) but this is unusual without some co-existing increase in pulmonary capillary pressure.

Lymphatic obstruction

Obstruction of the lymphatic drainage of all or part of the lung may produce a degree of local or generalized pulmonary oedema as part of the disturbance.

Increased capillary permeability

Interference with the competence of the capillary endothelial and alveolar lining layers may be produced by the direct effect of toxic agents or by other complex indirect effects.

TOXIC CHEMICAL AGENTS

Amongst these the commonest is acid gastric fluid. A florid form of pulmonary oedema may develop after inhalation of what may seem to be quite a modest amount of fluid. This is sometimes referred to as Mendelsohn's syndrome. Other harmful agents include smoke in those severely affected in fires and certain metal fumes. Harmful exposure to oxides of nitrogen may occur in welders working in extremely confined spaces and in silo-fillers encountering gases given off by stored grain or silage. In all of these forms the oedema may be delayed for some hours after the exposure.

BACTERIAL TOXINS

Some forms of acute septicaemia (e.g. due to gram-negative organisms) may be accompanied by pulmonary oedema. This is particularly likely to occur when there has been severe shock (see Shock lung and ARDS, p. 302).

VIRAL INFECTION

A severe infection by Influenza A virus may occasionally present as acute pulmonary oedema.

NEAR-DROWNING

Pulmonary oedema—sometimes delayed—may develop during resuscitation from near-drowning.

LUNG RE-EXPANSION

Pulmonary oedema may develop in a lung soon after relief of a large pleural effusion or pneumothorax. This is most likely to occur when a large amount of fluid or air has been removed and when the lung has been collapsed for more than a few days.

NEUROGENIC PULMONARY OEDEMA

This is a rare complication of serious intracranial disease (usually cerebral tumour or haemorrhage). The mechanism is unclear but it is known to be mediated via the nerve supply to the lungs. Pulmonary capillary pressure may be elevated.

NARCOTIC OVERDOSAGE

This generally arises as the result of miscalculation by a drug addict and may be produced by heroin or any other member of the opiate group of drugs. Onset may be abrupt or delayed and death may ensue. The mechanism is obscure.

ALTITUDE

Acute-pulmonary oedema may develop in unacclimatized individuals soon after arrival at altitudes in excess of 9000 feet. It is uncommon but can be life-threatening. The mechanism is poorly understood but it may be due to severe pulmonary arteriolar constriction, due to hypoxia, occurring with a patchy incomplete distribution so that an excessive fraction of the cardiac output is forced through a small proportion of scattered unconstricted areas. Pulmonary capillary pressure may be elevated.

Adult respiratory distress syndrome

This is an imprecise label which has been employed with increasing frequency in recent years to indicate respiratory inadequacy developing during severe acute illness or after trauma with the following features: rapid laboured breathing; increasing arterial hypoxaemia despite oxygen administration; generalized need for IPPV. Non-cardiac interstitial and alveolar oedema (with a normal pulmonary wedge pressure and greatly altered capillary permeability) is one component of this disorder, which is described more fully on p. 286.

CHAPTER 22 / PNEUMOTHORAX AND PLEURAL EFFUSION

PNEUMOTHORAX

Air may enter the pleural space from the lung or rarely from the outside as in the case of major chest trauma or thoracotomy. The intrapleural pressure is normally negative owing to the retractive force of lung elastic recoil (p. 12) so that once a communication is established between atmosphere and the pleural space the lung tends to deflate.

Spontaneous pneumothorax

The most common form of pneumothorax occurs spontaneously, usually in previously healthy young males. The source of the air leak is usually a tiny bleb on the surface of the lung near the apex.

The condition usually presents with the development of sudden unilateral pain which may be pleuritic and severe and accompanied by pallor, tachycardia and sweating. Breathlessness may follow if the pneumothorax is large or under tension (see below).

Physical signs

The principal physical sign is **diminution of breath sounds on the affected side**; in the absence of dullness to percussion this is usually most apparent anteriorly in the semirecumbent position. Hyper-resonance is usually unimpressive. Small left-sided pneumothoraces may give rise to a sticky clicking sound in time with the heart.

Chest X-ray

The diagnosis is confirmed by chest X-ray. When the pneumothorax is small a fine crescentic line is found almost parallel to the chest wall outside which no lung markings are seen.

Tension pneumothorax

Tension pneumothorax constitutes something of a medical emergency. It arises in a small proportion of spontaneous pneumothoraces in which

288

the communication between lung and pleural space acts as a valve, permitting air to enter the pleural space during inspiration but closing during expiration. This results in more and more air accumulating in the pleural space which compresses the affected lung to about the size of a hand. The pressure within the pleural space may become positive throughout almost all the breathing cycle. The mediastinum becomes pushed to the opposite side and expansion of the opposite lung becomes impeded. The high mean thoracic pressure begins to impede return of blood to the heart and shock develops. Death may ensue from the combined effects of acute ventilatory and circulatory failure.

Signs

The signs of tension pneumothorax are increasing respiratory distress, tachypnoea and tachycardia and evidence of mediastinal shift as judged by movement of the trachea or cardiac apex.

Treatment

No treatment is required for very small pneumothoraces. There is no need to hospitalize such patients provided they are intelligent and able to return rapidly for attention if worsening symptoms develop. Pneumothoraces in which the lung is less than 2 cm from the chest wall resolve in about 2 weeks.

Usually the pneumothorax occupies more than half of the chest and in this case active treatment is preferable as resolution is otherwise very protracted. Moderate pneumothoraces without tension and without features suggesting significant underlying lung disease can be dealt with satisfactorily by simple aspiration using a fine plastic 'intravenous' cannula, although a proportion prove impossible to aspirate or recur immediately. The technique is enjoying a return to popularity at present but intercostal drainage is still the most usual form of treatment.

Tension pneumothorax demands immediate treatment. An intercostal catheter of rubber or plastic is introduced in the mid clavicular line in the 3rd interspace or in the axilla in the 4th or 5th interspace and connected to an underwater seal (Fig. 22.1). (Some clinicians favour the use of a rubber and plastic flutter valve which is equally satisfactory and permits the patient to be mobile.) Air bubbles out at each expiration or cough and, if the lung perforation has sealed, bubbles soon stop. The fluid level is then seen to swing with each breath from about -3 to -10 cm water. If there is no further bubbling after 24 hours and the chest

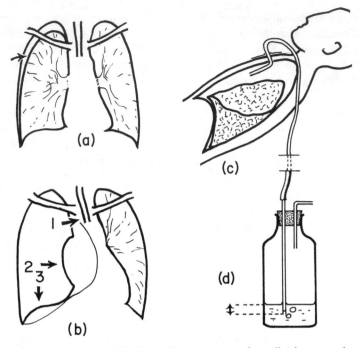

Fig. 22.1. *Pneumothorax.* (a) Radiographic appearances of a small right pneumothorax. (b) Radiographic appearances of a large tension pneumothorax on the right: 1, the trachea and mediastinum are displaced to the left; 2, the right lung has collapsed completely; 3, the diaphragm is depressed. (c) Intercostal tube in place. An anterior position of the chest drain is commonly used in treatment of pneumothorax but a mid-axillary line site is increasingly favoured. Drainage of any associated pleural fluid is assisted and trauma due to introduction is less likely to be important. (d) Underwater seal. The end of the tube is 2–3 cm below the level of the water in the bottle. If intrapleural pressure rises above 2–3 cm H_2O, air will bubble out. If intrapleural pressure becomes negative water rises up the tube, only to fall again when the intrapleural pressure falls towards atmospheric. The system operates as a simple one-way valve. When the pneumothorax has resolved, the water level will generally be slightly negative throughout the respiratory cycle reflecting the normal fluctuations in intrapleural pressure, and when the patient coughs air will no longer bubble out.

X-ray shows complete re-expansion of the lung the tube may be removed.

INDICATIONS FOR SURGICAL TREATMENT

In a few cases bubbling continues for 2–3 days. If it continues surgery is required to remove and oversew the lung perforation. About one in five spontaneous pneumothoraces recur, usually within the first year. If there are further recurrences or if an individual pneumothorax on the other side develops it is usual to recommend pleurodesis.

Pleurodesis

A pleural reaction is then generated with a view to producing fibrous obliteration of the pleural space. Some surgeons favour the use of talc and others favour stripping of part of the parietal pleural. Both methods give reliable security against subsequent pneumothorax.

Pneumothorax accompanying other lung disease

In the older age group pneumothorax most often results from rupture of an emphysematous bulla in an individual with established chronic airways obstruction. In this situation an already disabled patient may be rendered critically ill by a relatively small pneumothorax. Treatment by intercostal drainage is generally satisfactory, but a greater proportion continue to leak air for many days and eventually come to require thoracotomy and excision of the bullae.

A pneumothorax may result from rupture of lung cysts associated with advanced fibrosing alveolitis, other forms of lung fibrosis, eosinophilic granuloma, etc. A lung abscess or carcinoma may break down and lead to the development of a bronchopleural fistula. In this situation a pyopneumothorax is generally present and there is a well established persistent communication with the bronchial tree. Surgical treatment is always necessary.

Bronchopleural fistula

This term merely indicates that there is a persistent communication between the airways and the pleural space via a relatively large hole in the lung tissue. The communication may be with the pleural cavity as a whole as in a straightforward pneumothorax, or with a loculated section of an abnormal pleural cavity as in some empyemata. If a chest drain is inserted the size and permanence of the communication is evident from voluminous and persistent bubbling of the underwater seal. Surgical closure of the leak is almost always necessary.

Hydropneumothorax

This term is used to describe the presence of fluid and air together in the pleural space. The chest X-ray shows a pneumothorax bounded below by the horizontal surface of the pleural fluid. The air may have entered the pleural space from a break in the visceral pleura (e.g. a ruptured bleb or lung abscess) or may have been introduced inadvertently during chest aspiration. A rare cause of gas and fluid occurring together in the pleural space is infection by anaerobic gas-forming organisms, especially *Clostridium welchii*. The gas is usually present in small loculated collections.

Pyopneumothorax

This term describes the same situation as in hydropneumothorax except that there is pus instead of pleural fluid present together with air in the pleural cavity.

PLEURAL EFFUSION

Fluid dynamics

The two pleural surfaces are normally in close contact and the potential space between the two membranes contains only a very thin layer of fluid. Dryness of the pleural cavity is maintained principally by the osmotic pressure exerted by albumin in the intravascular space. Some forces influencing fluid movement within the pleural space are represented in Fig. 22.2. The oncotic pressure of plasma amounts to about 34 cm H_2O. Against this the small amount of protein in the pleural fluid exerts an osmotic pressure of about 8 cm H_2O. The hydrostatic pressure within capillaries tends to contribute water to the space. In the case of the pulmonary capillaries this pressure varies from the top to the bottom of the lung and with pulmonary artery and pulmonary venous pressure, but it is effectively about 11 cm H_2O. In the case of systemic capillaries of the parietal pleura, the mean pressure is probably of the order of 30 cm H_2O. Elastic recoil of the lungs makes the intrapleural pressure subatmospheric most of the time. The intrapleural pressure is influenced by a number of factors such as gravity and breathing pattern, but a mean value of -5 cm H_2O is usually accepted as an approximation in normals. In Fig. 22.2 it can be seen that the resultant gradients at the parietal and visceral surfaces are such that there tends to be contribution of fluid from the parietal surface and absorption of fluid by the visceral surface. In life other influences probably operate. The drying influence of pulmonary capillaries is probably the dominant effect because of the

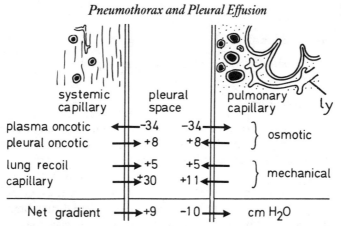

Fig. 22.2. *Fluid equilibrium in the pleural space.* Pressures influencing the movement of fluid are shown in cm H_2O. Positive values indicate forces encouraging entry of fluid into the space (and negative values the opposite effect). All values are crude approximations. Capillaries are profuse in the pulmonary subpleural layers and there is also a rich lymphatic drainage (ly); by contrast the parietal pleura is less vascular and less well supplied by lymphatics.

profusion and superficial distribution of these capillaries compared with those of the parietal pleura. The subpleural layer is very richly supplied with lymphatic channels which exert an active fluid extracting effect.

This analysis is a crude oversimplification of the operative factors, but it does allow an appreciation of the manner in which pleural effusion may accompany certain disturbances. For example:

1 Increased pulmonary capillary pressure secondary to raised pulmonary venous pressure.
2 Obstruction to the lymphatic drainage of a lung—for example, by malignant tumour.
3 Hypoproteinaemia.
4 Increased parietal pleural vascularity accompanying neoplasia.

The discovery of pleural fluid is always important and demands explanation. Pleural effusion may complicate a wide variety of pulmonary conditions but discussion will be limited here to pleural effusion apparently occurring in isolation.

Signs

Factors indicating pleural effusion are outlined on pp. 56–57.

Radiological features

Features apparent in radiology are outlined on p. 93.

Pleural aspiration

Useful information relating to the cause of the effusion can be obtained from pleural aspiration. Heavily-bloodstained fluid suggests pulmonary malignancy unless there is strong suspicion of pulmonary embolism and infarction. Pleural effusions fall into two main groups: transudates which as a rule accompany generalized oedematous states, and exudates which are derived from inflammation of the pleural membrane and adjacent tissues. It is not possible to discriminate between these groups completely, but fluid with a high protein content (above about half of the serum protein value) is likely to be an exudate.

A pleural fluid lactic dehydrogenase (LDH) level of greater than 200 IU or more than 60% of the serum LDH level is also characteristic of an exudate.

Cytological examination of the fluid is valuable if expertise is locally available. The patient should be tipped into various positions immediately before aspiration because cells tend to sediment into the dependent part of the pleural space and may not be sampled on aspiration. A large volume of fluid should be obtained and centrifuged and a smear of the sediment examined.

Cytogenetic. If the cause of the effusion is unknown, cytogenic study is probably the most discriminating procedure for the diagnosis of underlying malignancy. If examination of the fluid reveals dividing cells with an abnormal number of chromosomes, abnormal chromosomes or abnormal banding patterns on the chromosomes, malignancy is very likely. If the abnormality is seen in stereotyped form in a number of cells then an abnormal clone of cells is clearly present and malignancy is virtually certain. Failure to find cytogenetic abnormalities in dividing cells from a pleural effusion is weak evidence in support of a non-malignant cause.

Bacteriological examination is important in the presence of fever after pneumonia or in suspected tuberculosis.

Pleural biopsy. A pleural biopsy should be performed whenever a diagnostic pleural aspiration is undertaken (Fig. 19.6). This technique is particularly effective in the diagnosis of tuberculous and malignant pleural effusions.

Causes (see Table 22.1)

There may be difficulty in differentiating between exudates and transudates in practice.

Table 22.1. Causes of pleural effusion

Transudates (hydrostatic, osmotic)	Exudates (inflammatory, neoplastic)

Cardiovascular
  congestive failure
  constrictive pericarditis
  SVC obstruction
	Malignant
	  bronchial carcinoma
	  metastatic disease
	  mesothelioma
	  Pulmonary embolism

Hypoalbuminaemia
  cirrhosis
  nephrotic syndrome
  malnutrition
	Infective
	  tuberculosis
	  post pneumonic
	  empyema and lung abscess
	Inflammatory
	  rheumatoid arthritis
	  collagen vascular diseases
	Trauma
	  haemothorax
	  chylothorax
	  ruptured oesophagus

From peritoneal cavity (right-sided effusions)
  cirrhosis
  peritoneal dialysis
	Subdiaphragmatic
	  subdiaphragmatic abscess
	  pancreatitis (left-sided)

Although it is convenient for purposes of classification, the division into transudates and exudates is not a rigid one.

Measurement of fluid protein content plays little part in diagnosis.

Pleural transudates

Pleural effusions are common in florid right-heart failure and in constrictive pericarditis. They may less commonly accompany other generalized oedematous states; for example, renal failure or hypoproteinaemic states such as nephrotic syndrome or chronic hepatic failure. Right-sided pleural effusion may sometimes be due to ascitic fluid which may pass through congenital transdiaphragmatic communications on the right side. An ovarian fibroma may cause such a combination of ascites and pleural effusion (Meig's syndrome). Peritoneal dialysis fluid may produce a right-sided pleural effusion.

Pleural exudates

These are most commonly due to pulmonary malignant disease or infection. In the developed world the vast majority of very large effusions resulting in a radiological 'white out' of one hemithorax are due to underlying malignancy. Pulmonary tuberculosis may cause pleural effusion in the early post-primary phase (p. 123) but this presentation of tuberculosis is now rather rare. The effusion is generally large, has a high protein content and contains mainly lymphocytes. Pleural effusion may develop after almost any form of bacterial or viral pneumonia but is not usually massive. The cells may be largely either polymorphs or lymphocytes and the fluid is usually extensive. Persistent recurrence of effusion suggests that a neoplasm may have been the cause of the original pneumonia. Pleural effusion may accompany pulmonary embolism. It is sometimes haemorrhagic; the protein content may suggest exudate or transudate. Acute pancreatitis may be associated with a left-sided effusion. The fluid contains a high level of amylase and the effusion may be in fistulous communication with a pancreatic pseudocyst. A subdiaphragmatic abscess may sometimes result in the development of a 'sympathetic' pleural effusion without fistulous communication.

Pleural effusion is not uncommon amongst patients with rheumatoid arthritis. The effusion is usually small and sometimes asymptomatic. It usually resolves after some months. The diagnosis rests on clinical features of RA and on positive rheumatoid factor. Pleuritic pain and sometimes pleural effusion is one of the commoner features of systemic lupus erythematosus (SLE) in relapse. There may occasionally be underlying irregular lung infiltrations evident on the chest X-ray at this time. The diagnosis rests on other characteristic features of SLE, particularly skin rashes and arthritis, and on the finding of antinuclear factor and LE cells in the blood.

Treatment

The management of pleural effusion naturally depends upon treatment of the primary cause. Malignant pleural effusion may be very distressing and demoralising; treatment is discussed on p. 260.

Empyema

This term signifies the presence of pus in the pleural cavity. Usually it arises after severe pneumonia, rupture of a lung abscess or after thoracic surgery. Rupture of the oesophagus may lead to a left-sided empyema particularly when it is due to invasion by a malignant tumour. Actinomycosis is a rare cause of empyema. Sometimes it progresses to form a discharging chest wall sinus.

Empyema may complicate pulmonary tuberculosis. Whatever their origin, empyemata become the seat of anaerobic infection by a variety of organisms often occurring together.

The patient generally has a high swinging fever and is profoundly ill with high leucocytosis. The collection of fluid is often loculated and difficult to aspirate. The radiological appearances may vary from the usual appearance of an effusion because of fibrous adhesions and loculation.

The management of empyema depends upon antibiotic treatment, drainage and attention to the primary cause. Sometimes decortication (operative stripping of the pleura and pus-filled cavities) is necessary.

Haemothorax

Bleeding into the pleural cavity may complicate:
1 chest injury—especially with rib fracture;
2 rupture of pleural adhesions;
3 pulmonary infarction (usually not massive);
4 anticoagulant therapy especially with (1) or (2).

If massive intrapleural bleeding occurs and the patient becomes shocked, blood transfusion and even emergency surgical exploration to arrest bleeding may occasionally be required.

If repeated aspiration fails to remove the blood clot a fibrinous rind may develop which may become organized, lead to fibrosis and cause permanently restricted movement of the chest. In this situation a thoracotomy may be required for removal of the fibrinous rind.

Chylothorax

A rare phenomenon characterized by the accumulation of lymph in the pleural cavity. It is caused by leakage from the thoracic duct or other major lymphatic channel as a consequence of surgical trauma, other injury or malignant invasion. The chylous effusion reaccumulates rapidly after aspiration. Repeated aspiration leads to protein and lymphocyte depletion. Surgical treatment is required if it persists. Tying of the thoracic duct is generally effective.

Dry pleurisy

Pleurisy is a term used merely to indicate inflammation of the pleura and the characteristic pain that this causes. Any of the conditions which give rise to an exudative pleural effusion may cause dry pleurisy.

Bornholm disease
(Epidemic myalgia)

This uncommon condition is characterized by extremely severe immobilizing pleuritic chest pain and sometimes abdominal pain with variable symptoms of fever and sometimes sore throat. The condition persists for several days before spontaneously resolving. It is due to infection with Coxsackie B virus and the diagnosis may be confirmed by isolation of the virus from the throat or stool or, retrospectively, by observing a rising titre of specific antibody in the serum.

CHAPTER 23 / TRAUMA AND THE LUNGS

Penetrating wounds of the chest

Stabbing and similar penetrating injuries commonly cause a pneumothorax from lung perforation or sucking wound and may also result in intrathoracic haemorrhage. The management comprises infusion of blood and plasma, drainage of the pneumothorax and if there is evidence of continued bleeding emergency thoracotomy. Gaping sucking wounds of the chest may rapidly cause ventilatory failure.

Pneumothorax (p. 288).

Haemothorax (p. 297).

Rib fracture

Fracture of ribs is usually due to a fall or direct trauma to the chest but, in muscular patients with severe airways obstruction and those with oseteoporosis, ribs may be fractured by strenuous coughing. The cardinal sign is exquisite local tenderness. Distressing pain may lead to suppression of coughing and retention of bronchial secretions with subsequent pneumonia. Pain causes splinting of the affected side and progressive lung collapse may occur due to failure to take occasional deeper breaths.

Traumatic fracture

Fracture of ribs is usually due to a fall or direct trauma to the chest.

Cough fracture

Fracture of a rib sometimes develops apparently spontaneously without a history of trauma. Usually there is an association with vigorous or repetitive coughing due to acute tracheobronchitis or an exacerbation of underlying lung disease. Cough fractures are commonest in young women and middle-aged men and are particularly likely to occur in

299

those individuals with severe intractible asthma requiring long-term systemic corticosteroid therapy. The fracture is usually of the seventh rib or a near neighbour and situated laterally or at the angle of the rib.

Pathological fracture

This may be due to a local deposit of malignant disease which may or may not be painful and is sometimes associated with a palpable swelling. Local rib erosion is generally evident on X-ray. Rib fractures due to osteomalacia or osteoporosis are also referred to as 'pathological'; there are usually other clues of bone disease or of the underlying disease causing it.

DIAGNOSIS

The presence of a rib fracture may be revealed during examination of a patient with obscure pleuritic chest pain by compressing the chest laterally (tentatively to start with and never with more force than is required to produce slight movement). This will produce a sharp pain which can the be pursued by a careful search along the likely ribs. The cardinal sign is exquisite and reproducible local tenderness; occasionally—and undesirably—crepitus is elicited.

Acute fracture can be impossible to see on a chest X-ray if there is no displacement—even if special oblique views are taken. The diagnosis is primarily a clinical one. After a few weeks the development of callus at the site provides confirmation.

COMPLICATIONS

Distressing pain may lead to suppression of coughing and retention of bronchial secretions with subsequent pneumonia. Pain causes splinting of the affected side and progressive lung collapse may occur due to failure to take occasional deeper breaths. Rib fracture is a serious event in the elderly and those with advanced chronic obstructive lung disease. Pneumothorax and haemothorax may complicate rib fracture.

MANAGEMENT

A combination of adequate analgesia (sometimes with the help of intercostal block), antibiotic therapy and encouragement to cough and take occasional deep breaths may be all that is required but occasionally tracheostomy with or without IPPV is necessary. Pneumothorax and haemothorax may require drainage.

Multiple rib fractures—flail chest

Massive blunt injury to the chest occurs in car crashes and some industrial accidents and constitutes an immediate emergency. If more than two or three ribs are fractured in two places a substantial segment of the chest wall loses its rigidity and may flap in and out during breathing—this results in very inefficient ventilation and may be enough to cause acute respiratory failure with hypercapnia and hypoxia. IPPV is essential in this situation and, as it is required for a few weeks to ensure splinting of the chest whilst the ribs unite, it is usual to perform an elective tracheostomy at an early stage. In the early hours or days heavy sedation and curarization may be necessary to prevent respiratory distress and excessive displacement of the fractured ribs.

Rupture of the diaphragm

Severe injury to the lower chest or upper abdomen may lead to diaphragmatic rupture which is nearly always left sided. Diagnosis is sometimes difficult and centres on the radiological findings.

Injury to trachea and bronchi

Severe deceleration injury may cause rupture of the lower trachea or a major bronchus. The features which draw attention to the injury are surgical emphysema and perhaps pneumothorax, haemoptysis and lung or lobar collapse. Pneumomediastinum may be detected radiographically. The rupture may be confirmed by bronchoscopy. Large tears require early surgical repair.

Surgical emphysema

This term refers to the presence of air in the connective tissues. Air may enter from a surgical wound—particularly one in the chest and most commonly from an intercostal tube draining a pneumothorax. Sometimes it accompanies a tension pneumothorax when it is presumed air enters from a flaw in the parietal pleura. The phenomenon is sometimes seen in severe asthma (especially in small children) and occasionally during treatment with intermittent positive pressure ventilation. In these circumstances, the leak is thought to occur in some overdistended distal airspace with air tracking back along the bronchovascular connective tissue to the mediastinum. Air may also reach the mediastinum from rupture of the oesophagus.

Surgical emphysema is usually trivial, being detected by a peculiar downy crackling sensation on light palpation and also visible radiographically as air-defined fascial places. Occasionally it reaches alarming proportions with distension of the whole upper trunk, neck and face.

Rupture of the oesophagus

This usually results from trauma caused during intubation, bougienage or endoscopy and is occasionally due to a sharp swallowed object or vigorous vomiting. Rupture is particularly likely to occur if the oesophagus is involved by carcinoma. The rupture may communicate with the left pleural cavity leading to hydropneumothorax or it may communicate with the loose connective tissue of the mediastinum. One consequence of this may be acute mediastinitis, which is a serious condition characterized by collapse, high fever and substernal pain, sometimes with cyanosis and dyspnoea. Sometimes infection can be controlled by antibiotic treatment and interruption of oral feeding. Occasionally a mediastinal abscess or abscesses may form being recognized by unremitting swinging fever, leucocytosis and radiological displacement and widening of the mediastinum. This requires surgical drainage.

Crush injury to the lung

Blunt crushing injuries to the chest, with or without rib fractures, can cause profound pulmonary disturbance over the course of the first few days after injury. Widespread fluffy shadowing on the chest X-ray reflects alveolar haemorrhage and oedema and there is progressive dyspnoea and cyanosis. This sometimes proves fatal despite IPPV and oxygen.

Adult respiratory distress syndrome (ARDS)

This is a term which is used to describe diffuse lung injury which occurs in the course of acute catastrophic (usually non-pulmonary) illness. The term 'shock lung' was used until recently. Severe trauma, septicaemic shock, pulmonary aspiration and overwhelming infections are examples of the circumstances in which ARDS develops; the sufferer has often been completely healthy until the onset of the acute event. Diffuse intravascular coagulation (DIC) is a fairly common accompaniment. The lung disorder becomes evident with progressive rapid laboured breathing and later increasing hypoxaemia which is relatively resistant to oxygen administration. The chest X-ray shows diffuse fluffy or mottled shadowing suggesting pulmonary oedema. The pulmonary venous pressure assessed by wedged pulmonary arterial catheter is normal (unless there are other factors causing it to be raised).

Mechanisms
The nature of underlying mechanisms has not been resolved but is likely to be complex. There are many potential contributory causes for lung injury: inhalation of vomit, fat embolism, thromboembolism, haemorrhage, infection, oxygen toxicity, pulmonary oedema from infusion of electrolyte solutions and blood, and from reaction to blood products are a few broad categories. Impaired production of surfactant and increased pulmonary permeability accompany the disorder.

Management
Management almost always requires establishment of a tracheostomy since intermittent positive pressure ventilation is usually necessary and it may be needed for a prolonged period. It is generally agreed that maintenance of a positive end-expiratory pressure (PEEP) of 5–15 cm H_2O is helpful. Higher pressures may assist lung re-expansion but they impose a resistance to perfusion of the lungs which leads to circulatory embarrassment. Inspired oxygen concentrations are kept to the minimum which will prevent severe hypoxaemia. Inotropic agents with or without peripheral vasodilators may be required to manage circulatory failure. Corticosteroid treatment is commonly given but is of uncertain benefit.

Prognosis
Despite these supportive measures the mortality is about 60%. Paradoxically, pulmonary function may return to normal in those who survive.

CHAPTER 24 / OCCUPATIONAL LUNG DISEASE

The term pneumoconiosis is reserved for a group of occupational lung diseases characterized by a parenchymal reaction (which is usually fibrosis) to inhaled mineral dust. Although this group is the best-known form of occupational lung disease a variety of other reactions to dusts, gases, fumes and vapours are encountered. The character of the lung reaction depends upon the chemical nature of the substance, its physical form and the intensity and duration of exposure and it may also be influenced by the presence of pre-existing lung disease. The clinical features of occupational lung disease are in the main non-specific and the diagnosis depends to a large extent on obtaining a comprehensive occupational history.

Penetration, deposition and clearance of particles within the lung

The distance to which inhaled particles penetrate the respiratory tract depends principally upon their size. The nose is a surprisingly effective 'filter' and extracts almost all particles with a diameter greater than about 20 μm as well as a large proportion of particles which are smaller than this. Particles between 3 and 9 μm in diameter which are not deposited in the nose tend mainly to be deposited in the bronchial tree proximal to the respiratory bronchiole. They may then be removed by ciliary action within 12 hours or so. Particles smaller than 3 μm are most likely to penetrate as far as the alveoli and those of the order of 1 μm are most likely to be deposited there (see Fig. 4.1). Clearance of these particles is effected by alveolar macrophages. These cells are phagocytic and mobile; they engulf deposited particles and transport them to the terminal bronchiole from which they are carried on the 'mucociliary escalator' eventually to be swallowed or expectorated in the sputum. Some particles are toxic to macrophages, in which case transport to the terminal bronchiole is impaired. The particles tend to be liberated and re-engulfed repeatedly by macrophages and particles may accumulate in respiratory bronchioles. A proportion gain entry to the interstitial tissue of the lung and may ultimately be transported proximally via lymphatic channels. (See Fig. 24.1.)

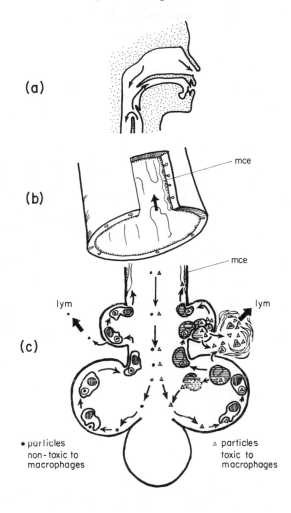

(a)

(b) — mce

— mce

lym   lym

(c)

• particles   △ particles
non-toxic to   toxic to
macrophages   macrophages

Fig. 24.1. *Removal of inhaled particles.* The arrows indicate the routes for disposal of inhaled particles (a) in the upper respiratory tract, (b) in the bronchi and (c) within the lobule. (c) Particles deposited in alveoli are ingested by phagocytic macrophages which migrate towards the terminal bronchiole. Most non-toxic particles (shown at the left) are successfully transported to the mucociliary escalator (mce). Some penetrate the alveolar wall if the inhaled load is heavy and are carried away by the lymphatics (lym). Particles (such as silica) which are toxic to macrophages may be liberated after death of the macrophage and be subsequently re-ingested. The particles may become covered with a proteinaceous coating. Damaged macrophages and particles tend to accumulate particularly in respiratory bronchioles. Coated particles which penetrate the alveolar walls appear to be capable of exciting a fibrous reaction.

Bronchial reactions

Acute tracheitis and bronchitis

These reactions are most likely to arise following rare accidental exposure to irritant fumes or gases or aerosols of irritant liquids (especially ammonia, chlorine).

Occupational asthma

The term is usually reserved for asthma induced by hypersensitivity to an agent encountered at work. Atopic individuals are particularly likely to become hypersensitive but, with higher levels of exposure, non-atopics may become sensitized. A wide range of inhaled substances may cause asthmatic responses. The subject is a difficult one since some irritant substances may cause obvious symptoms in individuals who already have hyper-reactive airways (p. 165) because of asthma. In true occupational asthma the hyper-reactive state develops along with the development of specific hypersensitivity to the agent in question; the agent itself should be known to be capable of sensitization, and disappearance or reduction in the hyper-reactive state can be expected in a high proportion of those who cease to be exposed.

Exposure to the agent in question may be followed by an immediate response (p. 166) or by a delayed response or by both. Where there is an immediate response, the relationship to work and to a particular agent is usually obvious to everyone. Where delayed response is more prominent the relationship may be more difficult to detect. Symptoms may then be worst when the subject is away from work; for example, during the night. Repeated delayed reactions induce a state of continuous asthmatic symptoms in which morning and nocturnal aggravation (p. 163) are more remarkable than worsening at work. The relationship to the work environment may then only become clear when improvement is noted at weekends or during holidays.

CAUSES
Exposure to the following:
Small laboratory animals—the sensitizing proteins are mainly in urine.
Locusts—highly antigenic to laboratory workers.
Proteolytic enzymes— manufacture of enzyme washing powders, brewing.
Grain, flour and contaminants—mites, weevils and mould may be the principal source of antigen.

Colophony—used as a flux for soft solder in the electronics industry.
Di-isocyanates—especially toluene di-isocyanate (TDI), used in manufacture of polyurethane foam, some spray paints which need an activator and in specialized printing, e.g. on plastic surfaces.
Acid anhydrides—used in special paints and adhesives.
Polyamines—used as hardening agents in plastic industry.
Platinum salts—released in refining.
All of the above are recognized as causes of occupational asthma under the UK Industrial Injuries Act; those affected are eligible for compensation for resulting physical disability and for hardship through termination of employment. There are numerous other causes of occupational asthma which are not yet included. These include *wood dusts* and *various pharmaceuticals*.

DIAGNOSIS
The diagnosis rests on an accurate history and an informed assessment of the occupational exposure. Important supporting evidence can be obtained by the use of peak flow recordings at 2 hourly intervals throughout the day, if necessary for a prolonged period. This can be a very subtle method of determining the potentially quite complex nature of the relationship between asthma and working environment (see above). Other evidence may come from skin-testing and measurement of specific immunoglobulin concentrations. Here interpretation rests on knowledge of the prevalence of positive results in other workers and the normal population. Only rarely will diagnosis depend on the result of inhalation challenge testing; this is difficult to do properly as control inhalations and prolonged observation and measurement are necessary.

MANAGEMENT
This is problematical. The simple solution of giving up the job may not be acceptable to the individual because of the economic consequences but, on the other hand, an employer may not be keen to accept responsibility for the long-term effects of continuing exposure. Suppression of the symptoms by treatment may be sought by the sufferer who wishes to remain at work, although the doctor will usually be unable to advise on the likelihood of long-term pulmonary damage through continued exposure with or without treatment. Information on prognosis after stopping work is slender. Roughly half can be expected to lose symptoms completely. Outlook may depend on duration of exposure.

Byssinosis

This disorder occurs in cotton workers employed in the card room after many years of heavy exposure to cotton dust. It is characterized by tightness in the chest and cough occurring promptly on entering the mill particularly after a few days' absence. The symptoms are particularly likely to develop in individuals who already have chronic bronchitis or asthma. There is no parenchymal lung involvement and no abnormalities are evident on the chest X-ray. There is some evidence to suggest that both Type I and Type III reactions may occur in the bronchi in response to an antigenic fraction of cotton dust.

Occupational causes of lung cancer (see p. 245)

Alveolar reactions

Extrinsic allergic alveolitis (see p. 199)

Most varieties of extrinsic allergic alveolitis arise as a consequence of heavy occupational exposure to allergenic dusts, e.g. Farmer's lung.

Humidifier fever

This takes the form of intermittent influenzal symptoms usually unaccompanied by significant respiratory features. It is due to hypersensitivity to the products of microbial growth occurring in the water contained in humidifiers which form part of air-conditioning plants. Air tends to be recirculated in order to retain heat and this encourages build up of organisms in the water as organic dust from the workplace provides nutrition.

Affected individuals develop delayed symptoms which may only ease on stopping work. Radiological changes are not seen. Functional changes are minimal or absent. Serum precipitins against extracts of humidifier water are usually identifiable. The contaminating microbial flora is commonly complex. Legionnaire's disease is another condition which may be propagated by air-conditioning plants (p. 115).

Pulmonary oedema

Acute pulmonary oedema may occur following inhalation of some toxic gases including sulphur dioxide, chlorine and ammonia. The reaction may be prompt or delayed.

Welding yields a variety of oxides of nitrogen and, if it is undertaken in very confined spaces, exposure to the gases may result in the development of acute pulmonary oedema with cough, tightness, dyspnoea, widespread crepitations and radiological shadowing. This may resolve slowly and reappear later, sometimes after an interval of some weeks. Fresh silage yields nitrogen dioxide and workers entering silo towers may develop similar pulmonary oedema which may be delayed in appearance.

Metal fume may cause pulmonary irritation and pulmonary oedema or pneumonia. Cadmium workers may develop severe reactions with subsequent lung destruction. Lesser reactions follow exposure to magnesium, vanadium, zinc and tungsten fume. 'Metal fume fever' is a term used to describe generalized symptoms of malaise which may accompany exposure.

Pneumoconiosis

Coal-worker's pneumoconiosis

There are about 40 000 persons in the UK at the present time with established coal-workers pneumoconiosis. The development of pneumoconiosis is directly related to the total exposure to dust which is determined by the particular working conditions experienced by the individual. Dust exposure varies in different parts of the coal mine and is heaviest at the coal-face. Strenuous efforts have been made to reduce dust exposure during the last 20 years and there has been some reduction in the incidence of new cases. There is an important distinction to be made between the two major categories of coal-worker's pneumoconiosis.

SIMPLE PNEUMOCONIOSIS
This term refers to the accumulation within the lung tissue of relatively small (up to 5 mm diameter) aggregations of coal particles which are fairly uniformly dispersed and evident on the chest X-ray as a delicate micronodular mottling. A series of X-rays is published by the International Labour Office which allows standardized categorization of the

radiological appearances. Numerals (0, 1, 2, 3, 4) are used to indicate the profusion of opacities and letters to indicate size (p, q, r, for rounded opacities and s, t, u for irregular opacities). Examination of the lungs may show localized dilatation of the air spaces immediately adjacent to the aggregations of coal (sometimes referred to as focal emphysema). **Simple pneumoconiosis causes no important symptoms, signs or physiological impairment.** There is to date no strong evidence that its presence influences subsequent health or life expectancy. The benign nature of simple pneumoconiosis is sometimes not appreciated and there is a widespread tendency to attribute almost any respiratory symptoms to pneumoconiosis once simple pneumoconiosis has been recognized from the chest X-ray. An alternative explanation—usually in the shape of chronic bronchitis, asthma or heart disease—should always be suspected in such individuals.

PROGRESSIVE MASSIVE FIBROSIS (PMF)

In PMF, larger opacities are evident on the chest X-ray. The ILO classifications A, B and C are used to indicate opacities of greater than 1 cm in diameter.

A = Sum of diameters of opacities less than 5 cm.

B = Sum of diameters of opacities more than 5 cm but the opacities occupy less than one-third of the area of the right lung field.

C = Greater than B.

Category C is more commonly accompanied by symptoms of breathlessness and detectable physiological impairment in the form of a restrictive ventilatory defect and a variable reduction in transfer factor. On the other hand, extensive PMF may be present without notable symptoms or important physiological impairment. Categories B and C do carry a higher than expected risk of subsequent respiratory illness and premature death.

The lungs contain condensed masses of fibrous tissue heavily infiltrated with collections of coal dust particles. Sometimes the centres of these masses becomes softened and they rupture into the lung tissue. Large amounts of black material may be coughed up and part of the radiological shadowing may be found to have disappeared.

It is not clear why some coal workers develop PMF whilst others equally exposed to coal dust do not. The condition is not closely related to the silica content of the workings or to pulmonary tuberculosis and it may perhaps depend on obscure individual differences in reticuloendothelial function.

CAPLAN'S SYNDROME (RHEUMATOID COAL PNEUMOCONIOSIS)

Coal workers with rheumatoid arthritis may develop multiple nodular pulmonary opacities, usually about 0.5–2 cm in diameter, which may superficially resemble PMF. Usually, however, the nodules are accompanied by only very modest evidence of simple pneumoconiosis and there may be no background stippling at all. Sometimes the manifestations of rheumatoid arthritis are very slight or even absent but rheumatoid factor is always present in the serum. The radiological appearances may sometimes be misinterpreted as being due to multiple pulmonary metastases.

Silicosis

Silicosis is now relatively uncommon because of the widespread recognition of the hazards of respirable silicaceous dust. There is still a risk of harmful exposure in certain quarrying, mining and sandblasting operations. Foundry workers are exposed to silica dust from the sand used in forming moulds. Sand particles become partly fused and adherent to the castings and removal of this material (fettling and blasting) is hazardous. Workers involved in maintaining the refactory lining of kilns and furnaces are also at risk, as are workers in the ceramic industry involved in dry-milling of ingredients or dry-finishing of fired articles.

Clinical features

Simple nodular silicosis, like simple coal-worker's pneumoconiosis, is not usually accompanied by symptoms and may be apparent only from the chest X-ray appearances. With advance of the disease a troublesome cough tends to develop. Advanced nodular silicosis with widespread confluent radiological shadowing or large masses and streaky lung fibrosis is accompanied by increasing breathlessness, a restrictive ventilatory defect and impairment of gas transfer. Another form of silicosis takes the form of diffuse interstitial fibrosis. Occasionally after relatively short but heavy exposure to silical dust the disease may progress rapidly, resulting in widespread fibrosis and honeycomb change within a matter of months (acute silicosis). Silicosis shows a general tendency to progress long after removal from exposure. Silicosis seems to predispose to pulmonary tuberculosis and leads to a particularly vicious fibrous reaction to the infection.

Pathological features

Microscopic examination of silicotic nodules shows them to be composed of concentric whorls of densely arranged collagen fibres showing varying amounts of hyaline change. Silica particles may be found in these nodules as well as within macrophages and the alveoli, where there may be proliferation of adjacent cells. The most proximal alveoli opening off respiratory bronchioles seem to be most heavily involved.

Siderosis

Dust containing iron and its oxides is encountered in haematite mines, at various stages in the iron and steel industry and in welding. It gives rise to a simple pneumoconiosis (siderosis) which produces a striking mottled appearance on the chest X-ray because of high radiodensity of iron, but which is not accompanied by symptoms, signs or physiological defect. Other metals such as antimony and tin may produce a similar picture.

Asbestos

Asbestos is a collective term which refers to a number of naturally occurring fibrous mineral silicates which have found widespread use throughout the civilized world on account of their ability to bind other materials together, and because of striking resistance to heat and corrosive agents. The most important forms of asbestos are:

Chrysotile (white asbestos)
This is a 'serpentine' form of asbestos; the fibres are wispy, flexible and often relatively long. Chrysotile accounts for most of the asbestos used. It appears as a bonding agent in asbestos-cement product—pipes, tiles, roofing materials, etc.—and is also included in asbestos-paper insulating materials and brake-linings.

The amphibole group
These forms have straighter, more brittle fibres. Crocidolite (blue asbestos), amosite and anthophyllite are the most important members of the group. Longer fibres can be carded, spun and made into heat-resistant fabric; shorter fibres tend to be used in other forms of insulation and a filler and reinforcing agents in a variety of plastic, rubber and paint products. Despite its universal presence the great bulk

of asbestos is safely bound within composite materials and important exposure is still largely confined to certain occupations in which actual dust is produced. Amongst those at risk are pipe laggers and industrial plumbers who come into contact with asbestos insulation, and workers in the construction industries who process asbestos-cement products, laminated asbestos materials used in fireproof partitions and sprayed wall coverings. In some industries (e.g. shipbuilding) heavy environmental contamination may result in exposure of other workers.

Consequences of heavy exposure

ASBESTOSIS

The term 'asbestosis' is usually reserved for the description of diffuse parenchymal pulmonary fibrosis. This is only seen after heavy occupational exposure to asbestos; the worker will certainly have been handling asbestos as part of the job and exposure is generally over many (say 10) years; casual or short term contact with asbestos does not lead to asbestosis.

Diffuse fibrosis may be evident on the chest X-ray as a fine basal haziness or mottling, sometimes accompanied by streaky shadows. Clinically the disease presents with cough and slowly progressive dyspnoea which may later be accompanied by cyanosis and clubbing. The earliest clinical sign is usually fine basal crepitations. Tests of pulmonary function reveal reduction in vital capacity and lung compliance and a progressive impairment of gas transfer. The condition may progress even after exposure has ceased.

BRONCHCIAL CARCINOMA

A high proportion of individuals with established pulmonary asbestosis die from bronchial carcinoma. Carcinoma occuring in this situation qualifies for compensation under the Industrial Injuries Acts.

There appears to be an increased incidence of bronchial carcinoma amongst those exposed to asbestos but without asbestosis. Cigarette smoking and asbestos may exert a synergistic effect in its causation.

Consequences of even trivial exposure

PLEURAL CALCIFICATION

Calcified pleural plaques are very common in workers exposed to asbestos and are also found amongst members of their families and those who have had quite trivial exposure. The plaques are visible on the

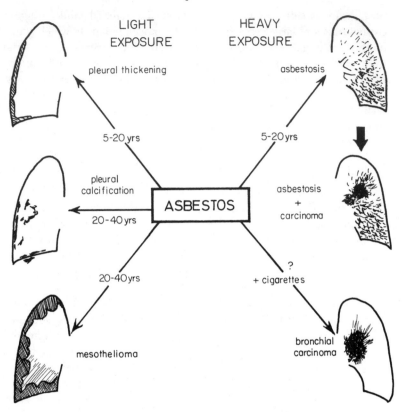

Fig. 24.2. *Pulmonary diseases relating to exposure to asbestos.*

chest X-ray but are quite harmless. They serve as a 'marker' of asbestos exposure and may develop many years later.

PLEURAL THICKENING

Localized or occasionally diffuse thickening of the pleura may be seen with or without notable calcification. Small areas are without effect. Diffuse involvement may be associated with reduced exercise tolerance or even a restrictive ventilatory defect. Sometimes there are strands of subpleural fibrosis extending into the lungs.

MESOTHELIOMA

This malignant pleural tumour is most commonly seen in occupationally-exposed individuals but it is probable that only relatively light exposure is necessary. Mesothelioma generally develops some 20–40 years after exposure. The condition presents with pleurisy and perhaps a small pleural effusion. Progressive pleural thickening follows due to tumour extension and this may show a lobulated appearance on the chest X-ray (Fig. 24.2). Progressive restriction of chest movement and severe persistent chest pain are features of the advanced disease and death follows within a year or two of diagnosis. Metastasis is very rare but surgery is generally useless because of diffuse chest wall and mediastinal invasion.

ASBESTOS BODIES

After deposition in the lungs, asbestos fibres become engulfed by macrophages which deposit a proteinaceous material on their surface. Repeated ingestion, liberation and reingestion probably results in the production of asbestos bodies with their characteristic bulbous ends. They may be present in the sputum and a small proportion may gain access to the interstitium. Asbestos bodies are thought to be produced from fibres of the amphibole group. They serve as another 'marker' of previous asbestos exposure but they are not essential to the diagnosis of the asbestos-related conditions. Asbestos bodies are found fairly commonly in the lungs and sputum in industrial societies.

CHAPTER 25/DRUG-INDUCED LUNG DISEASE

Adverse drug reactions affecting the lung are not common but they are nevertheless important because they are generally avoidable, sometimes dangerous and they can cause diagnostic difficulty. The clinical features may be quite indistinguishable from those of naturally occurring disease if the possibility of a drug-induced effect is not considered.

Drug-induced bronchoconstriction

The most vigorous drug-induced bronchial effects are seen in asthma. The control of bronchial smooth muscle tone and some of the factors involved in the asthmatic process are reviewed in Chapter 15 (p. 157).

PROTEIN PREPARATION

Individuals may become sensitized to protein preparations and develop bronchoconstriction as part of a response on re-exposure. The preparations responsible include:

Antisera produced in animals.

Pituitary snuff used in the treatment of diabetes insipidus (but being superseded).

Skin-testing solutions used in the diagnosis of allergic disorders.

Solutions of antigens used in desensitizing treatment of allergic disorders.

Blood and blood products in transfusion treatment.

PENICILLIN ALLERGY

Acute 'asthmatic' reactions may form part of an anaphylactic response to penicillin; circulatory collapse is usually a more prominent feature. Anaphylactic reactions are rare but very dangerous. Penicillin allergy is much more common amongst asthmatic subjects than amongst others and the possibility of its existence should be constantly considered when treating infections in patients with asthma. All of the penicillins can provoke the reaction in a hypersensitive subject and there is commonly cross-reaction with the cephalosporins and erythromycin and these should also be avoided in severe pencillin allergy.

DEXTRAN

Acute bronchospasm may accompany anaphylactic reactions due to dextran infusion.

CONTRAST MEDIA

Acute 'asthmatic' reactions to contrast media used in X-ray diagnosis are occasionally seen, particularly during intravenous cholangiography. Some authorities recommend pre-treatment with hydrocortisone and antihistamines if contrast media are to be used in cases of severe asthma. Bronchography may cause serious aggravation of asthma.

HISTAMINE

Bronchial hypersensitivity to histamine is one of the hallmarks of asthma, and occasional unintended severe reactions may be seen when histamine is used as a bronchial challenge test or as a test of gastric acid secretion.

CHOLINERGIC DRUGS

Carbachol and related drugs may be used in the management of urinary retention and can lead to aggravation of asthma and other forms of chronic airways obstruction.

BETA-BLOCKING DRUGS

All beta-blockers can produce some increase in airways obstruction in asthma but some such as practalol and acebutolol have a relatively selective effect on cardiac receptors with only a minor effect on the bronchi. Propranolol and oxprenolol are relatively unselective and can cause important aggravation of asthma or other forms of chronic airways obstruction.

PROSTAGLANDINS

Prostaglandin $F_{2\alpha}$ has a bronchoconstrictor effect and subjects with asthma are generally very sensitive to its effect.

ASPIRIN SENSITIVITY

A small proportion of asthmatic patients (but perhaps 15% of severe asthmatics) are extremely hypersensitive to aspirin so that dangerous or even fatal attacks may follow ingestion of a small dose. Aspirin hypersensitivity may accompany any form of asthma at any age but it is particularly seen in those with nasal polyposis and 'intrinsic' asthma and seems commoner in middle-aged female subjects. Patients with these features who do not know themselves to be tolerant of aspirin should be warned never to take aspirin (in any form) or any of the other antipyretic analgesic drugs.

The mechanism of the reaction seems to be related to the suppression of prostaglandin synthesis and it is possible that sensitive individuals are unduly dependent upon the bronchodilator effect of prostaglandins E_1 and E_2. Other non-steroid anti-inflammatory drugs (NSAIDs) provoke asthma in aspirin-sensitive patients. Their ability to provoke a reaction is in proportion to their effectiveness in suppressing prostaglandin synthesis.

TARTRAZINE SENSITIVITY

Individuals who are sensitive to aspirin are commonly also sensitive to tartrazine and other agents used to provide a yellow colour in confectionery, cooking and drug manufacture. Aspirin-sensitive asthmatic patients should be advised to avoid all orange or yellow artificial colouring agents in food.

ADVERSE EFFECTS FROM BRONCHODILATOR AEROSOLS

These effects have mainly been encountered with the use of isoprenaline aerosols. They include: 'rebound' bronchoconstriction, tachyphylaxis, acute overdosage, lowering of arterial oxygen tension and the masking of severe uncontrolled asthma. These adverse effects are discussed on p. 176.

ANAESTHESIA

Wheezing which develops during anaesthesia is commonly due to the reflex effects of mechanical stimulation of the airways, particularly in individuals with airways obstruction. Rarely a very severe bronchoconstrictive reaction may follow administration of thiopentone or succinyl choline. Sometimes the reaction takes the form of acute anaphylaxis with immediate shock and sometimes the bronchial obstruction itself leads to respiratory arrest and subsequent cardiac arrest. Severe or fatal reactions are almost confined to those with asthma, but there is no close relationship between the severity of the asthma preceding anaesthesia and predisposition to adverse reaction.

HYPOTONIC INHALATIONS

Nebulized water causes bronchoconstriction in asthmatic subjects but inhalation of nebulized isotonic saline does not. Hypotonic preparations for inhalation or inappropriate dilution of preparations for inhalation can provoke bronchoconstriction.

Drug effects on the pulmonary vasculature

PULMONARY THROMBOEMBOLISM

There is a small but significant increased risk of pulmonary thrombo-embolism amongst women taking oral contraceptive agents. There is no known means of forecasting this tendency.

OTHER FORMS OF EMBOLIZATION

These include foreign material contaminating infusion fluids and certain forms of oily radiocontrast material, especially that used in lymphangiography.

PULMONARY OEDEMA

Acute pulmonary oedema may be produced by:
1   Over-transfusion or infusion of excessive quantities of intravenous fluid.
2   Hypersensitivity to transfused blood—usually to infused IgA, white cells or platelets.
3   Narcotic overdosage.
4   Rare reactions to phenylbutazone and hydrochlorothiazide.
5   Hypersensitivity to contrast media used in right-sided angiocardi-ography and pulmonary arteriography.
6   Reaction to bleomycin.

Drug-related opportunistic pulmonary infections (see p. 117)

Corticosteroids, antineoplastic agents and other immunosuppressive drugs may predispose to pulmonary infection. This may take a variety of forms of which the following are noteworthy:
1   Pulmonary tuberculosis.
2   Infection by *Pseudomonas aeruginosa* and other gram-negative bacteria.
3   Cytomegalovirus and other viruses such as varicella.
4   Infection by *Pneumocystis carinii.*

Pulmonary infiltrations due to drugs

SYSTEMIC LUPUS ERYTHEMATOSUS (SLE)

Over twenty drugs have been recorded as causing this phenomenon, those most commonly to blame being hydrallazine, procainamide, isoniazid and phenytoin. The pulmonary manifestations include cough, dyspnoea and sometimes pleuritic chest pain associated with patchy pulmonary infiltration and sometimes pleural effusion. SLE follows a more favourable course when secondary to drug administration.

PULMONARY EOSINOPHILIA

Irregular or diffuse radiological shadowing in the lung fields accompanied by a high blood eosinophil count may be produced by reactions to sulphonamides (including salazopyrine and the sulphonyl urea oral hypoglycaemic agents), sodium aminosalicylate (PAS), and nitrofurantoin.

REACTIONS TO METHOTREXATE

This antineoplastic antimetabolite may produce a variety of pulmonary reactions including pulmonary eosinophilia, diffuse pneumonia or patchy pulmonary consolidation.

Pulmonary infiltration leading to fibrosis

Some forms of diffuse drug-induced pulmonary infiltration are followed by fibrosis. Drugs which may cause this include:

Amiodarone, a fairly new and very effective anti-arrhythmic agent.

Hexamethonium, a little-used ganglion blocker.

Busulphan, used in the treatment of chronic myeloid leukaemia.

Melphalan, used in the treatment of multiple myeloma.

Cyclophosphamide, widely used as an immunosuppressive and anti-mitotic agent.

Bleomycin, an antineoplastic antibiotic.

Fibrosis may complicate the pulmonary reaction in oxygen toxicity (see p. 329).

Pleural inflammation

Methysergide, a drug used in the treatment of intractible migraine, may produce a diffuse pleural thickening with or without pleural effusion. Practalol has produced a similar phenomenon but its long-term use has now been discontinued. Pleural effusion may accompany various pulmonary drug reactions especilly those of the SLE type. Haemothorax should be suspected in patients on anticoagulants who present with obscure pleural effusion, shock or anaemia.

Control of ventilation

Any sedative drug may produce depression of ventilation and this is particularly likely to occur in patients with pre-existing chronic ventilatory failure or hepatic failure. Sedative drugs predispose to inhalation of gastric contents in patients who vomit.

Muscular paralysis

Prolonged apnoea and hypoventilation due to muscular weakness may occur in certain individuals who receive succinyl choline and other muscle relaxants. Patients being treated with polymyxin antibiotics are especially vulnerable. The aminoglycoside antibiotics can also produce neuromuscular weakness, particularly where renal failure results in sustained high blood levels. Patients with myasthenia gravis are at increased risk of all the above effects.

CHAPTER 26 / HYPOXIA AND OXYGEN THERAPY

Hypoxia

Hypoxia is ultimately a cellular phenomenon. Mitochondrial activity continues by aerobic metabolism until very low intracellular oxygen tensions are reached (of the order of 0.15 kPa or about 1 mmHg P_{CO_2}) after which anaerobic metabolism appears. This is inefficient and leads to accumulation of lactic acid which is a by-product.

Tissues vary greatly in their susceptibility to hypoxia. Broadly, those tissues with a high extraction rate are the most susceptible (brain, heart). Hypoxia becomes important when:

1   It causes reduction in function of the organ with remote adverse effects which could themselves worsen hypoxia (the positive-feedback situation).

2   It threatens to cause irreversible damage to the organ.

It is often difficult to estimate when these two situations exist. The diagnosis of hypoxia relies heavily on the overall assessment of the factors known to be important in determining the rate of oxygen delivery to the tissues. These factors are summarized in Fig. 26.1.

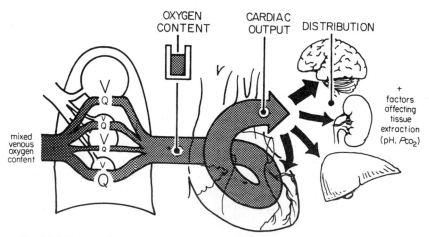

Fig. 26.1. *Factors to be considered in the assessment of hypoxia.*

Arterial oxygen content

This is determined by:
1   Haemoglobin concentration.
2   Factors affecting the shape of the dissociation curve such as pH and PCO_2.
3   Ventilation/perfusion relationships within the lung. When these include an important shunt component the mixed venous oxygen content influences arterial oxygen and venous content is itself determined by oxygen delivery to the tissues.

Cardiac output

Oxygen delivery to the body (or oxygen flux) is determined by:

Arterial oxygen content × Cardiac output

Circulatory impairment is potentially a much more potent cause of hypoxia than pulmonary impairment.

Distribution

Local vasoconstriction or vasodilatation is determined by reflex and local metabolic factors which can have a marked effect on oxygen delivery. The effect can be in the direction of aggravating hypoxia or ameliorating it (for example hypercapnia, hypoxia and hypotension all have a vasodilator effect in the cerebral circulation).

Other factors

Other factors which are of some importance include those affecting tissue oxygen extraction. Increase in H^+, PCO_2 and temperature all shift the oxygen dissociation curve to the right and facilitate the unloading of oxygen.

From the foregoing discussion it should be evident that:
1   **The arterial oxygen content is only one factor which determines the development and severity of hypoxia.**
2   **The only part of the oxygen delivery system which can readily be influenced by oxygen administration is the arterial oxygen content.**

Oxygen therapy

Indications

The indications for oxygen therapy are difficult to define rigidly. Broadly speaking, oxygen should be given when arterial hypoxaemia is an important threat to the patient's security provided that it is safe to do so.

Limiting factors

The two main considerations limiting the use of oxygen are:

1   The danger of inducing hypoventilation in patients with poor respiratory drive who may be relying on the ventilatory stimulus of hypoxia.

2   The danger of oxygen toxicity with the administration of high concentrations.

CORRECTION OF ARTERIAL HYPOXAEMIA

Arterial hypoxaemia arises as a consequence of underventilation of all or part of the circulating blood.

1   *Alveolar hypoventilation*

This results in hypoxaemia and reciprocal hypercapnia (p. 21). Oxygen administration may completely reverse the hypoxaemia. The problem of underventilation remains.

2   *Disturbed ventilation/perfusion relationships* (p. 23)

Oxygen administration may completely reverse the arterial hypoxaemia from this cause as the blood perfusing underventilated areas then encounters adequate oxygen tensions.

4   *Right–left shunts*

Such shunts may be regarded as an extreme form of (2) except that the blood passing to the shunt is inaccessible to the increased oxygen tension. A small amount of oxygen can be carried in the plasma of the blood traversing the lungs—about 2 ml per 100 ml for every 101 kPa (760 mmHg) partial pressure of oxygen—and this can be useful in the critically placed patient.

Other indications

Oxygen administration is desirable in situations where the cardiac output is seriously low even if arterial oxygen saturation is normal. A high concentration may increase the oxygen content of blood slightly by virtue of plasma solubility. Very severe anaemia and carbon monoxide poisoning constitute further indications for oxygen administration.

Method of administration

100% OXYGEN

Most of the masks in general use, although supplied by 100% oxygen, in fact achieve much lower inspired concentrations. An inspired concentration of 100% oxygen can only be achieved with apparatus which provides a complete seal from the outside air and a non-return valve; in the clinical situation this only occurs in the context of artificial ventilation. One hundred per cent oxygen may be indicated in exceptional circumstances; prolonged use is attended by the risk of oxygen toxicity.

MASKS DELIVERING 40–60%

A variety of masks achieve inspired levels of this order and two are shown in Fig. 26.2. The actual inspired concentration depends upon a number of factors which include: rate of oxygen flow, breathing pattern (tidal volume, frequency and inspiratory flow rate) and the amount of rebreathing permitted by the mask. The effective concentration of oxygen is also influenced by the position of the mask on the face.

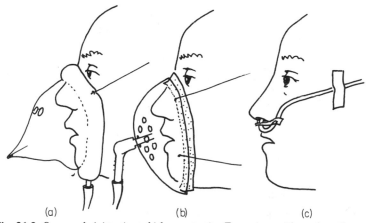

(a)   (b)   (c)

Fig. 26.2. *Oxygen administration—high concentration.* For patients with good ventilatory drive. (a) Pneumask; (b) MC mask (Henleys Medical Supplies Ltd). These masks can deliver the equivalent of an inspired concentration of 40–60% depending on oxygen flow rate and a number of other factors. (c) Nasal catheters. A short catheter is situated in each nostril penetrating only as far as the anterior nares.

Application

Masks in this group are appropriate in patients with good respiratory drive—severe asthma, infiltrative lung disorders, pneumonia, pulmonary oedema, etc.

MASKS DELIVERING LOW OXYGEN CONCENTRATIONS

These masks produce a fast-flowing stream of fixed low oxygen concentration (Fig. 26.3). Air is entrained by a jet of oxygen, exploiting the venturi principle. The inspired oxygen concentration is independent of breathing pattern, no rebreathing occurs and the position of the mask is less critical than is the case with some other masks. The concentration delivered is also relatively independent of the oxygen flow-rate, being determined by the geometry of the air-entrainment mechanism. A selection of masks giving 24, 28, and 35% oxygen is available. In general these masks are well tolerated; some patients appreciate the breeze they produce but others are distressed by the noise.

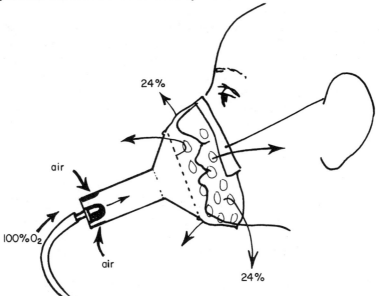

Fig. 26.3. *Oxygen administration—controlled low concentration.* ('Ventimask Mk. 1', Vickers Medical shown above; other masks employing the same principle are available). **Suitable** for patients with impaired ventilatory drive. **Unsuitable** for patients with arterial hypoxaemia in other situations. A low concentration of oxygen is produced by the oxygen-driven air-entraining venturi and a high flow rate is maintained through the mask so that no room air or exhaled air is inspired. Note that masks are available which produce other higher concentrations (24, 28 and 35%).

Application

The only indication for the use of masks in this group (controlled low concentration) is the presence of severe chronic ventilatory failure in which there is already serious underventilation (high arterial Pco$_2$) and a **poor drive to breathe** (but see p. 237).

Note

Although these masks limit the extent of hypoventilation which may accompany oxygen administration they do not prevent it altogether. Even 24% oxygen increases the inspired Pco$_2$ by about 2.8 kPa (21 mmHg) so that, if a patient was heavily dependent upon the hypoxic drive, the alveolar Pco$_2$ could theoretically rise by 2.3–2.8 kPA (17–21 mmHg) as he reduced ventilation until the arterial Pco$_2$ reached its former level. In the case of a mask delivering 28% the Pco$_2$ could conceivably rise by 5 or 6 kPa (say 40 to 50 mmHg).

NASAL OXYGEN ADMINISTRATION

Some patients do not tolerate covering of the face with a mask. Nasal administration overcomes this difficulty and also permits feeding and expectoration without interruption. Oxygen can be delivered by means of two short catheters which enter only the anterior nares or by means of a longer soft catheter reaching to the nasopharynx. Inspired levels of the order of 40% may be obtained. Some patients breathe through the mouth but nasal administration even with the short catheters is often surprisingly effective nevertheless. This is the usual means of administering long-term near-continuous oxygen (p. 330).

OTHER METHODS

Oxygen tents provide an oxygen-rich environment but it is extremely difficult to maintain a constant inspired oxygen concentration. Oxygen tents severely limit ease of access to the patient for nursing purposes. Their main application is in childhood; children do not tolerate masks well.

A head-tent (Vickers Ltd) is occasionally useful in patients who require a low concentration of oxygen but are intolerant of masks. It comprises a transparent plastic curtain which surrounds the head and shoulders but is open at the bottom. A high flow of low oxygen concentration is directed downwards through the tent by means of an oxygen-driven air-entraining venturi housed in a dome from which the curtain is suspended.

MASKS INCORPORATING A NEBULIZER

It is rarely necessary to humidify the oxygen supplied to masks. However, masks which incorporate a gas-driven nebulizer are sometimes employed to supersaturate the inspired air with an aerosol of water droplets with the aim of wetting the tracheal and bronchial secretions.

These masks, which are described in Fig. 15.10, also provide a useful means of administering larger doses of bronchodilator drug to individuals who are either too ill to use pressurized aerosols or unfamiliar with them. Used with oxygen, these are effectively high-concentration masks. They may be driven by compressed air in ventilatory failure if the patient is intolerant of oxygen.

Oxygen therapy in exacerbations of chronic bronchitis (p. 237)

Hazards of oxygen therapy

1 HYPOVENTILATION (see above)

2 WITHDRAWAL OF OXYGEN

If oxygen is being given to a patient with severe hypoventilation it may be dangerous to withdraw it.

The dotted line in Fig. 2.7 shows the relationship beteen alveolar P_{O_2} and P_{CO_2} when breathing air. The extent to which hypoventilation can progress is limited by hypoxia. For example, if the P_{CO_2} rises to 12 kPa (90 mmHg) the P_{O_2} falls to about 4.7 kPa (35 mmHg). Survival is unusual if the arterial P_{O_2} falls much below 25 mmHg. When oxygen is administered much more severe hypoventilation can be tolerated. If oxygen is then withdrawn the patient will be plunged into catastrophic hypoxia. Even if ventilation is then increased, the body reserves of accumulated CO_2 will ensure that the alveolar P_{CO_2} remains elevated for some time.

If oxygen is being administered to a patient with severe hypoventilation of whatever cause, it must be administered **continuously** until ventilation has been improved.

3 RETROLENTAL FIBROPLASIA

Administration of high concentrations of oxygen (sufficient to produce an arterial P_{O_2} of over 19 kPa or approximately 140 mmHg) may produce retrolental fibroplasia in the neonatal period leading subsequently to variable degrees of blindness.

4 PULMONARY OXYGEN TOXICITY

High concentrations of oxygen cause damage to the alveoli. The earliest changes are those of capillary proliferation followed by intra-alveolar haemorrhage and exudation and the formation of hyaline membranes. Areas of collapse develop, lung compliance falls and gas transfer becomes progressively impaired leading ultimately to arterial hypoxaemia despite the high inspired concentration. Inhalation of 100% oxygen causes reversible symptoms in 48–72 hours but changes may be irreversible after exposure for many days. The rate of development of the pulmonary reaction is influenced by a number of metabolic and pharmacological factors as well as by the inspired concentration. Prolonged exposure to concentrations in excess of 50% appears to be necessary. Interruption of the exposure by periods breathing lower concentrations appears to have a protective effect. In practice uninterrupted administration of really high concentrations of oxygen is mainly confined to patients with tracheostomies or endotracheal tubes who are receiving artificial ventilation. Clinically overt oxygen toxicity is almost unheard of as a consequence of oxygen administration using conventional masks. Whenever patients require high concentrations of oxygen, care must be taken to ensure that the inspired level is maintained at the lowest compatible with a safe arterial oxygen tension. Once the condition is established, no treatment other than lowering of the oxygen concentration is of any avail—and this may be impossible.

5 FIRE

The hazard of fire should not be underestimated. Many materials which are normally relatively nonflammable burn furiously in an oxygen-rich atmosphere. Naked flames and smoking must be absolutely forbidden in the vicinity of oxygen administration.

Domiciliary oxygen therapy

There are a few instances in which oxygen therapy may be valuable at home.

1 TO AID EXERCISE IN THE HOME

Oxygen therapy can be used, for example, when climbing stairs, washing, or moving from room to room. The cylinder should be situated strategically and long lengths of low-pressure plastic tubing used to make oxygen available at a distance.

2 PORTABLE OXYGEN

In a few patients exercise is much extended by use of oxygen and they may find it useful out of doors. It is very desirable to test a patient's response to oxygen under controlled conditions before supplying portable equipment; detailed instruction is required. In practice, most systems are too cumbersome and heavy and, although the idea of portable oxygen therapy appeals to disabled patients, it is found useful in only a few cases.

3 LONG-TERM OXYGEN THERAPY

The long-term administration of oxygen in the home has a place in the management of patients with severe airways obstruction accompanied by chronic hypoxia. Typically the patient is of the blue-bloater type and there is an element of underventilation also present. The aim of this treatment is to give oxygen for as many hours of the day and night as is possible. This is not to say that treatment is required for minute-to-minute survival; the patient is able to interrupt treatment for modest periods to travel, visit shops and friends. It has been found in controlled trials conducted in the UK by the MRC and in the USA by the NIH that survival is increased if at least 15 of the 24 hours are spent breathing oxygen-enriched air. Furthermore, it seems that the results are proportionately better if more than 15 hours are spent breathing oxygen and best of all if oxygen is breathed more or less continuously. For the first year or so of treatment mortality in most studies has been similar in treated and control groups, suggesting that there may be some patients who are so deteriorated that oxygen breathing will not materially extend life. After a year, treated and untreated mortality rates become increasingly different. With near-continuous oxygen it is probable that the untreated mortality of 70% at 5 years could be approximately halved.

Protection from severe nocturnal hypoxia and relief of severe pulmonary hypertension may be responsible for improved survival. Increased well-being, and improvement in sleep patterns and mood are also observed. Progressive CO_2 retention is not a problem in patients in a steady state who are not in a severe exacerbation.

A number of practical problems must be overcome in order to achieve near-continuous oxygen breathing. The only practical form of oxygen delivery is the oxygen concentrator. This is an electrically powered instrument which compresses air and then releases it through a molecular filter which retains nitrogen. Continuous supply of about 90% oxygen is achieved at a flow rate of between 1 and 3 litres per minute by switching compression and release between twin sets of reservoirs and filters. Lightweight transparent nasal cannulae are used, together with long lengths of non-kinkable tubing which lead around the house. The patient uses oxygen throughout the night and throughout the day whilst ordinary quiet domestic activities are carried out.

Suitable patients should have documented day-time chronic hypoxaemia, severe airways obstruction (FEV$_1$ usually well below 1 litre), and they should have been shown (by two separated measurements of carboxyhaemoglobin or expired carbon monoxide concentration) to be current non-smokers. The treatment is expensive but much cheaper than the use of cylinders. It should only be invoked in the specific circumstances described. It is being made available on prescription through the National Health Service in the UK.

4 PLACEBO EFFECT

All oxygen administration exerts a strong placebo effect. Where advanced disease is causing great anguish the availability of oxygen may do much to relieve the worst moments even if its use seems illogical. The hazards of inappropriate use may sometimes be acceptable under these circumstances.

CHAPTER 27 / MULTIPLE-CHOICE
QUESTIONS

ANSWERS BEGIN ON PAGE 356

Many examinations now include a section comprised of multiple choice questions (MCQs) and, whilst the following section will certainly offer some practice in answering MCQs, a few points should be noted:
1   The questions are intended to be an interesting means of instruction rather than a means of self-assessment.
2   Some of the questions cover areas beyond the scope of this book.
3   The majority of the MCQs are in the 'multiple true/false' format favoured in most examinations; each of the answers may be either true or false and it is possible for all five to be true (or false).
4   Some questions are uncued where the material is best suited to this mode.
5   Where 'q.v.' appears in the answers section the reader is invited to refer to the pages dealing with the subject by using the index.
6   The numbering of the questions indicates the chapter dealing with the subject.

QUESTIONS

1.1   The following statements are true:
   a The left main bronchus lies in front of the left pulmonary artery.
   b The bronchial arteries arise from the internal mammary arteries.
   c The right pulmonary artery lies behind the ascending aorta.
   d The right main bronchus is more directly in line with the trachea than the left.
   e The right recurrent laryngeal nerve loops round the arch of the aorta.

1.2   In the alveoli:
   a Type I pneumocytes form the major part of the surface.
   b Type II pneumocytes produce surfactant.
   c Type III pneumocytes contain concentric lamellated bodies.
   d Gas flow is highly turbulent.
   e Macrophages are usually present.

2.1 Lung compliance is:
  a A measure of airways resistance.
  b Measured with the use of an oesophageal balloon.
  c Increased in pulmonary fibrosis.
  d Increased in severe emphysema.
  e Measured in litres per kilopascal (or $1/cm\ H_2O$).

2.2 The following statements are true:
  a The volume of CO_2 produced at rest is generally greater than the volume of O_2 consumed.
  b Increase in ventilation on exercise is stimulated by the fall in arterial oxygen content.
  c The alveolar air equation relates ventilation to CO_2 production.
  d The P_{CO_2} of expired air towards the end of expiration is normally of the order of 5.3 kPa (40 mmHg).
  e 30% oxygen (dry) has a P_{O_2} of about 230 mmHg (about 30 kPa).

2.3 In normal lungs:
  a In the upright posture ventilation is greater at the apex than at the base.
  b In the upright posture perfusion is greater at the base than at the apex.
  c 90% of the total airways resistance resides in airways of less than 2 mm in diameter.
  d Residual volume is less than 35% of total lung capacity.
  e Airways resistance falls during expiration.

2.4 The partial pressure of:
  a Oxygen in ambient air at sea level is about 20 kPa (150 mmHg).
  b A gas is the pressure that the gas would exert if present alone without the other gases in a mixture.
  c Oxygen in a 5% mixture will be found to be less than that of carbon dioxide in a mixture containing 5% of CO_2.
  d Carbon dioxide has an almost linear relationship with content in blood over the usual physiological range.
  e Oxygen has an almost linear relationship with content in blood over the usual physiological range.

2.5   Arterial P_{CO_2}:
    a Can be measured directly using an electrode.
    b Is usually low in diabetic ketoacidosis.
    c Can be estimated by analysis of end-expired air.
    d Normally increases during exercise.
    e Is directly proportional to alveolar ventilation under steady-state conditions.

2.6   In inspiration:
    a The abdomen moves outwards.
    b The costal margin moves outwards and upwards.
    c Central venous pressure increases.
    d Airways resistance is less than during expiration.
    e Intrapleural pressure is subatmospheric.

2.7   The presence of areas of low V/Q (i.e. regional underventilation) inevitably causes:
    a Hypercapnia.
    b Decrease in plasma bicarbonate.
    c Reduced arterial pH.
    d Reduced tidal volume.
    e Arterial hypoxia.

3.1   Surfactant:
    a Produces a greater lowering of surface tension in small bubbles than in large bubbles.
    b Activity in a surface is enhanced by transient increase in area or radius of curvature of the surface.
    c Is produced from concentric lamellar bodies within type II pneumocytes.
    d Is present within foetal lungs from the twentieth week of gestation.
    e Production is dependent upon pulmonary perfusion.

4.1   The following statements are true:
    a Particles deposited on the walls of the bronchial tree are largely cleared within 24 hours.
    b Particles of 10 μm or less (aerodynamic diameter) tend to penetrate to alveolar level.
    c The surface of the terminal bronchiole is predominantly made up of ciliated epithelial cells.

d Fluid is absorbed from respiratory secretion as it moves up the airways.

e The nose does not remove an appreciable proportion of particles below 25 μm in aerodynamic diameter.

6.1 Match the physical signs described below (*a–e*) with the diagnoses (1–5). Assume that features not mentioned are either normal or unhelpful:

a Tachypnoea; absent or very distant breath sounds all over the left chest; trachea deviated to the right; apex beat not palpable; no dullness on percussion.

b Reduced movement of right side of chest; very dull at right base up to the mid-zone posteriorly; trachea deviated to the left; absent vocal fremitus on the right; greatly reduced or absent breath sound at the right lower zone.

c Normal respiratory rate; bovine cough; reduced movement of left side of chest; trachea deviated to the left; apex beat in 4th intercostal space in the anterior axillary line; gastric resonance detected at and below 5th intercostal space in mid-clavicular line; reduced air entry on left side; dull on percussion posteriorly and in the axilla on the left.

d Tachypnoea, fine pan-inspiratory crepitations (crackles) in both lower zones; clubbing; cyanosis on light exercise.

e Tachypnoea; rattling cough; slight dullness left lower zone posteriorly; and in the left lower axillary region.

  1 Left lower lobe pneumonia
  2 Left pneumothorax
  3 Right pleural effusion
  4 Fibrosing alveolitis
  5 Collapse of left lung

6.2 Pulses

The following statements are true:

a The jugular venous pressure falls during inspiration.

b In pericardial effusion the jugular venous pressure may rise in inspiration.

c In pulsus paradoxicus the pulse becomes weaker during expiration and fuller in inspiration.

d Pulsus paradoxicus is commonly observed in severe asthma.

e In sinus arrhythmia the pulse rate quickens in inspiration and slows in expiration.

6.3 Clubbing is a recognized complication of:
     a Bronchiectasis.
     b Chronic liver disease.
     c Gout.
     d Psoriasis.
     e Fibrosing alveolitis.

6.4 In auscultation of the chest the following statements are true:
     a The presence or absence of rhonchi (wheezes) gives a reliable indication of the presence or absence of airways obstruction.
     b Crepitations (crackles) are commonly heard throughout inspiration in the presence of airways obstruction.
     c Consolidated lung transmits high frequency sound well and low frequency sound poorly.
     d Bronchial breathing tends to be heard over consolidated lung.
     e Breath sounds are loud and 'ringing' in quality over a pneumothorax.

6.5 Cyanosis:
     a Would be expected with an arterial P_{O_2} of 9 kPa (67.5 mmHg).
     b Will be recognized when there is 5 g of reduced haemoglobin per 100 ml of blood.
     c May be produced by methaemoglobinaemia.
     d Secondary to lung disease is most commonly due to alveolar underventilation.
     e Of central type indicates a requirement for oxygen therapy.

7.1 Definitions
     What is:
     a The peak expiratory flow rate?
     b The FEV_1?
     c The vital capacity?
     d Functional residual capacity?
     e Residual volume?

7.2 Transfer factor measured by the single-breath technique:
     a Is reduced in the presence of anaemia.
     b Is reduced in emphysema.
     c Is reduced in atrial septal defect.

d Is reduced in individuals who have undergone pneumonectomy.

e Allows an estimate of alveolar wall thickness.

7.3 The following statements are true:

a Blood with a haemoglobin of 14.8 g/100 ml can carry
approximately 20 ml of oxygen (at STPD) per 100 ml.

b The affinity of haemoglobin for oxygen is decreased by increase in temperature above 37°C.

c At normal body pH and temperature the saturation of blood
with a Po_2 of 7.7 kPa (58 mmHg) is about 60%.

d In arterial blood with a Po_2 of 12.5 kPa (94 mmHg) the oxygen
dissolved in plasma amounts to about 0.3 ml per 100 ml of
blood.

e A shift of the oxygen dissociation curve to the left may be said
to facilitate loading of O_2 in the lungs and to make unloading of
O_2 in the tissues more difficult.

7.4 Vital capacity

a Is reduced in airways obstruction.

b Is reduced in diffuse lung fibrosis.

c Can normally be expelled in about 1.5 seconds.

d Increases after middle life.

e Is commonly larger if measured with a slow expiration than
with a forced expiration.

7.5 A 63-year-old man who is a heavy smoker and known to suffer
from chronic obstructive pulmonary disease is admitted to hospital acutely ill. On examination he is confused and cyanosed and
breathing is extremely laboured. Arterial blood gas analysis
reveals the following values:

Pco_2 4.3 kPa (32 mmHg)
pH 7.18
bicarbonate (actual) 11 mmol/l.
Po_2 3.9 kPa (29 mmHg).

a Administration of oxygen would be dangerous in this patient.

b Acute left ventricular failure might account for the clinical and
blood-gas features.

c Acute bacteraemic shock might account for the clinical and
blood-gas features.

    d Administration of a sedative drug might account for the
clinical and blood-gas features.

    e An acute exacerbation of chronic bronchitis and worsening
ventilatory failure is the most likely cause of the clinical and
blood-gas features.

7.6 A raised arterial P_{CO_2}:

    a Tends to cause vasodilatation in the skin.

    b Tends to cause lowering of blood pressure.

    c Is commonly seen at altitudes above 5000 feet (1500 metres).

    d Causes cerebral vasoconstriction.

    e Will tend to rise higher during oxygen with spontaneous
ventilation.

7.7 The FEV_1:

    a Is directly related to the effort applied during the manoeuvre.

    b Usually comprises more than 70% of the vital capacity.

    c Increases with age in normal subjects.

    d Usually increases after a bronchodilator aerosol is administered in patients with chronic bronchitis.

    e Is typically normal in patients with diffuse pulmonary fibrosis.

7.8 The FEV_1:

    a Is measured with a peak flow meter.

    b Is the volume of air expired in the first second of a maximal
forced expiration.

    c Is highly reproducible.

    d Is 3.5 litres in normal subjects.

    e Is reduced in the presence of airways obstruction.

7.9
$$P_{CO_2}\ 9.0\ \text{kPa (68 mmHg)}$$
$$pH\ 7.22$$
$$\text{bicarbonate (actual) 25 mmol/l.}$$
$$P_{O_2}\ 12.0\ \text{kPa (90 mmHg)}$$

These values:

    a Suggest chronic ventilatory failure.

    b Are compatible with the consequences of heavy postoperative
sedation.

    c Suggest impending danger of severe hypoxia in a spontaneously breathing patient.

    d Are compatible with the effects of acute salicylate poisoning.

    e In a patient who is unrousable suggest a respiratory cause for
the coma.

7.10 Match the following blood-gas analysis (*a–e*) with the clinical situations described below (1–5).

	P_{CO_2} (kPa)	P_{CO_2} (mmHg)	pH	Actual bicarbonate (mmol/l.)	P_{O_2} (kPa)	P_{O_2} (mmHg)
a	8.5	(64)	7.36	35	5.1	(38)
b	4.4	(33)	7.28	15	7.7	(58)
c	9.3	(70)	7.20	26	16	(120)
d	8.1	(61)	7.13	18	7.2	(54)
e	2.4	(18)	7.64	19	12.8	(96)

1 Acute respiratory acidosis.
2 Acute metabolic acidosis.
3 Acute respiratory alkalosis.
4 Chronic (compensated) respiratory acidosis.
5 Mixed respiratory and metabolic acidosis.

8.1 *a* Sugggest four of the commoner causes of a 'miliary mottling' pattern on the chest X-ray.
   b Suggest four of the commoner causes of an isolated round shadow on the chest X-ray.

8.2 The following statements may be confirmed by inspection of the normal chest X-ray:
   a The right diaphragm is higher than the left.
   b The trachea passes to the left of the aortic arch.
   c The pulmonary arterial shadow appears above that of the aortic arch.
   d The horizontal fissure delineates the superior border of the right middle lobe.
   e Kerley 'B' lines are commonly visible at the lung bases.

8.3 The following are accepted causes of multiple rounded shadows 0.5 to 1 cm in diameter visible on the chest X-ray:
   a Rheumatoid arthritis.
   b Wegener's granuloma.
   c Tuberculosis.
   d Haematoma.
   e Metastatic carcinoma.

9.1 Croup
   a Is most often caused by parainfluenza viruses.

b Is sometimes caused by *Haemophilus influenzae* type B.
c Is characterized by an audible wheeze.
d Usually lasts 3–4 weeks.
e Is usually associated with a normal chest X-ray.

9.2 Acute bronchiolitis:
  a Occurs most commonly between 2 and 3 years of age.
  b Is due to infection by adenovirus.
  c Produces airways obstruction.
  d Is accompanied initially by high fever.
  e Sometimes requires treatment by IPPV.

9.3 Ampicillin (and the related antibiotics amoxycillin and talampicillin) is active against:
  a *Haemophilus influenzae.*
  b *Mycoplasma pneumoniae.*
  c *Streptococcus pneumoniae.*
  d *Candida albicans.*
  e *Chlamydia psittaci.*

10.1 Match the following cases of pneumonia (*a*-*e*) with the anti-biotics which you would not expect to be omitted from their treatment (1-5).
  a *Staphylococcus aureus.*
  b *Mycoplasma pneumoniae.*
  c *Pseudomonas aeruginosa.*
  d *Legionella pneumophilia.*
  e *Chlamydia psittaci.*
  1 Tetracycline
  2 Gentamycin (or Ceftazidime)
  3 Erythromycin
  4 Flucloxacillin—or cloxacillin
  5 Amoxycillin

10.2 Pneumonia. Suggest the name(s) of the missing organism(s).
  a In a previously well individual who is severely ill during an influenza epidemic, pneumonia is commonly due to ————.
  b Pneumonia affecting one lobe of the lung and associated with the identification of gram-negative rods in the sputum is probably due to ————.
  c Pneumonia of the right lower lobe in a man with bulbar palsy is commonly due to ————.

d Pneumonia in an adult with irregular shadowing at the right upper zone may be due to ————.

e Pneumonia which is unresponsive to either amoxycillin or cotrimoxazole and which is accompanied by the finding of cold agglutinins in the serum is probably due to ————.

10.3 What conditions are suggested by sputum?
  a Containing large numbers of iron-laden macrophages.
  b Containing solid brown plugs of amorphous material.
  c Containing macrophages laden with oily globules.
  d Containing abundant eosinophils.
  e Which is always copious and greenish in colour.

11.1 In tuberculosis:
  a It is extremely rare for active infection to be accompanied by a negative tuberculin test.
  b Sputum culture is only positive in cases in which acid- and alcohol-fast bacilli have been identified.
  c Primary infection by tuberculosis nearly always leaves a visible lesion on the chest X-ray.
  d The following are different forms of tuberculin test: Heaf, Mantoux, Tine test.
  e Tuberculin testing consists in the subcutaneous injection of old tuberculin.

11.2 In the management of pulmonary tuberculosis:
  a Children living in the same household should have a tuberculin skin test.
  b Patients with smear positive (for AAFBs) sputum should be treated in hospital for the first 2 weeks of treatment.
  c All persons employed at an infected person's place of work should have a chest X-ray.
  d Persons who are close household contacts of a patient with smear positive (for AAFBs) sputum should have chest X-rays at 6 months and 1 year from the start of the patient's treatment.
  e AAFBs may be produced in the sputum for 2 months after starting an approved treatment regimen which includes rifampicin.
  (AAFBS = acid- and alcohol-fast bacilli).

11.3 Atypical mycobacteria:

    a Are responsible for about one-quarter of newly-diagnosed cases of tuberculosis in the UK.

    b Are responsible for minor epidemics of tuberculous disease in closed communities.

    c May cause cervical lymphadenopathy.

    d May cause infection in the apex of the lung.

    e Are commonly resistant to available antituberculous drugs.

11.4 Match each of the side-effects (*a–e*) listed below with one antituberculous drug.

    a Peripheral neuritis.

    b Impaired visual acuity.

    c Red coloration of the urine.

    d Nerve deafness.

    e Altered liver function tests.

    1 Rifampicin.

    2 Ethambutol.

    3 Isoniazid.

    4 Streptomycin.

12.1 Bronchiectasis:

    a Is a common cause of haemoptysis.

    b Is generally treated surgically.

    c Is diagnosed by bronchoscopy.

    d Is almost inevitably accompanied by impaired ventilatory performance.

    e In the UK is usually the legacy of childhood whooping cough.

12.2 The following are accepted clinical features of bronchiectasis:

    a Inspiratory rhonchi.

    b Clubbing.

    c Coarse basal crepitations.

    d Copious green sputum.

    e Normal chest X-ray.

12.3 The following features are common accompaniments of cystic fibrosis:

    a Meconium ileus.

    b Abnormally low sodium concentration in the sweat.

    c Nasal polyps.

d Airways obstruction.

e Clubbing.

13.1 In cystic fibrosis:

    a Both parents are carriers of the disease.

    b All affected individuals are sterile.

    c The gene for the disease is carried by about 1 in 20 of the population.

    d Unaffected sibs of an affected individual have a 1 in 4 chance of being carriers.

13.2 The following have an established place in the management of cystic fibrosis:

    a Forced expiratory manoeuvres.

    b Long-term inhalation of nebulized water at night.

    c Oral treatment with pancreozymin.

    d Vitamin treatment.

    e Intravenous antibiotic treatment.

14.1 Lung abscess:

    a Is a recognized complication of staphylococcal pneumonia.

    b Is usually treated by surgical drainage.

    c Is commonly due to inhalation of food or other foreign material.

    d Due to tuberculosis is almost always readily confirmed by the finding of acid- and alcohol-fast bacilli on direct examination of a sputum smear.

    e Is generally accompanied by characteristic physical signs: local hyper-resonance and 'amphoric' breath sounds.

14.2 Suggest four conditions of clinical situations associated with a high risk of aspiration pneumonia and lung abscess.

14.3 Sputum:

    a Is expectorated by the act of coughing in normal individuals in quantities of up to 50 ml daily.

    b Which is yellow inevitably signifies active bronchial infection.

    c Is abnormally viscid in cystic fibrosis.

    d Usually contains excessive numbers of eosinophils in un-treated asthma.

    e Which is offensive and dark green in colour commonly harbours anaerobic bacteria.

15.1 The following statements are true:
  a The term 'reagin' refers to IgE.
  b Type II hypersensitivity (Gell and Coombs) plays an important part in extrinsic allergic alveolitis.
  c Hay fever is commonly associated with extrinsic asthma.
  d Nasal polyposis is commonly associated with intrinsic asthma.
  e Atopic individuals tend to have higher than average circulating levels of IgE.
  f Atopic individuals tend to have lower than average levels of IgA in early years.

15.2 The following either produce or accompany bronchoconstriction in asthma.
  a Beta-sympathetic blockade.
  b Administration of a phosphodiesterase inhibitor.
  c Rising intercellular levels of cyclic GMP (guanine monophosphate).
  d Administration of prostaglandin F_2 alpha.
  e Cholinergic agents.

15.3 Mechanisms in asthma.
  The following statements are true:
  a Degranulation of mast cells is discouraged by administration of beta-sympathomimetic drugs.
  b Degranulation of mast cells is discouraged by sodium cromoglycate.
  c Fall in intracellular levels of cyclic AMP within bronchial smooth muscle cells is associated with bronchodilatation.
  d Beta-blocking drugs tend to cause bronchoconstriction.
  e Prostaglandin E_1 acts as a bronchodilator.

15.4 Exercise-induced asthma:
  a Can be prevented by prior administration of salbutamol aerosol.
  b Can be demonstrated in almost 25% of asthmatic children.
  c Can be prevented by prior administration of sodium cromoglycate.
  d Is much less readily induced by swimming than by equivalent exercise performed running.
  e Is mediated by lactic acidosis.

15.5   Asthma:

   a Has a negligible mortality.

   b May develop at some time in the life of about 5% of the population.

   c Is commoner in boys than in girls.

   d Is virtually unknown after the age of 70 years.

   e Is commoner amongst the higher social classes.

15.6   Asthma.

   a Suggest three common allergies which may be important in extrinsic asthma.

   b Describe three characteristic physiological abnormalities which may be identified in persons with airways obstruction.

   c What is meant by 'reversibility' in the context of physiological measurements made in airways obstruction.

15.7   An episode of acute severe asthma (status asthmaticus) is usually accompanied by:

   a Lowered Po_2.

   b Lowered Pco_2.

   c Lowered heart rate.

   d Lowered respiratory rate.

   e Relative resistance to the bronchodilator effect of beta-sympathomimetic drugs.

15.8   Aerosol preparations:

   a Of bronchodilator drugs in pressurized form have been associated with a continuing rise in mortality from asthma dating from the time of their introduction.

   b Of salbutamol and terbutaline are more specific beta-1-adrenoceptor stimulants than isoprenaline.

   c Of bronchodilator drugs usually result in spirometric values returning to normal in asthma.

   d Of bronchodilator drugs are available for inhalation in dry powder form.

   e Of bronchodilator drugs may produce a fall in arterial oxygen tension after use.

15.9   In asthma:

   a Oral steroid therapy should be avoided unless the patient is *in extremis.*

    b Short courses of prednisolone are given with a progressively reducing dose because of the risk of adrenal suppression.

    c Steroid aerosol treatment should be maintained in patients with severe asthma who require continuous treatment with oral steroids.

    d Antibiotics need not necessarily be given in an acute exacerbation.

    e Morning levels of plasma cortisol are low.

15.10 In childhood:

    a Asthma is generally associated with positive skin tests.

    b Asthma may produce stunting of growth.

    c Asthma may produce a deformity of the chest wall known as pectus excavatum.

    d Steroid therapy may suppress growth.

    e Exercise-induced attacks may be averted by taking an inhalation of steroid aerosol immediately before the exercise.

15.11 *Aspergillus fumigatus:*

    a Spores are widely disseminated and a common component of inspired air.

    b May be recovered from the sputum in some patients with asthma.

    c May be associated with the development of a proximal form of bronchiectasis.

    d May produce haemoptysis.

    e May be associated with lobar collapse.

15.12 The use of a nebulizer to administer a beta-agonist bronchodilator:

    a Results in about 40% of the inhaled dose reaching beyond the trachea.

    b Achieves a greater effect than the same dose of bronchodilator administered with a metered dose (pressurized) inhaler.

    c Leads to important hypoxia if oxygen is not used as the driving gas.

    d Is contraindicated in patients taking a long-acting theophylline preparation.

    e Is the only way of achieving bronchodilatation in a child of under 12 months.

15.13 Regular exposure to the following may be associated with the development of extrinsic allergic alveolitis:
a Phthallic anhydride.
b A budgerigar in the home.
c Talc.
d Stored hay.
e Mushroom compost.

16.1 The following features are common accompaniments of established fibrosing alveolitis:
a Nasal polyps.
b Exclusively early-inspiratory crepitations (crackles).
c Cyanosis on exertion.
d Clubbing.
e Polycythaemia.

16.2 Physiological disturbance accompanying fibrosing alveolitis includes:
a Reduction in lung volumes.
b Reduced transfer factor.
c Reduced lung compliance.
d Reduced FEV_1: FVC ratio.
e Reduced arterial PO_2.

16.3 Fibrosing alveolitis:
a Is commoner in the elderly than in young adults.
b Is almost always fatal within 5 years of diagnosis.
c Leads to 'honeycomb lung'.
d Is commonly associated with symptoms of polyarthritis or frank rheumatoid arthritis.
e May only be diagnosed by lung biopsy.

16.4 The following pulmonary phenomena are associated with rheumatoid arthritis:
a Kartagener's syndrome.
b Intrapulmonary nodules.
c Diffuse pulmonary fibrosis.
d Pleural effusion.
e Pulmonary oedema.

16.5 The following conditions are associated with diffuse pulmonary fibrosis:
   a Polyarteritis nodosa.
   b Sarcoidosis.
   c Systematic sclerosis.
   d Agammaglobulinaemia.
   e Tuberose sclerosis.

16.6 Bronchoalveolar lavage:
   a In the normal yields fluid in which about 90% of the cells are macrophages.
   b In the smoker yields fluid with an increased proportion of neutrophils.
   c In sarcoidosis typically yields fluid with an increased proportion of lymphocytes.
   d Can be used to confirm the diagnosis of *Pneumocystis carinii* infection.
   e Can be used to confirm the diagnosis of fibrosing alveolitis.

17.1 Sarcoidosis commonly presents with pain:
   a After alcohol.
   b In the neck.
   c In the eye.
   d In the abdomen.
   e Below the knees.

17.2 In sarcoidosis there may be enlargements of:
   a Spleen.
   b Liver.
   c Testes.
   d Parotid.
   e Fingers.

17.3 Erythema nodosum:
   a Is confined to the lower limbs.
   b In the UK is most commonly due to sarcoidosis.
   c Never recurs.
   d In sarcoidosis is associated with poor prognosis.
   e Is painful.

18.1 Chronic obstructive pulmonary disease shows an association with:

a Atmospheric pollution.

b Social class.

c Cigarette smoking.

d Urbanization.

e Alcoholism.

18.2 Amongst patients with severe chronic obstructive pulmonary disease the following features help to distinguish the Type A (Pink puffer) pattern from the Type B (Blue bloater) pattern:

a Normal PCO_2.

b Reduced PO_2.

c Reduced transfer factor.

d Radiological evidence of emphysema.

e Past history of smoking.

18.3 Cigarette smoking has been shown to be significantly associated with increased risk of developing:

a Adenocarcinoma of the stomach.

b Adenocarcinoma of the lung.

c Emphysema.

d Duodenal ulcer.

e Ischaemic heart disease.

18.4 In patients with chronic obstructive pulmonary disease the probability of co-existing asthma (treatable with corticosteroid preparations) is increased by the presence of the following factors:

a Family history of wheezing or 'bronchitis'.

b Prominent nasal symptoms.

c Prominent nocturnal symptoms.

d Eosinophilia in sputum or blood.

e Life-long abstinence from smoking.

18.5 A 59-year-old man who is a heavy smoker with chronic obstructive pulmonary disease becomes unwell following a cold and describes the expectoration of an increased volume of sputum which is yellow in colour. Suitable treatment would be:

a Flucloxacillin.

b Clindamycin.

    c Cotrimoxazole.
    d Amoxycillin.
    e Treatment with antibiotics should be withheld until results of
       sputum culture are available.

18.6 Patients with ventilatory failure (respiratory failure) complicating
    chronic obstructive pulmonary disease commonly have:
    a Peripheral oedema.
    b Jerky tremor.
    c Hypotension.
    d Somnolence.
    e Headache.

18.7 *a* Define respiratory failure.
     b Outline the measures you would take to assess and treat a
       patient in an acute exacerbation of chronic obstructive
       pulmonary disease with presumed or suspected respiratory
       failure.

18.8 Chronic ventilatory failure is regularly encountered in:
    a Cystic fibrosis.
    b Heroin addiction.
    c 'Pickwickian syndrome'.
    d Superior vena caval obstruction.
    e Kyphoscoliosis.

19.1 Carcinoma of the bronchus.
    The following statements are true:
    a Carcinoma of the bronchus is largely due to cigarette smoking.
    b Carcinoma of the bronchus is the cause of approximately 3500
       deaths per annum in the UK.
    c Even if an individual stops smoking the risk from lung cancer
       remains the same as if he had continued to smoke.
    d The mortality rate from lung cancer is now beginning to fall in
       all groups in the UK.
    e The risk of carcinoma of the bronchus is much less in pipe and
       cigar smokers than in cigarette smokers.

19.2 Suggest six non-metastatic manifestations of carcinoma of the
    bronchus.

19.3 Describe the clinical syndromes which may be produced by a carcinoma encroaching upon:
   a The apex of the left lung.
   b The root of the left lung.
   c The root of the right lung.
   d Thoracic sympathetic fibres.

20.1 Deep venous thrombosis in the legs:
   a Is more likely to lead to pulmonary embolism if the local signs are florid than if they are slight.
   b May be excluded by ultrasonic testing.
   c After operation is encouraged by hyper-coagulability of the blood.
   d Should usually be confirmed by venography before instituting anticoagulant therapy.
   e May be confirmed or excluded by measuring local uptake of I^{125} fibrinogen.

20.2 Pulmonary embolism.
   a Thrombolytic activity is reduced in patients with malignant disease.
   b The presence of varicose veins increases the risk of post-operative deep venous thrombosis.
   c A peak incidence of pulmonary embolism occurs at about 10 days after surgical operations.
   d Pulmonary embolism is almost always accompanied by clinical signs of deep venous thrombosis in the legs.

20.3 In a patient who has just sustained massive pulmonary embolism:
   a Elevation of the jugular venous pressure would be expected.
   b The ECG is commonly normal in appearance.
   c There will generally be a large wedge-shaped opacity visible on the chest X-ray.
   d Pulmonary function tests are helpful in demonstrating an enlarged physiological deadspace.
   e There will generally be arterial hypoxia.

20.4 Radioisotope lung scanning techniques:
   a May include breathing air containing $Xenon^{133}$ using a closed circuit spirometer.

b Are generally accepted as the best means of distinguishing between pulmonary infarction and pneumonia.

c Employing Technetium-labelled albumin results in a radiation dose to the patient roughly equivalent to that of five standard full-size chest X-rays films.

d Virtually exclude acute pulmonary embolism as a cause of breathlessness and chest pain if a normal pattern of perfusion is demonstrated.

e May reveal local areas of defective perfusion in patients with well-controlled asthma.

20.5 Treatment of acute pulmonary embolism with urokinase or streptokinase:

a Is contained for at least 4 days.

b Is monitored by measurement of prothrombin time.

c Is strikingly more effective if administered by a catheter direct into the pulmonary artery.

d Is of little value in pulmonary embolism of over 1 week's standing.

e Carried a risk of secondary haemorrhage if employed in the first 3 days after a surgical operation.

20.6 Pulmonary hypertension:

a Is generally accepted as being present if the mean pulmonary artery pressure is above 20 mmHg.

b May present clinically with episodes of syncope.

c Is commonly caused by diffuse lung disease.

d Is characteristically accompanied by ECG changes as follows: QS pattern in leads II, III and AVF with ST elevation and T wave inversion.

e May be the consequence of repeated pulmonary embolism.

20.7 The following features contribute towards an electrocardiographic diagnosis of right ventricular hypertrophy:

a Tall R wave in lead I with deep S wave in leads III and AVF.

b Deep S wave in leads V_5 and V_6.

c Inverted T waves in V_1-V_3.

d QRS duration in excess of 0.12 seconds.

e A dominant R wave in lead V_1.

21.1   Pulmonary oedema:
    a May be defined as the condition in which fluid transudate from plasma crosses into the alveoli.
    b Only develops when there is an increase in pulmonary capillary pressure.
    c Commonly causes widespread crepitations (crackles).
    d Commonly causes widespread rhonchi.
    e Is commonly associated with Cheyne–Stokes' respiration.

21.2   Mitral stenosis regularly produces:
    a Kerley 'B' lines.
    b Pulmonary hypertension
    c Spirometric features of airways obstruction.
    d Haemoptysis.
    e Recurrent episodes of cough and sputum production.

21.3   Accepted radiological features of pulmonary oedema include:
    a Kerley 'B' lines.
    b Kerley 'Λ' lines.
    c Unilateral lung mottling.
    d Prominent, distended upper lobe vessels.
    e Prominent pulmonary arterial shadow.

21.4   The following are potential causes of pulmonary oedema:
    a Altitude.
    b Head injury.
    c Anaesthesia with nitrous oxide.
    d Influenza A virus.
    e Drainage of pleural effusion.

22.1   Pneumothorax usually causes:
    a Pleuritic pain on the same side.
    b Tachypnoea.
    c Cyanosis.
    d Reduced or absent breath sounds.
    e Deviation of the trachea to the same side.

23.1   What are the clinical consequences of the following—and what treatment may be required?
    a Infection in the pleural space.
    b Rib fracture with damage to an intercostal artery.

    c Damage to the thoracic duct.
    d Bronchial rupture.
    e Rupture of the oesophagus.

23.2   What is meant by the term 'Shock lung' or adult respiratory distress syndrome?

24.1   *a* Name three occupational causes of asthma.
    b Name three occupational causes of widespread miliary mottling on the chest X-ray.
    c Name three substances which are encountered in the course of occupation and which are known to be associated with increased risk of lung carcinoma.

24.2   Diffuse pulmonary fibrosis is a recognized sequel of exposure to:
    a Nickel carbonyl.
    b Mouldy hay dust.
    c Silica dust.
    d Chrysotile
    c Western Red Cedar dust.

24.3   A 57-year-old coal worker presents with cough and gradually progressive shortness of breath of about 10-years duration. He smokes 20 cigarettes daily. Spirometry shows the following results: FEV_1 1.5 litres; FVC 2.75 litres. The chest X-ray shows normal heart size and shape with fine nodular shadowing (average size 1–2 mm) scattered throughout the upper two-thirds of both lung fields.
    a He will probably have been a coal-face worker for more than 10 years of his life.
    b His symptoms are due to coal-workers' pneumoconiosis.
    c He will be eligible for compensation under the National Insurance (Industrial Injuries) Act.
    d It is probable that within a further 10 years he will develop progressive massive fibrosis.
    e He has above average risk of developing bronchial carcinoma.

24.4   Occupational asthma occurs after exposure to:
    a Silica.
    b Toluene di-isocyanate.
    c Asbestos.

d Proteolytic enzymes.

e Silica dioxide.

24.5 Mesothelioma:

  a Is virtually confined to workers subjected to heavy industrial exposure to asbestos.

  b Commonly presents as an obscure pleural effusion.

  c May develop more than 40 years after asbestos exposure.

  d Is readily diagnosed by pleural biopsy.

  e Is resistant to radiotherapy.

25.1 Bronchoconstriction is a recognized adverse effect of the following drugs:

  a Carbachol.

  b Propranolol.

  c Succinyl choline.

  d Nitrofurantoin.

  e Sodium salicylate.

25.2 Diffuse pulmonary shadowing may accompany adverse reactions to the following drugs:

  a Diazepam.

  b Methotrexate.

  c Chlorpropamide.

  d Busulphan.

  e Bleomycin.

26.1 Oxygen masks.

  a Describe briefly the features of a mask which provides a high concentration of inspired oxygen (in excess of 40%).

  b Describe briefly the features of a mask which provides a low, controlled concentration of inspired oxygen.

  c Outline the circumstances in which these two types are most appropriate.

ANSWERS

1.1 *a* False.
    b False; from the aorta.
    c True.
    d True.
    e False; the left does.
(If you found this question at all difficult you need more basic revision in anatomy than is offered in this book. You will have a great deal of difficulty in interpreting chest X-rays if you do not understand the relationship of the principal structures in the mediastinum.)

1.2 *a* True.
    b True.
    c False.
    d False; gas movement is mainly by diffusion; linear velocity is very low.
    e True.

2.1 *a* False.
    b True.
    c False. Compliant lungs comply—move easily.
    d True.
    e True.

2.2 *a* False; the reverse is generally true (see RQ).
    b False; there is little or no change in PO_2 during most exercise.
    c False; it is an equation expressing the relationship between alveolar PO_2 and PCO_2.
    d True; it approximates to 'ideal' alveolar PCO_2 in the normal.
    e True; at atmospheric pressure at sea level 30% of 760 mmHg = 228 mmHg.

2.3 *a* False
    b True.
    c False; most of the total airways resistance is produced by flow through the larger airways and upper airway where flow rates are highest.
    d True; usually less than 30% in younger individuals.
    e False; increases.

2.4   *a* True.
     b True.
     c False; the pressure for each would be 5% of ambient pressure.
     d True (See Fig. 2.8).
     e True (See Fig. 2.8).

2.5   *a* True; Severinghaus CO_2 electrode.
     b True.
     c True; end-expired air as a P_{CO_2} approximating to arterial P_{CO_2}.
     d False; P_{CO_2} usually changes very little during exercise. There is variation in the changes seen but a decrease is rather more common than an increase.
     e True.

2.6   *a* True
     b True.
     c False.
     d True.
     e True.

2.7   *a* False; hypercapnia is not inevitable but is compensated for by increase in level of ventilation of other areas.
     b False.
     c False.
     d False.
     e True (Fig. 2.10).

3.1   *a* True (Fig. 3.1).
     b True.
     c True; strong body of albeit indirect evidence.
     d False; from 30th to 35th week.
     e True; probably explains collapse of areas deprived of pulmonary arterial blood supply experimentally and in pulmonary embolism.

4.1   *a* True.
     b False; significant penetration does not occur above about 3 μm.
     c False.

    d True; the effect of convergence of the airways is such that it has been suggested that, if it were not for absorption, fluid would be gushing from the trachea like a fountain!

    e False; it removes almost all above 20 μm and makes a major reduction in particles of all sizes down to about 4 μm.

6.1 *a* 2.
    b 3.
    c 5.
    d 4.
    e 1.

6.2 *a* True.
    b True; Kussmaul's sign (different from Kussmaul's breathing but same gentleman).
    c False; the reverse is true.
    d True.
    e True.

6.3 *a* True.
    b True.
    c False.
    d False.
    e True.

6.4 *a* False.
    b False.
    c True.
    d True.
    e False.

6.5 *a* False; this gives a saturation of about 93.5% at normal temperature and pH.
    b True.
    c True.
    d False: it is most commonly due to abnormal ventilation/perfusion relationships (see Figs 2.9 and 2.10).
    e False; it certainly raises the question but is not an absolute indication.

7.1   See index entries for answers.

7.2   *a* True.
       b True.
       c False; generally normal or high because of the increased
            pulmonary capillary blood volume.
       d True.
       e False.

7.3   *a* True.
       b True; the oxygen dissociation curve (Fig. 2.8) is shifted to the
            right.
       c False.
       d True.
       c True; (something of an oversimplification).

7.4   *a* True; see p. 67. Although the reduction in FEV$_1$ is propor-
            tionately greater in airways obstruction, the vital capacity is
            inevitably reduced also.
       b True.
       c False; normally takes 3–4 seconds; generally abnormal above
            5 seconds.
       d False; it decreases during adult life.
       e True.

7.5   *a* False; he clearly has good ventilatory drive.
       b True.
       c True.
       d False: sedation might lead to hypoventilation—the values
            shown here indicate hyperventilation in response to a severe
            metabolic acidosis.
       e False; (see *d* above).

7.6   *a* True.
       b False; BP generally slightly increased.
       c False; hypocapnia is the rule.
       d False; causes cerebral vasodilatation.
       e True.

7.7   *a* False. It remains constant over a wide range of effort given
            minimum cooperation, so not directly related.
       b True.

   c False; gradually declines from mid-twenties.
   d True (see Fig. 15.6).
   e False; diffuse fibrosis typically causes a restrictive ventilatory defect in which the FEV_1 is reduced in proportion to the reduction in vital capacity.

7.8 *a* False.
   b True.
   c True.
   d False; normal values very dependent upon age, height and sex (see Figs 7.1 and 7.2).
   e True.

7.9 *a* False; this is uncompensated acute respiratory acidosis.
   b True.
   c True; have you noticed that this patient must be breathing oxygen-enriched air? (Partial pressures of oxygen and carbon dioxide add up to more than PO_2 of air.) If we suppose that the patient was in fact breathing from a high concentration mask there must be a severe defect of ventilation: perfusion matching to give such a modest arterial PO_2 and severe hypoxia is quite probable if the mask is removed.
   d False.
   e False; this PCO_2 might be the cause of confusion but not coma.

7.10 *a* 4.
   b 2.
   c 1.
   d 5.
   e 3.

8.1 *a* Miliary tuberculosis, haemosiderosis, pneumoconiosis and other occupational causes, sarcoidosis, lymphangitis carcinomatosa, acute viral pneumonia, pulmonary eosinophilia, etc.
   b Carcinoma, tuberculoma, abscess, hamartoma, rheumatoid nodule, arteriovenous aneurysm, infarct, etc.

8.2 *a* True.
   b False; to the right.
   c False; below (Fig. 8.1).
   d True.
   e False; not seen in normal chest X-ray (but see Fig. 21.3).

8.3 *a* True, q.v.
       b True, q.v.
       c True.
       d False; almost always solitary.
       e True.

9.1 *a* True.
       b True.
       c False.
       d False.
       e True.

9.2 *a* False.
       b False.
       c True.
       d False.
       e True.

9.3 *a* True.
       b False.
       c True.
       d False.
       e False.

10.1 *a* 4.
        b 1.
        c 2.
        d 3.
        e 1.

10.2 *a* Staphylococcus.
        b *Klebsiella pneumoniae.*
        c Pseudomonas, staphylococcus and anaerobic species.
        d Tuberculosis!
        e *Mycoplasma pneumoniae.*

10.3 *a* Any cause of recurrent haemoptysis; any cause of intra-
            alveolar haemorrhage (left-heart failure, mitral stenosis,
            idiopathic pulmonary haemosiderosis).
        b Allergic aspergillosis.
        c Lipoid pneumonia, q.v.

    d Asthma (and some cases of pulmonary eosinophilia, q.v.).
    e Bronchiectasis or chronic lung abscess or cystic fibrosis.

11.1   *a* True; non-reactive tuberculosis is rare.
    b False.
    c False.
    d True.
    e False; injection is intradermal.

11.2   *a* True.
    b False.
    c False; except where very few individuals work in a very confined space, circumstances at the place of work are rarely such as to make other workers significantly close contacts.
    d True; disease may not reveal itself till then and there is a significant yield of new cases from late X-rays.
    e True; for even longer than this but they are not viable.

11.3   *a* False; about 1–2%.
    b False; transmission between humans is not reliably recorded.
    c True.
    d True.
    e True.

11.4   *a* 3.
    b 2.
    c 1.
    d 4.
    c 1.

12.1   *a* True.
    b False.
    c False; bronchoscopy may show abnormal appearances but it is not a satisfactory method for diagnosis. Bronchography, although not obligatory, is the most satisfactory method for confirming the diagnosis.
    d False; sometimes accompanied by airways obstruction but ventilatory function is often quite normal even in the presence of quite marked bronchiectasis.
    e True.

12.2 *a* False.

   b True; though usually only in severe long-standing bronchiectasis.

   c True.

   d True; the 'hallmark' of bronchiectasis.

   e True. Normal X-ray common.

12.3 *a* True.

   b False; abnormally *high* sodium concentration in sweat.

   c True; polyps much more common than would be expected.

   d True.

   e True.

13.1 *a* True.

   b False; females have reduced fertility if malnourished but they are not sterile.

   c True.

   d False; a 2 out of 3 chance.

13.2 *a* True.

   b False.

   c False; pancreatic extracts.

   d True.

   e True.

14.1 *a* True.

   b False. Most resolve with antibiotic treatment—often prolonged.

   c True.

   d True.

   e False.

14.2 (See Chapter 14).

14.3 *a* False; normal individuals do not cough daily. About 10–20 ml of mucoid respiratory secretion passes through the larynx from the lungs each day.

   b False; yellow coloration most often does indicate the presence of infection but yellow sputum in asthma is sometimes due to the presence of large numbers of eosinophil cells.

    c False; it is produced in excessive quantities but is not specially viscid despite the name 'mucoviscidosis' sometimes applied to the condition.

    d True.

    e True.

15.1 *a* True.

    b False.

    c True.

    d True.

    e True.

    f True.

15.2 *a* True.

    b False; produces bronchodilatation.

    c True.

    d True.

    e True.

15.3 *a* True (see 'mast cell').

    b True.

    c False; the reverse is true.

    d True; this is particularly the case in asthmatic subjects.

    e True.

15.4 *a* True.

    b False; it can be demonstrated in the vast majority.

    c True.

    d True. Almost certainly because of the very limited scope for respiratory heat loss when breathing fully-saturated air at water level—usually in a heated pool in colder climates.

    e False.

15.5 *a* False; in the UK it is responsible for about 1500 deaths annually.

    b False; the fraction is probably in excess of 5%.

    c True.

    d False; asthma can become manifest for the first time at any age.

    e False; there is only a slight influence of social class upon prevalence which most studies show operating in the reverse direction.

15.6 *a* House dust mite, grass pollen, other pollens, domestic animals, etc.

b Reduced FEV_1/FVC ratio, reduced peak flow rate, reduced maximum mid-expiratory flow rate, prolonged forced expiratory time, increased residual volume, increased functional residual capacity, etc.

c See index 'reversibility'.

15.7 *a* True; hypoxia of some degree is inevitable.

b True; patients presenting in status asthmaticus usually respond to the intense respiratory drive produced by the asthmatic process in the bronchi by achieving a higher alveolar ventilation than normal.

c False; tachycardia is the rule.

d False.

e True.

15.8 *a* False; the rise in mortality so soon after the introduction of pressurized aerosols in the 1960s has been followed by a steady fall back to former levels.

b False; beta-2 stimulants, not beta-1 (but, yes, they are selective).

c False; values rarely return to normal.

d True.

e True; thought to be due to pulmonary arteriolar dilatation allowing increased perfusion of relatively underventilated areas; not usually an important fall.

15.9 *a* False; this idea probably contributes to the continuing substantial mortality rate from asthma.

b False; short courses are too short to produce important pituitary/adrenal suppression.

c True; there is some merit in ensuring that maximal effect is being achieved by the direct route so that minimal doses of oral steroid are used to treat remaining unacceptable asthma.

d True.

e False; they are highest in the morning as in normals. The diurnal variation in asthma bears no relationship to variations in cortisol levels.

15.10 *a* True.

   b True.

   c False; the chest-wall deformity which may result from severe uncontrolled asthma is a pigeon-chest deformity (Fig. 15.14). Pectus excavatum refers to depression of the sternum.

   d True. *Systemic* therapy may do so but only if more or less continuous and prolonged.

   e False.

15.11 *a* True.

   b True; whether or not they are sensitive to it.

   c True (see Fig. 15.15).

   d True; often the presenting feature of aspergilloma (mycetoma).

   e True; see 'mucoid impaction'.

15.12 *a* False; only about 10% of the dose reaches the lungs.

   b False; metered dose aerosols used with a spacer attachment produce the same or better bronchodilatation if the same dose is used.

   c False.

   d False.

   e False; beta-agonists are ineffective below the age of about 18 months.

15.13 *a* False; a cause of occupational asthma.

   b True.

   c False; causes a simple pneumoconiosis.

   d True; see farmer's lung.

   e True; mushroom spores of respirable size.

16.1 *a* False.

   b False; (see Fig. 6.5).

   c True.

   d True.

   e True.

16.2 *a* True.

   b True.

   c True; i.e. the lungs are stiffer.

   d False; the ratio is normal or increased.

   e True.

16.3 *a* True.
    b False.
    c True; (see Fig. 16.1).
    d True; (see Fig. 16.2).
    e False; confident diagnosis often possible without.

16.4 *a* False; Caplan's syndrome (q.v.) is associated with rheumatoid arthritis. (For the curious, Kargatener's syndrome is a rarity: bronchiectasis accompanying dextrocardia—of interest because the bronchiectasis is a consequence of immotile cilia.)
    b True.
    c True.
    d True.
    e False.

16.5 *a* False.
    b True.
    c True.
    d False; it leads to suppurative lung disease both in childhood and in adult life.
    e True; also called Adenoma sebaceum, a proportion of individuals affected by this condition develop pulmonary fibrosis.

16.6 *a* True.
    b True.
    c True.
    d True; by retrieval of the organism which is identifiable by microscopic examination.
    e False; the increased proportion of neutrophils usually seen is not specific for fibrosing alveolitis.

17.1 *a* True.
    b False.
    c True; acute uveitis is a not uncommon mode of presentation.
    d False.
    e True; erythema nodosum is usually painful.

17.2 *a* True.
    b True.
    c False.
    d True.

    e True; bone cysts due to sarcoidosis are particularly common in the fingers and generally accompanied by local swelling.

17.3 *a* False; sometimes it affects the arms—usually the skin overlying the triceps.
    b True.
    c False; persistence or recurrence is unusual but occurs.
    d False; generally good prognosis in acute sarcoidosis which is the form usually associated with erythema nodosum.
    e True.

18.1 *a* True.
    b True.
    c True.
    d True.
    e False.

18.2 *a* True; hypoventilation is a principal feature of the Type B pattern.
    b False.
    c True.
    d True.
    e False; both forms are usually associated with cigarette smoking.

18.3 *a* False.
    b False; other forms of lung (bronchial) carcinoma *are* associated with smoking.
    c True.
    d True.
    e True.

18.4 *a* True.
    b True.
    c True.
    d True.
    e True.

18.5 *a* False.
    b False.
    c True.

    d True.
    e False.

18.6   *a* True.
    b True.
    c False.
    d True.
    e True.

18.7   *a* q.v.
    b q.v.

18.8   *a* True.
    b False; *acute* hypoventilation is seen; other pulmonary complications include pulmonary oedema, lung abscess and talc granuloma.
    c True; q.v.
    d False.
    e True; especially when it is associated with even mild airways obstruction.

19.1   *a* True.
    b False; the figure is in excess of 35 000.
    c False; it comes down quite rapidly, halving very 3–5 years.
    d False; mortality rate is still rising in women.
    e True.

19.2   See p. 248.

19.3   *a* See Pancoast's tumour.
    b Include collapse left lung, recurrent laryngeal nerve paralysis.
    c Include collapse of right lung and early progress to superior vena caval obstruction in some tumours.
    d Horner's syndrome.

20.1   *a* False.
    b False.
    c True.
    d False.
    e False. May miss major venous thrombosis.

20.2 a True.
    b True.
    c True.
    d False; an unfortunately widespread misconception.

20.3 *a* True.
    b True.
    c False.
    d False.
    e True.

20.4 *a* True.
    b False.
    c False. Less.
    d True.
    e True.

20.5 *a* False; haemorrhagic complications are increasingly common if treatment is continued beyond 2 days.
    b False.
    c False.
    d True.
    e True.

20.6 *a* False.
    b True.
    c True.
    d False.
    e True.

20.7 *a* False; the described features are those of left axis deviation. Right axis deviation would contribute to a diagnosis of RVH.
    b True.
    c True.
    d False; this duration is conventionally interpreted as reflecting bundle branch block.
    e True; (see Fig. 20.3 and related text).

21.1 *a* False; see beginning of Chapter 21.
    b False; see end of Chapter 21.
    c True.

d True.

e True; when pulmonary oedema is the result of severely compromised left ventricular function—especially where the cardiac output is low.

21.2 *a* True.

b True.

c True; but rarely severe.

d True.

e True.

21.3 *a* True.

b True; these are harder to recognize and less commonly seen. They comprise fine streaks radiating from the hilum and probably represent distended lymphatic channels.

c True.

d True.

e False.

21.4 *a* True.

b True.

c False.

d True.

e True; confined to the side of the re-expansion but can be potentially threatening nevertheless.

22.1 *a* True.

b True.

c False.

d True.

e False.

23.1 *a* See empyema.

b See haemothorax.

c See chylothorax.

d See pneumomediastinum and surgical emphysema.

e See mediastinitis.

23.2 q.v.

24.1   *a* See occupational asthma.

      b Coalworker's pneumoconiosis, antimony, haematite, welder's siderosis, silicosis, asbestosis, etc.

      c Nickel, chromates, arsenic, coal gas, radioactive gases, asbestos.

24.2   *a* False; incriminated as a risk factor in development of lung cancer.

      b True; advanced stages of farmer's lung.

      c True.

      d True; one of the commonest forms of asbestos used in industry.

      e False; causes asthma in woodworkers—often of delayed type.

24.3   *a* True.

      b False; the condition described is simple coalworkers' pneumoconiosis. This is not associated with symptoms of physiological impairment. He has airways obstruction and this is likely to be related to smoking (or asthma).

      c True; generally compensation is offered to those with shadowing of this sort involving over one-third of the lung fields. The compensation is increased in the presence of important symptoms from bronchitis and airways obstruction.

      d False; only a small proportion (perhaps 1% per annum) progress to PMF—this varies between different coalfields.

      e True; but because of cigarette smoking. It is uncertain whether the presence of coalworkers' pneumoconiosis confers additional risk of carcinoma.

24.4   *a* False.

      b True; q.v.

      c False.

      d True; see p. 306.

      e False.

24.5   *a* False; trivial contact may lead to mesothelioma.

      b True.

      c True; an interval of this order is usual.

      d False; diagnosis by this means is notoriously difficult.

      e True.

25.1   *a* True.
         b True.
         c True.
         d False.
         e False.

25.2   *a* False.
         b True.
         c True.
         d True.
         e True.

26.1   *a* See Fig. 26.2.
         b See Fig. 26.3.
         c See neighbouring text.

APPENDIX: SI UNITS OF PRESSURE

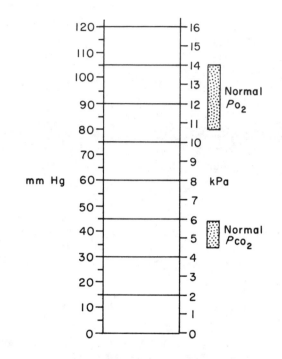

Nomogram relating mmHg and kPa
Even numbers of kPa relate exactly to convenient values of mmHg at intervals of
15 mmHg and some of these values may be worth remembering.

$$1 \text{ kPa} = 7 \cdot 5 \text{ mmHg}$$
$$1 \text{ mmHg} = 0 \cdot 13 \text{ kPa}$$

FURTHER INFORMATION

The reader seeking more information on a subject may find it in one of the reference textbooks listed below or in one of the monographs or reviews which are grouped according to subject. Respiratory topics of general importance are the subject of editorials at regular intervals in the mainstream general medical journals such as the *British Medical Journal*, *Lancet*, the *New England Medical Journal*, etc. A wealth of more detailed information is contained in specialist respiratory journals. In addition to original research these journals also publish review articles which provide an easy means of gaining access to the relevant literature. Under this heading *Thorax*, *British Journal of Diseases of the Chest*, the *American Review of Respiratory Disease* and *Chest* will probably be found most helpful. If a particular subject is being explored the reader can work back through the indexes of recent years' bound volumes of these and other respiratory journals, or turn to *Index Medicus*. Alternatively, a computer search can be commissioned but this may be costly and, unless the searcher has a particularly well defined target, it may yield too much (or too little) to be useful.

Reference Textbooks

CROFTON J. & DOUGLAS A. (1981) *Respiratory Diseases*, 3rd edition. Oxford, Blackwell Scientific Publications.
(This excellent reference work will usually provide what is required or give suitable source references.)
EMERSON P.A. (ed) (1981) *Thoracic Medicine*. London, Butterworth.
(A very clear large textbook; useful lists of diagnostic possibilities.)
FRASER R.G. & PARE J.A.P. *Diagnosis of Diseases of the Chest*. Vols 1 (1977), 2 (1978), 3 & 4 (1979). Philadelphia, Saunders.
(Encyclopaedic work based on radiological diagnosis.)
GUENTER C.A. & WELCH M.H. (1977) *Pulmonary Medicine*. Philadelphia, Lippincott.
(A high quality reference work, well illustrated and with a very good introductory section on structure and function.)
PHELAN P.D., LANDAU L.I. & OLINSKY A. (1982) *Respiratory Illness in Children*, 2nd edition. Oxford, Blackwell Scientific Publications.
(Excellent textbook. Readable, well illustrated and well referenced.)

Examination of the chest

FORGACS P. (1978) *Lung Sounds*. London, Balliere Tindall.
(Strongly recommended; only 65 pages. Combines an understanding of basic physiology and acoustics in making sense of auscultatory signs.)

Respiratory physiology and pulmonary function tests

BATES D.V., MACKLEM P.T. & CHRISTIE R.V. (1971) *Respiratory Function in Disease*. Philadelphia, Saunders.
(Notable for worked examples correlating clinical and physiological findings.)

CAMPBELL E.J.M., AGOSTONI E. & NEWSOM DAVIS J. (1970) *The Respiratory Muscles*, 2nd edition. London, Lloyd-Luke.
(Excellent review of lung mechanics and comprehensive review of ventilatory control.)

COMROE J.H. Jr, FORSTER R.E., DUBOIS A.B., BRISCOE W.A. & CARLSEN E. (1962) *The Lung*. Chicago, Year Book Medical Publishers.
(Basic text on pulmonary physiology and function testing; good diagrams. An ageless classic.)

COTES J.E. (1979) *Lung Function*, 4th edition. Oxford, Blackwell Scientific Publications.
(Essential reference work on laboratory investigation of pulmonary function. Normal values.)

CUMMING G. & SEMPLE S.G. (1980) *Disorders of the Respiratory System*, 2nd edition. Oxford, Blackwell Scientific Publications.
(First 155 pages; gas transport and control of ventilation particularly well done.)

FENN W.O. & RAHN H. (eds) (1964) *Handbook of Physiology, Section 3, Respiration*, Vols 1, 2. Washington, American Physiological Society.
(Monumental reference work; very valuable despite age.)

GIBSON G.J. (1984) *Clinical Tests of Respiratory Function*. London, Macmillan.
(Critical review of pulmonary function tests used in clinical practice and research accompanied by review of underlying physiological principles. Lung mechanics especially strong.)

NUNN J.F. (1977) *Applied Respiratory Physiology, with Special Reference to Anaesthesia*, 2nd edition. London, Butterworth.
(Clear and comprehensive.)

WEST J.B. (1977) *Ventilation/Blood-flow and Gas Exchange*, 3rd edition. Oxford, Blackwell Scientific Publications.
(Readable essay with exposition of O_2—CO_2 diagram.)
WEST J.B. (1979) *Respiratory Physiology—the Essentials*, 2nd edition. Oxford, Blackwell Scientific Publications.
(Concise, clear and inexpensive.)

Radiology

SIMON G. (1978) *Principles of Chest X-ray Diagnosis*, 4th edition. London, Butterworth.
(Informative, systematic approach.)
SQUIRE L.F., COLIACE W.M. & STRUTYNSKY N. (1970) *Exercises in Diagnostic Radiology, I: The Chest*. Philadelphia, Saunders.
(Well illustrated, stimulating question and answer format.)

Respiratory infections

GARROD L.P., LAMBERT H.P. & O'GRADY F. (1981) *Antibiotic and Chemotheraphy*, 5th edition. Edinburgh, Churchill Livingstone.
(First part; review of the antibiotics; second part: their application in disease.)
KNIGHT V. (1973) *Viral and Mycoplasmal Infection of the Respiratory Tract*. Philadelphia, Lea and Febiger.
(Thorough, systematic, many references.)

Tuberculosis

JOINT TUBERCULOSIS COMMITTEE OF THE BRITISH THORACIC SOCIETY. (1983) Control and Prevention of Tuberculosis: A Code of Practice. *Brit. med. J.* 287, 1118–21.
(Recommendations regarding segregation, management of contacts, vaccination, etc.)
ROSS J.D. & HORNE N.W. (1983) *Modern Drug Treatment in Tuberculosis*, 6th edition. London, Chest, Heart and Stroke Association.
(Invaluable inexpensive practical handbook likely to contain the answer to most questions about management.)

Cystic fibrosis

ANDERSON C.M. & GOODCHILD M.C. (1976) *Cystic Fibrosis; Manual of Diagnosis and Management*. Oxford, Blackwell Scientific Publications.
(Extremely sensible. Best available summary of the subject.)

Asthma

CIBA FOUNDATION GUEST SYMPOSIUM (1971) *Identification of Asthma.* Edinburgh, Churchill Livingstone.
(Useful review of the problem of definition and of pathogenesis.)

CLARK T.J.H & GODFREY S. (eds) (1983) *Asthma,* 2nd edition. London, Chapman Hall.
(22 authors contributing a series of in-depth reviews of different aspects of asthma. Physiology, pharmacology and exercise-induced asthma especially useful.)

LICHENSTEIN L.M. & AUSTEN K.F. (eds) (1977) *Asthma, Physiology, Immunopharmacology and Treatment.* New York, Academic Press.
(Excellent review of some underlying mechanisms.)

LANE D.J. & STORR A. (1979) *Asthma: The Facts.* Oxford, Oxford University Press.
(Straightforward account of asthma and its management written to be understood by the layman. Recommended reading for patients with chronic asthma who want to find out more as well as for those who treat asthma.)

CLARKE S.W. & PAVIA D. (1984) *Aerosols and the Lung: Clinical and Experimental Aspects.* London, Butterworth.
(Detailed account of physical properties and clearance of inhaled aerosols and their research, diagnostic and therapeutic applications.)

Fibrosing alveolitis

HANCE A.J. & CRYSTAL R.G. (1983) Idiopathic pulmonary fibrosis. In: Flenley D.C. (ed) *Recent Advances in Respiratory Medicine,* pp. 249-287. Edinburgh, Churchill Livingstone.
(Authoritative review with almost 300 references.)

LIVINGSTONE J.L., LEWIS J.G., REID L. & JEFFERSON K. (1964) Diffuse interstitial pulmonary fibrosis, *Quart. J. Med.,* 33, 71.
(Very informative account of large series.)

TURNER-WARWICK M. (1972) Cryptogenic fibrosing alveolitis, *Brit. J. Hosp. Med.,* 7, 697.
(Good all-round description.)

TURNER-WARWICK M. (1978) *Immunology of the lung.* London, Arnold.

Sarcoidosis

SCADDING J.G. (1967) *Sarcoidosis.* London, Eyre and Spottiswoode.
(Definitive reference work.)

FANBURG B.L. (ed) (1983) *Sarcoidosis and other Granulomatous Diseases* (Lung Biology in Health and Disease, Vol 20), New York, Marcel Dekker.
(Collection of 17 reviews of specialised aspects of sarcoidosis. Vol 20 of a series of high quality monographs on respiratory disease.)

Chronic bronchitis, airways obstruction and emphysema

CUMMING G. & HUNT L.B. (eds) (1968) *Form and Function in the Human Lung.* Edinburgh, Livingstone.
(Symposium centred upon chronic airways obstruction and emphysema.)
FILLEY G.F. (1967) *Pulmonary Insufficiency and Respiratory Failure.* Philadelphia, Lea and Febiger.
(Lucid, readable account. Ageless.)
FLETCHER C., PETO R., TINKER C., SPEIZER F.E. (1976) *The Natural History of Chronic Bronchitis and Emphysema.* Oxford, Oxford University Press.
(Detailed presentation of major longitudinal study. Important but not light reading.)
HEARD B.E. (1969) *Pathology of Chronic Bronchitis and Emphysema.* London, Churchill.
(Beautiful account of pathology; worth looking at if only for illustrations.)
ROYAL COLLEGE OF PHYSICIANS
(Reports on smoking—see below.)
SYKES M.K., McNICHOL M.W. & CAMPBELL E.J.M. (1976) *Respiratory Failure,* 2nd edition. Oxford, Blackwell Scientific Publications.
(Physiological and practical aspects clearly dealt with.)

Carcinoma of the bronchus

HANSEN H.H. & RORTH M. (1983) Small cell cancer of the lung. In: Flenley D.C. (ed) *Recent Advances in Respiratory Medicine.* Edinburgh, Churchill Livingstone.
HANDLE K.R. & DES PREZ R.M. (1983) Non-small cell cancer of the lung. In: Flenley D.C. (ed) *Recent Advances in Respiratory Medicine,* Edinburgh, Churchill Livingstone.
STRADLING P. (1981) *Diagnostic Bronchoscopy,* 4th edition. London, Livingstone.
(Worth looking at if only for illustrations.)

Smoking

ROYAL COLLEGE OF PHYSICIANS (1977) *Smoking or Health.* Tunbridge Wells, Pitman Medical.
(Very useful assimilation of evidence.)
ROYAL COLLEGE OF PHYSICIANS (1983) *Health or Smoking.* Tunbridge Wells, Pitman Publishing.

Pulmonary embolism and pulmonary hypertension

HARRIS P. & HEATH D. (1977) *The Human Pulmonary Circulation,* 2nd edition. Edinburgh, Churchill Livingstone.
(Illustrated readable comprehensive reference work.)

Occupational lung disease

MORGAN W.K.C & SEATON A. (1984) 2nd edition. *Occupational Lung Diseases.* Philadelphia, Saunders.
(Comprehensive and well-referenced. Useful introduction and pathology.)
MUIR D.C.F. (ed) (1972) *Clinical Aspects of Inhaled Particles.* London, Heinemann.
(Useful sections on deposition and clearance, also asbestos-induced diseases.)
PARKES W.R. (1981) *Occupational Lung Disorders,* 2nd edition. London, Butterworth.
(Definitive reference work.)

Drug-induced lung disease

BREWIS R.A.L. (1980) *Respiratory Disorders,* Chapter in *Textbook of Adverse Drug Reactions* (ed. Davies D.M.). 2nd edition, Oxford, Oxford University Press.
(Review with numerous references.)

Oxygen therapy

SYKES M.K., MCNICHOL M.W. & CAMPBELL E.J.M. (1976) *Respiratory Failure,* 2nd edition. Oxford, Blackwell Scientific Publications.
GREEN I.D. (1967) Choice of method for administration of oxygen, *Brit. med. J.* 3, 593.
(Informative assessment of performance of different masks.)

INDEX

381